Advances in Neurosurgery 5

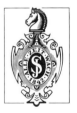

Head Injuries

Tumors of the Cerebellar Region

Edited by
R. A. Frowein O. Wilcke
A. Karimi-Nejad M. Brock M. Klinger

With 205 Figures and 74 Tables

Springer-Verlag
Berlin Heidelberg New York 1978

Proceedings of the 28th Annual Meeting
of the Deutsche Gesellschaft für Neurochirurgie
Köln, September 18–21, 1977

ISBN 3-540-08964-0 Springer-Verlag Berlin Heidelberg New York
ISBN 0-387-08964-0 Springer-Verlag New York Heidelberg Berlin

Library of Congress Cataloging in Publication Data. Deutsche Gesellschaft für Neurochirurgie. Head injuries. (Advances in neurosurgery; 5) "Proceedings of the 28th annual meeting of the Deutsche Gesellschaft für Neurochirurgie, Köln, September 18–21, 1977." Bibliography: p. Includes index. 1. Cerebellum-Tumors-Congresses. 2. Brain damage-Congresses. 3. Head-Wounds and injuries-Congresses. I. Frowein, Reinhold A. II. Title. III. Series. RC280.C4D48 1978 616.9'92'81 78-15592

This work is subject to copyright. All rights are reserved, whether the whole or part of the material is concerned, specifically those of translation, reprinting, re-use of illustrations, broadcasting, reproduction by photocopying machine or similar means, and storage in data banks.
Under § 54 of the German Copyright Law, where copies are made for other than private use, a fee is payable to the publisher, the amount of the fee to be determined by agreement with the publisher.

© by Springer-Verlag Berlin Heidelberg 1978
Printed in Germany

The use of registered names, trademarks, etc. in this publication does not imply, even in the absence of a specific statement, that such names are exempt from the relevant protective laws and regulations and therefore free for general use.

Offsetprinting and Binding: Beltz Offsetdruck, Hemsbach/Bergstr.
2127/3140-543210

Preface

The 28th annual conference of the German Society for Neurosurgery was held in Cologne, West Germany, from the 18th to the 21st of September 1977. The conference dealt with problems concerning craniocerebral injuries and space-occupying processes in the posterior cranial fossa as well as general topics on clinical practice and research with special attention paid to the work of younger neurosurgeons. This volume is a presentation of the conference results.

Within the scope of the **general topics**, special interest was directed toward the question of the current status of cytostatic treatment for brain tumors. In addition to experimental investigations, the results concerning cerebral tumors and medulloblastomas are reported.

Cerebellar tumors represent two further focal points:
1. From the diagnostic viewpoint, specific results from computerized tomography are discussed, especially with regard to the more extensive anatomic difficulties involved in the posterior cranial fossa.
2. With emphasis on cerebellar processes, the results of long-term measurements of intracranial pressure during the postoperative follow-up period are reported.

Computerized tomography and the measurement of intracranial pressure are also of aid in determining the course after severe **craniocerebral trauma**. Therefore, in addition to the primarily traumatic brain tissue damage that cannot be treated, the subsequent changes in the swelling of the brain and the possible complications are presented, especially hemorrhages that affect the prognosis. However, since many other factors determine the special, individual course, a certain "confusion of goals" prevails, as KAUTZKY in a citation from EINSTEIN appropriately termed the situation, which should be cause for reflection. These considerations should be placed on the same footing as the attempts "to clarify the limits of the well-founded prospects for recovery."

It is in just this field that several of our foreign colleagues – BRIHAYE, BRAAKMAN, JENNETT, EVANS, DIEMATH – have accomplished commendable spadework; indeed, appropriate measures are being investigated everywhere to optimally utilize the limited time and energy of personnel. In this connection, our Society once again extends its thanks and expresses recognition of the daily and nightly services rendered by the nurses and attendants on all wards and their physical and mental self-sacrifice in the interest of our patients.

Based on decades of experience, TÖNNIS and FROWEIN (among others) presented a study in 1968 on the personnel and equipment necessary for the diagnosis and treatment of severe craniocerebral injuries. These recommendations must be put further into effect, even if at a rate slower than previously envisioned, since the new accident statistics released by the Ministry of the Interior have by no means shown any decline. The acute care of the seriously injured and severely ill patients cannot be dismissed by neurosurgeons.

The topic of acute treatment and acute examination, therefore, also represents a focal point for research and the theoretical instruction of our specialty. We would like to thank both the Rector and the Chancellor of the University of Cologne, West Germany, and also the city of Cologne, West Germany, for their understanding cooperation in this sphere. Nevertheless, the longstanding problem of understaffing, especially for the acute care of our patients, has continued to remain unsolved, and I feel compelled to once again call attention to the serious consequences for patients and personnel.

The limitations to our prospects and activities are also of ethical nature, as GROSS, HILGER, KAUFMANN, and SCHEUERLEN reported in detail in their symposium "Medical Ethics" (Schattauer-Verlag, 1978).

The broad spectrum and large number of contributions to this conference are due to our apprehension that this speciality will be fragmented into highly specialized fields. On the one hand, our Society must continue to support further developments through new specialized research since the Society itself was created due to the specialization of its pioneers. On the other hand, we should not overlook the danger of isolating these newer specialized fields. Therefore, we have made every effort at this conference to offer as many colleagues as possible the opportunity to report on their specialized results in the various fields of pressure measurements, intensive therapy, vertebral tumors and trauma, microsurgery, pediatric neurosurgery etc.

I wish to thank Springer-Verlag for once again making the presentation of the results of this conference possible in such a precise manner, and to SHARP and DOHME Company as well as other sponsors for their generous support, which will enable us to reach a large audience.

R. A. Frowein

Rede zur Eröffnung der 28. Jahrestagung der Deutschen Gesellschaft für Neurochirurgie

Meine Damen und Herren,
sehr verehrter Herr Professor Tönnis!

Es ist für mich eine besondere Freude und Ehre, gerade bei der Jahrestagung in Köln als derzeitiger Vorsitzender der Deutschen Gesellschaft für Neurochirurgie meine Grußworte an Sie richten dürfen. Denn es bietet sich an, hier an der langjährigen Wirkungsstätte unseres hochverehrten Lehrers Rückschau zu halten auf die Entwicklung der Deutschen Neurochirurgie und unserer Gesellschaft, die auf das Engste mit dem Namen Wilhelm Tönnis verbunden ist. Genau vor 40 Jahren, im Jahre 1937, zeichnen sich Marksteine der raschen Entfaltung unseres Fachgebietes ab. Professor Tönnis übernahm das planmäßige Extraordinariat für Neurochirurgie in Berlin, den ersten Lehrstuhl in Deutschland und in Personalunion die Leitung der Abteilung für Tumorforschung und Experimentelle Pathologie am Kaiser-Wilhelm-Institut für Hirnforschung in Berlin-Buch, dessen Direktor Hugo Spatz war. Im gleichen Jahr fand eine Tagung mit der Britischen Gesellschaft für Neurologische Chirurgie in Berlin und Breslau mit der Besichtigung der neu eingerichteten Neurochirurgischen Klinik in Berlin und des Neurologischen Forschungsinstitutes von Otfrid Foerster in Breslau statt. Am ersten Tag des Treffens operierte Professor Tönnis zwei Patienten mit Großhirntumoren und demonstrierte anschließend eine übersichtlich zusammengestellte Sammlung von Ventrikulogrammen und Arteriogrammen, die den Wert dieser Hilfsmethoden zeigen sollten, wobei nicht nur auf die Aussagekraft hinsichtlich der Lokalisation und der Ausdehnung des Prozesses, sondern auch schon auf die Möglichkeit artdiagnostischer Vorhersagen hingewiesen wurde. Am letzten Tag der Berliner Sitzung hatte Ferdinand Sauerbruch in seine Klinik eingeladen. Er demonstrierte einige Operationen nach Auswahl der Gäste und stellte einige von ihm wegen Hirngeschwülsten operierte Kranke vor. Diese historische Reminiszenz mag ahnen lassen, daß sich die Emanzipation der Neurochirurgie nicht ohne Schwierigkeiten und Widerstände vollzog. Im Jahre 1937 fand auch der Kongreß der Gesellschaft Deutscher Neurologen und Psychiater in München statt, auf dem der ganze erste Tag dem Thema „Klinik, Pathologie und Therapie der Hirngeschwülste" gewidmet war. Bemerkenswert ist, daß Prof. Tönnis bereits damals in seinem Referat, das sich auf Erfahrungen an 596 bestätigten Hirntumoren stützen konnte, vornehmlich das Problem des Hirndrucks, seiner Entstehung und Behandlung herausstellte; auch heute noch beschäftigen uns diese Fragen vorrangig, wie das Programm unserer morgen beginnenden Tagung ausweist. Unmittelbar im Anschluß an diesen Neurologen-Kongreß 1937 trafen sich deutsche Neurochirurgen in der neu geschaffenen Neurochirurgischen Abteilung an der Chirurgischen Universitätsklinik in München.

Nach dem Kriege wurde mit sogen. Schülertreffen und Kolloquien das wissenschaftliche Gespräch wieder aufgenommen, bevor an ihre Stelle die Tagungen der Deutschen Gesellschaft für Neurochirurgie traten. Insgesamt siebenmal fanden diese Veranstaltungen in Köln statt, wobei der Kölner Karneval in manchem Jahr dazu beitrug, persönliche Kontakte zwischen der Vor- und Nachkriegsgeneration zu fördern, wie der Chronist H. W. Pia festhielt.

Neurologen und Psychiater hatten nach dem Krieg die Gesellschaft Deutscher Neurologen und Psychiater gegründet. Auf der gemeinsamen Tagung für Neurochirurgie und Neurologie in Bonn wurde am 13. 9. 1950 unter dem Vorsitz von Prof. Tönnis die Deutsche Gesellschaft für Neurochirurgie gegründet und in einer ersten Mitgliederversammlung von sieben Anwesenden die Satzung verabschiedet; als Mitglieder des Vorstandes zeichneten die Herren Tönnis, Okonek, Röttgen, Zülch und Häusler. Gleichzeitig wurde auch ein Antrag auf Abhaltung von Fedor Krause- und Otfrid Foerster-Gedächnisvorlesungen gestellt. Prof. Tönnis begründete seinen Antrag mit dem Hinweis auf die Pionierleistungen für die Entwicklung unseres Fachgebietes und führte u. a. aus: „Deshalb sollten die Namen von drei deutschen Ärzten in der Erinnerung jedes deutschen Neurochirurgen festgehalten werden: Ernst von Bergmann, Fedor Krause und Otfrid Foerster". Die Gedächtnisvorlesungen für Fedor Krause und Otfrid Foerster sind die höchsten Ehrungen, welche die Deutsche Gesellschaft für Neurochirurgie zu vergeben hat; sie sind mit der Verleihung der Fedor-Krause- bzw. Otfrid Foerster-Medaille sowie einer Urkunde verbunden. Schon in allernächster Zeit hoffen wir, wieder zwei prominente Neurochirurgen damit auszeichnen zu können. – Der Initiative Heinrich Pettes ist es zu danken, daß sich die Einzeldisziplinen der Nervenheilkunde zum Gesamtverband Deutscher Nervenärzte zusammenschlossen. Der erste Präsident war Prof. Tönnis und der erste Kongreß des Gesamtverbandes fand 1959 in Köln statt.

In den 50iger Jahren kamen auch erste Kontakte mit ausländischen Neurochirurgischen Gesellschaften zustande und in den letzten zehn Jahren wurden jeweils neben unserer Jahrestagung oder einem internationalen oder europäischen Kongreß gemeinsame Tagungen mit ausländischen Fachgesellschaften veranstaltet; so werden wir im kommenden Jahr im Frühjahr mit unseren niederländischen und britischen Kollegen in Berlin tagen und im Herbst in München unsere Jahrestagung mit der American Academy of Neurological Surgery abhalten.

Aus der Arbeit unserer Gesellschaft sind ferner die Verhandlungen zu erwähnen, die mit dem Präsidium des Deutschen Ärztetages zur Einführung des Facharztes für Neurochirurgie in den Jahren 1949 und 1950 aufgenommen wurden. 1951 erfolgte die Empfehlung des Ärztetages zur Annahme des Vorschlages, aber nur im Bundesland Niedersachsen wurde der Facharzttitel eingeführt. Erst im Jahre 1956 wurde auf dem Deutschen Ärztetag die Einführung des Facharztes für Neurochirurgie beschlossen. Unterdessen sind über 180 Fachärzte für Neurochirurgie ordentliche Mitglieder unserer Gesellschaft. Weitere Bemühungen in diesen und in folgenden Jahren galten der Errichtung und Struktur Neurochirurgischer Kliniken und Abteilungen sowie der Organisation der Versorgung von schweren Schädel-Hirnverletzungen. – Den Forderungen und dem Trend unserer Zeit entsprechend befassen sich zahlreiche Kommissionen unserer Gesellschaft mit übergeordneten Fragen der Organisation, der Aus- und Weiterbildung; der Verbundforschung usw. Arbeitsgemeinschaften für Intensivmedizin, Stereotaxie und funktionelle Neurochirurgie sowie pädiatrische Neurochirurgie haben die Aufgabe, spezielle Entwicklungen im Rahmen der Neurochirurgie zu fördern. Im Jahre 1970 wurde die Wilhelm-

Tönnis-Stiftung ins Leben gerufen, die Stipendien an junge Neurochirurgen zur Ausbildung an Forschungs- und Lehrstätten im Ausland vergibt.

Weniger erfreulich haben sich die Dinge um das Zentralblatt für Neurochirurgie entwickelt, das als erste Fachzeitschrift der Welt im Jahre 1936 von Prof. Tönnis gegründet wurde und seitdem in einem Leipziger Verlag erscheint. Den westdeutschen Herausgebern wurde in diesem Jahr die Mitarbeit gekündigt, ohne daß stichhaltige sachliche Argumente hervorgebracht werden konnten. Wenn die Zusammenarbeit von Ost und West nicht einmal auf einem so unpolitischen Gebiet wie der Neurochirurgie möglich ist, dann dürfte das ein weiteres Beispiel dafür sein, wie einseitig Entspannungspolitik gehandhabt wird. Den westdeutschen Herausgebern des Zentralblattes, vor allen Dingen den Bemühungen seines langjährigen Chefredakteurs, Herrn Zülch, ist es zu danken, daß ein Nachfolgeblatt in diesen Tagen aus der Taufe gehoben werden kann.

Versuchen wir, die Entwicklung der Deutschen Neurochirurgie in Zahlen auszudrücken, so ergibt sich folgendes: Es existieren in der Bundesrepublik zur Zeit insgesamt 51 selbständige Neurochirurgische Einrichtungen, 22 Ordinariate, 39 außeruniversitäre Abteilungen; davon sind in den letzten acht Jahren zwei Ordinariate und zwölf selbständige Abteilungen entstanden. Zusätzlich wurden vier selbständige Abteilungen für stereotaktische bzw. funktionelle Neurochirurgie geschaffen. Die Berufsaussichten für unseren Nachwuchs sind also offenbar gar nicht so ungünstig wie mancher annehmen mag. Die bisherige Entwicklung hat gezeigt, daß auch unsere Befürchtungen, sich einer zu weitgehenden Spezialisierung gewidmet zu haben, nicht zu Recht bestanden. Die Neurochirurgie ist unterdessen ein fest eingefügter, nicht mehr wegzudenkender Bestandteil der klinischen Medizin geworden und die stets neu auf uns zukommenden operativen Aufgaben deuten darauf hin, daß die Entwicklung nach wie vor in starker Bewegung ist.

So dürfen wir hoffen, auch in den nächsten Tagen Neues zu lernen. Darüber hinaus freue ich mich auf Köln und die Begegnung mit früheren Kollegen und Mitarbeitern, mit denen mich Erinnerungen an die Kölner Zeit verbinden, in denen wir noch neurochirurgische Kinderpantoffeln trugen und versuchten, sie abzustreifen.

Ich wünsche Ihnen gute und schöne Tage und unserem Kongreß-Präsidenten, Herrn Frowein, und seinen Mitarbeitern einen erfolgreichen Verlauf seiner Tagung.

F. Marguth

Contents

Craniocerebral Trauma

Increase Intracranial Pressure

H. Vogelsang and C. Rieck: Prognosis of Severe Head Injuries in Relation to the Flow Speed of Contrast Medium in Cerebral Angiography   1

M. Gaab, O. E. Knoblich, K. Dietrich, and P. Gruss: Miniaturized Methods of Monitoring Intracranial Pressure in Craniocerebral Trauma Before and After Operation   5

Classification and Prognosis

R. Braakman: Interactions Between Factors Determining Prognosis in Populations of Patients With Severe Head Injury   12

R. A. Frowein, H. W. Steinmann, K. auf der Haar, D. Terhaag, and A. Karimi-Nejad: Limits to Classification and Prognosis of Severe Head Injury   16

W. Lanksch, Th. Grumme, and E. Kazner: Correlations Between Clinical Symptoms and Computerized Tomography Findings in Closed Head Injuries . .   27

H. W. Pia, H. Abtahi, and R. Schönmayer: Epidemiology, Classification, and Prognosis of Severe Craniocerebral Injuries: Computer-Assisted Study of 9038 Cases   31

W. I. Steudel and J. Krüger: Using the Frequency Analysis of the EEG for Prognosis in Severe Brain Injuries   36

H. E. Nau and W. J. Bock: Electroencephalographic (EEG) Differentation of the Apallic Syndrome in Severe Craniocerebral Injuries   44

D. Kühne and H. Arnold: Diagnosis of Brain Death by Means of Computerized Tomography   52

J. Brihaye: Classification and Prognosis of Coma: Summary and Conclusion . . .   54

Hematomas

E. Hamel and A. Karimi-Nejad: Traumatic Intracerebral Hematomas   56

K. Weigel, Chr. B. Ostertag, and F. Mundinger: CT Follow-Up Control of Traumatic Intracerebral Hemorrhage   62

H. Huttarsch and G. Cardauns: Clinically Nonmanifest Hematomas   68

Frontobasal Injuries

I. SCHÖTER: Head Injuries in Young Motorcyclists 71
H. E. DIEMATH, B. RICHLING, and G. SORGO: Safety Helmets and Craniocerebral Injuries 75
R. A. PACHAY: Catamneses of Frontobasal Head Injuries 78

Prolonged Unconsciousness

F. MILTNER and J. WICKBOLDT: Effects of Anti-Parkinsonian Drugs on Behavior and EEG of Comatose Patients 83
O. LEITHOLF and E. KNECHT: Long-Term Observation of Patients With Closed Head Injuries and a 24 h Period of Unconsciousness 88
B. WIDER, H. LANGE-COSACK, and H. J. SCHLESENER: Late Sequelae of Head Injury in Infancy and Early Childhood, With Special Reference to Child Abuse 91
M. LANGER and D. TERHAAG: Follow-Up Studies After Craniocerebral Injury in Children 98
S. TODOROW and E. HEISS: The "Fall-Asleep-Syndrome" – A Kind of Secondary Disturbance of Consciousness After Head Injury in Children 102
A. VIOLON, J. DEMOL, and J. BRIHAYE: Memory Sequelae After Severe Head Injuries 105

Clinical Aspects and Research

J. P. EVANS: Notes on the Development of Interest in North America in Head Injury 108
W. REICHMANN, J. ROSENBERGER, and B. HORTEN: Schedule for the Care of Extremity Fractures in Patients With Serious Brain Injuries 112
N. FRECKMANN, K. SARTOR, and K. MATSUMOTO: Angiographic Demonstration of Vascular Injuries Following Head Injury and Its Significance 116
A. LAUN: Traumatic Aneurysms 124
L. AUER, E. MARTH, W. PETEK, H. HOLZER, and G. GELL: The Prognostic Value of Biochemical Data From Blood and CSF: Analysis in Patients With Severe Head Injury 132
R. PREGER: Changes in Lipid Metabolism in Experimentally Produced Head Injury: Qualitative and Quantitative Studies of Lipids 138

Cerebellum

Positive Ventriculography

ST. KUNZE and W. HUK: Ventriculography With Resorbable Contrast Media: Field of Indication and Experience 147

H.-P. Richter and P. C. Potthoff: Ventriculography With Amipaque (Metrizamide) 150
H. Altenburg and W. Walter: Value of Central Ventriculography With Dimer-X in the Differentiation Between Cerebellar Tumors and Caudal Brain Stem Tumors Before and After Radiation Therapy of So-Called Inoperable Midline Tumors 155

Computer Tomography

Th. Grumme, A. Aulich, E. Kazner, K. Kretschmar, W. Lanksch, and W. Meese: Typical Findings With Computerized Tomography in Tumors of the Posterior Fossa 159
E. Kazner, Th. Grumme, W. Lanksch, and J. Wilske: Limitations of Computerized Tomography in the Detection of Posterior Fossa Lesions 166
W. Ischebeck, H. U. Thal, and R. Nabakowski: Computerized Tomography of the Posterior Fossa and the Upper Cervical Spine 171
W. Mauersberger: Vascular Deformity of the Basilar Artery Which Gave the Clinical and Computerized Tomographic Impression of a Tumor 176

Intracranial Pressure

K. E. Richard: Long-Term Measuring of Ventricular CSF Pressure With Tumors of the Posterior Fossa 179
M. Brock, W. M. Tamburus, C. R. Telles Ribeiro, and H. Dietz: Circadian Occurrence of Pathologic Cerebrospinal Fluid Pressure Waves in Patients With Brain Tumor 188
B. Böhm, M. Mohadjer, and R. Hemmer: Preoperative Continuous Measurements of Ventricular Pressure in Hydrocephalus Occlusus With Tumors of the Posterior Fossa: The Value of Ventriculoauricular Shunt 194
P. Gruss, M. Gaab, and O. E. Knoblich: Disorders of CSF Circulation After Interventions in the Area of the Posterior Cranial Fossa With Prior Shunt Operation 199
J. Zierski: Ventricular Drainage in Patients With Posterior Fossa Tumors and the Problem of Intracranial Decompensation 203
N. O. Ameli and H. Rahmat: A Safe and Simple Method of Ventricular Drainage . 209
E. C. Fuchs: Quantitative CSF Drainage in Cases of Posterior Fossa Tumor . . . 211
M. Schäfer, C. Lapras, and H. Ruf: Catheterization of the Aqueduct in Certain Lesions of the Posterior Fossa 216

Clinical Aspects and Anatomy

D. Linke: Electromyographic Analysis of Brain Nerve Reflexes in Posterior Fossa Processes 221
H. Stefan, J. Wappenschmidt, and W. Fröscher: Prepontine and Parapontine Tumors 224

K. Sartor, E. Fliedner, N. Freckmann, and K. Matsumoto: The Role of Angiotomography in the Evaluation of the Posterior Fossa 229

Medulloblastomas

W. Müller, F. Slowik, and R. Schröder: Studies on the Biology of Medulloblastoma 232
D. K. Böker, W. Entzian, and F. Gullotta: Immunoelectrophoretic Evaluations in Posterior Fossa Tumors 236
O. Wilcke and U. Fuhrmann: The Clinic of Medulloblastoma 239
N. Klug: Management and Prognosis of Medulloblastomas: Review Series of 80 Cases 245
H. Arnold, G. Grubel, H. Franke, I. Grosch, and G. Marsmann: Results of Medulloblastoma Treatment Under the Influence of Modern Therapy . . . 253
P. Gutjahr and D. Voth: Successful Treatment of Childhood Medulloblastoma – and What Thereafter? 257
J. Menzel, H. J. Denecke, and H. Penzholz: Surgery of Extensive Glomus Jugulare Tumors 259
H. Miltz and H.-U. Thal: Catamnestic Examinations of Patients With Cerebellar Tumors 266
F. Oppel, Ch. Zeytountchian, G. Mulch, and H.-D. Kunft: Endoscopy of the Cerebellopontine Angle: Its Diagnostic and Therapeutic Possibilities 269

Free Communications

K. J. Zülch: Principles of the New WHO Classification of Brain Tumors 279
W. Heienbrock, M. Roters, and W. A. Linden: Objective Characterization of Proliferation and Malignancy in Human Brain Tumors 285
H. D. Mennel and J. Szymas: Chemotherapy of Brain Tumors – Experimental Results 289
J. N. Petrovici and H.-W. Ilsen: Chemotherapy of Brain Tumors 292
E. Markakis, R. Heyer, L. Stoeppler, and J. Taegert: Agenesis of the Perisylvian Region (Temporal Lobe Agenesis): Neurologic Symptoms and Therapy . . 297
G. Graef: Interhemispheric Subdural Empyema 302
J. Krüger, A. Ritz, and W. Ingunza: A Case of Intraventricular Hydatid Cyst . . . 306
D. Voth, P. Gutjahr, and J. Spranger: Benign Osteoblastoma of the Skull With Secondary Aneurysmal Bone Cyst Formation, With Special Reference to the Differential Diagnosis of Osteogenic Sarcoma 311
A. Grimmer: EEG-Changes With Acute Secondary Mesencephalic Lesions Accompanied by Disturbances of Consciousness 313
R. Müke: Value of Measuring the Cranial Circumference 320
M. Samii and W. Draf: Neurosurgical-ENT Treatment of Lesions of the Base of the Skull 324

Increase in Intracranial Pressure

M. HOLZGRAEFE and O. SPOERRI: Elucidation and Histologic Technique: An Aid in Determining Pathologic Changes in Bones as Exemplified by Hydrocephalus in the C57 Black Murine Strain 331
O. E. KNOBLICH, M. GAAB, U. FUHRMEISTER, F. HERRMANN, K. DIETRICH, and P. GRUSS: Comparison of the Effects of Osmotherapeutic Agents, Hyperventilation, and Tromethamine (THAM) on Brain Pressure and Electric Activity of the Brain in Experimental and Clinical Brain Edema 336
R. SCHRÖDER: Chronomorphology of Brain Death 346

Intensive Therapy

R. NESSLER: Catheterization of the Superior Vena Cava With the ALPHA System 349

Vascular Surgery

W. WALTER and H. ALTENBURG: Operative Treatment of Giant Basal Intracranial Aneurysms 351
V. OLTEANU-NERBE, H. INGRISCH, F. MARGUTH, and H. STEINHOFF: Therapeutic Embolization of the External Carotid Artery 354
J. DE PREUX: Multipurpose Bipolar Forceps 360

Spine and Spinal Cord

H. COLLMANN, R. WÜLLENWEBER, CH. SPRUNG, M. BOROWSKI, and R. DUISBERG: Alteration of Spinal Cord Blood Flow in the Area Surrounding an Experimental Injury 362
J. SCHRAMM, K. HASHIZUME, H. TAKAHASHI, and T. FUKUSHIMA: Histologic Findings in Graded Experimental Spinal Cord Compression in the Cat 368
K. ROOSEN, W. GROTE, J. LIESEGANG, and U. LINKE: Epidural Temperature Changes During Anterior Cervical Interbody Fusion With Polymethylmethacrylate . 373
J. WICKBOLDT and F. MILTNER: Value of EMG Monitoring in Percutaneous Chordotomy 376
H. TAKAHASHI, M. STRASCHILL, and L. KÜTER: Value of the F Wave in the Diagnosis of Cervical and Lumbosacral Root Compression Syndromes 382
H. ASSMUS: Diagnostic Value of the Somatosensory Evoked Response (SER) in Peripheral Nerve Lesions 389

Subject Index 393

List of Senior Authors

ALTENBURG, H.: Lehrstuhl für Neurochirurgie, Chirurgische Klinik der Westfälischen Wilhelms-Universität, Jungeblodtplatz 1, D-4400 Münster (FRG)

AMELI, N. O.: Dariush Kabir Medical School, Teheran (Iran)

ARNOLD, H.: Neurochirurgische Abteilung der Neurologischen Universitätsklinik, Martinistrasse 52, D-2000 Hamburg (FRG)

ASSMUS, H.: Neurochirurgische Abteilung des Chirurgischen Zentrums der Universität, Im Neuenheimer Feld 110, D-6900 Heidelberg (FRG)

AUER, L.: Landeskrankenhaus, A-8036 Graz (Austria)

BÖHM, B.: Neurochirurgische Universitätsklinik, Hugstetter Strasse 55, D-7800 Freiburg (FRG)

BÖKER, D. K.: Neurochirurgische Universitätsklinik, D-5300 Bonn-Venusberg (FRG)

BRAAKMAN, R.: Academisch Ziekenhuis, Dr. Molewaterplein 40, Rotterdam 3002 (The Netherlands)

BRIHAYE, J.: Clinique Neurochirurgicale, 1, rue Heger Bordet, B-1000 Bruxelles (Belgium)

BROCK, M.: Neurochirurgische Klinik der Medizinischen Hochschule Hannover, Karl-Wiechert-Allee 9, D-3000 Hannover 61 (FRG)

COLLMANN, H.: Neurochirurgische Klinik der Freien Universität Berlin, Klinikum Charlottenburg, Spandauer Damm 130, D-1000 Berlin (FRG)

DE PREUX, J.: Neurochirurgische Universitätsklinik, Gosslerstraße 10, D-3400 Göttingen (FRG)

DIEMATH, H. E.: Abteilung für Neurochirurgie der Landesnervenklinik, Ignaz Harrerstrasse 79, A-5020 Salzburg (Austria)

EVANS, J. P.: Assistant Director Amer. College of Surgeons, 55 East Erie Street, Chicago, Illinois (USA)

FRECKMANN, N.: Strahlendiagnostische Abteilung, Allgemeines Krankenhaus Altona, Paul-Ehrlich-Strasse 1, D-2000 Hamburg 50 (FRG)

FROWEIN, R. A.: Neurochirurgische Universitätsklinik Köln, Joseph-Stelzmann-Strasse 9, D-5000 Köln (FRG)

FUCHS, E. C.: Neurochirurgische Klinik und Poliklinik, Spandauer Damm 130, D-1000 Berlin 19 (FRG)

Gaab, M.: Neurochirurgische Klinik der Universität Würzburg, Kopfklinik, Josef-Schneider-Strasse 11, D-8700 Würzburg (FRG)

Graef, G.: Neurochirurgische Klinik im Klinikum Charlottenburg der Freien Universität Berlin, Spandauer Damm 130, D-1000 Berlin 19 (FRG)

Grimmer, A.: Neurochirurgische Abteilung, Klinikum Westend, Freie Universität Berlin, Spandauer Damm 130, D-1000 Berlin-Westend (FRG)

Grumme, Th.: Neurochirurgische Klinik der Freien Universität Berlin, Klinikum Westend, Spandauer Damm 130, D-1000 Berlin 19 (FRG)

Gruss, P.: Neurochirurgische Universitätsklinik, Josef-Schneider-Strasse 11, D-8700 Würzburg (FRG)

Gutjahr, P.: Universitäts-Kinderklinik, Langenbeckstrasse 1, D-6500 Mainz (FRG)

Hamel, E.: Neurochirurgische Universitätsklinik, Gleueler Strasse 12, D-5000 Köln 41 (FRG)

Heienbrock, W.: Neurochirurgische Abteilung der Neurologischen Universitätsklinik, Martinistrasse 52, D-2000 Hamburg 20 (FRG)

Holzgraefe, M.: Neurochirurgische Universitätsklinik, Gosslerstrasse 10, D-3400 Göttingen (FRG)

Huttarsch, H.: Institut für Anästhesiologie, Medizinische Universitätsklinik, Joseph-Stelzmann-Strasse 9, D-5000 Köln (FRG)

Ischebeck, W.: Neurochirurgische Klinik der Universität, Moorenstrasse 5, D-4000 Düsseldorf 1 (FRG)

Kazner, E.: Neurochirurgische Klinik im Klinikum Grosshadern der Ludwig-Maximilians-Universität, Marchioninistrasse 15, D-8000 München 70 (FRG)

Klug, N.: Neurochirurgische Universitätsklinik, Klinikstrasse 29, D-6300 Giessen (FRG)

Knoblich, O. E.: Neurochirurgische Klinik der Universität Würzburg, Kopfklinik, Josef-Schneider-Strasse 11, D-8700 Würzburg (FRG)

Krüger, J.: Abteilung für Allgemeine Neurochirurgie im Zentrum der Neurologie und Neurochirurgie des Klinikums der J. W. Goethe-Universität Frankfurt am Main, Schleusenweg 2–16, D-6000 Frankfurt am Main 71 (FRG)

Kühne, D.: Neuroradiologische Abteilung des Universitätskrankenhauses, D-2000 Hamburg-Eppendorf (FRG)

Kunze, S.: Neurochirurgische Universitätsklinik, Krankenhausstraße 12, D-8520 Erlangen (FRG)

Langer, M.: Neurochirurgische Universitätsklinik, Joseph-Stelzmann-Strasse 9, D-5000 Köln 41 Lindenthal (FRG)

Lanksch, W.: Neurochirurgische Klinik im Klinikum Grosshadern der Ludwig-Maximilians-Universität, Marchioninistrasse 15, D-8000 München 70 (FRG)

Laun, A.: Zentrum für Neurochirurgie am Klinikum der Justus-Liebig-Universität Giessen, Klinikstrasse 37, D-6300 Giessen (FRG)

LEITHOLF, O.: Neurologische Kliniken Dr. Schmieder, D-7704 Gailingen (FRG)

LINKE, D.: Neurochirurgische Universitätsklinik, Annaberger Weg, D-5300 Bonn-Venusberg (FRG)

MARKAKIS, E.: Neurochirurgische Klinik der Medizinischen Hochschule Hannover, Karl-Wiechert-Allee 9, D-3000 Hannover 61 (FRG)

MAUERSBERGER, W.: Neurochirurgische Klinik im Klinikum Charlottenburg der Freien Universität Berlin, Spandauer Damm 130, D-1000 Berlin 19 (FRG)

MENNEL, H. D.: Pathologisches Institut der Universität, Albertstrasse 19, D-7800 Freiburg (FRG)

MENZEL, J.: Neurochirurgische Abteilung des Chirurgischen Zentrums der Universität, Im Neuenheimer Feld 110, D-6900 Heidelberg 1 (FRG)

MILTNER, F.: Neurochirurgische Universitätsklinik, Josef-Schneider-Strasse 11, D-8700 Würzburg (FRG)

MILTZ, H.: Neurochirurgische Universitätsklinik, Moorenstrasse 5, D-4000 Düsseldorf (FRG)

MÜKE, R.: Neurochirurgische Abteilung der Neurologischen Universitätsklinik, Martinistrasse 52, D-2000 Hamburg 20 (FRG)

MÜLLER, W.: Pathologisches Institut der Universität Köln, Joseph-Stelzmann-Strasse 9, D-5000 Köln 41 (FRG)

NAU, H. E.: Neurochirurgische Universitätsklinik, Hufelandstrasse 55, D-4300 Essen 1 (FRG)

NESSLER, R.: Paracelsusstrasse 24, D-3320 Salzgitter 51 (FRG)

OLTEANU-NERBE, V.: Neurochirurgische Klinik der Universität München, Klinikum Grosshadern, Marchioninistrasse 15, D-8000 München 70 (FRG)

OPPEL, F.: Neurochirurgische Klinik, Klinikum Steglitz der Freien Universität Berlin, Hindenburgdamm 30, D-1000 Berlin 45 (FRG)

PACHAY, R. A.: Neurochirurgische Universitätsklinik, Gleueler Strasse 12, D-5000 Köln 41 (FRG)

PETROVICI, J. N.: Neurologische Klinik der Städtischen Krankenanstalten Merheim, Ostmerheimer Strasse 200, D-5000 Köln 91 (FRG)

PIA, H. W.: Neurochirurgische Universitätsklinik, Klinikstrasse 29, D-6300 Giessen (FRG)

PREGER, R.: Eichendorffstrasse 13, D-7400 Tübingen 5 (FRG)

REICHMANN, W.: Abteilung für Unfallchirurgie in der Chirurgischen Universitätsklinik Köln, Joseph-Stelzmann-Strasse 9, D-5000 Köln 41 (FRG)

RICHARD, K. E.: Neurochirurgische Universitätsklinik Köln, Joseph-Stelzmann-Strasse 9, D-5000 Köln 41 (FRG)

RICHTER, H.-P.: Neurochirurgische Abteilung des Bezirkskrankenhauses, Reisenburger Strasse 2, D-8870 Günzburg (FRG)

Roosen, K.: Neurochirurgische Universitätsklinik, Hufelandstrasse 55, D-4300 Essen (FRG)

Samii, M.: Neurochirurgische Universitätsklinik, Langenbeckstrasse 1, D-6500 Mainz (FRG)

Sartor, K.: Strahlendiagnostische Abteilung, Allgemeines Krankenhaus Altona, Paul-Ehrlich-Strasse 1, D-2000 Hamburg 50 (FRG)

Schäfer, M.: Abteilung für Allgemeine Neurochirurgie im Klinikum der Universität, Schleusenweg 2–16, D-6000 Frankfurt/Main (FRG)

Schramm, J.: Neurochirurgische Klinik, Klinikum Steglitz der Freien Universität Berlin, Hindenburgdamm 30, D-1000 Berlin 45 (FRG)

Schröder, R.: Pathologisches Institut der Universität Köln, Joseph-Stelzmann-Strasse 9, D-5000 Köln 41 (FRG)

Schöter, I.: Neurochirurgische Universitätsklinik Venusberg, Annaberger Weg, D-5300 Bonn (FRG)

Stefan, H.: Universitäts-Nervenklinik, Annaberger Weg, D-5300 Bonn (FRG)

Steudel, W. I.: Neurochirurgische Universitätsklinik, Schleusenweg 2, D-6000 Frankfurt/Main (FRG)

Takahashi, H.: Neurochirurgische Universitätsklinik im Klinikum Steglitz, Hindenburgdamm 30, D-1000 Berlin 45 (FRG)

Todorow, S.: Neurochirurgische Abteilung im Zentrum für Chirurgie der Universität, Calwer Strasse 7, D-7400 Tübingen (FRG)

Violon, A.: Service de Neurochirurgie, 1, rue Heger Bordet, Bruxelles (Belgium)

Vogelsang, H.: Abteilung für Neuradiologie der Medizinischen Hochschule, Karl-Wiechert-Allee 9, D-3000 Hannover 61 (FRG)

Voth, D.: Neurochirurgische Universitätsklinik, Langenbeckstrasse 1, D-6500 Mainz (FRG)

Walter W.: Neurochirurgische Abteilung der Chirurgischen Universitäsklinik, Jungeblodtplatz 1, D-4400 Münster (FRG)

Weigel, K.: Neurochirurgische Universitätsklinik, Hugstetter Strasse 55, D-7800 Freiburg (FRG)

Wickboldt, J.: Neurochirurgische Universitätsklinik, Josef-Schneider-Strasse 11, D-8700 Würzburg (FRG)

Wider, B.: Jagowstrasse 9, D-1000 Berlin 21 (FRG)

Wilcke, O.: Neurochirurgische Universitätsklinik Köln, Joseph-Stelzmann-Strasse 9, D-5000 Köln (FRG)

Zierski, J.: Neurochirurgische Klinik, Klinikstrasse 29, D-6300 Giessen (FRG)

Zülch, K. J.: Max-Planck-Institut für Hirnforschung, Ostmerheimer Strasse 200, D-5000 Köln 91 (FRG)

Craniocerebral Trauma

Increase in Intracranial Pressure

Prognosis of Severe Head Injuries in Relation to the Flow Speed of Contrast Medium in Cerebral Angiography[1]

H. VOGELSANG and C. RIECK

Apart from its diagnostic possibilities, cerebral angiography is also helpful in deciding on the prognosis in severe head injuries. The retardation of circulation as a result of increased intracranial pressure - by a hematoma or an acute, localized, or generalized brain edema - demonstrates this clearly. This had already been shown by TÖNNIS and his school in the 1950s (c.f. 5, 9). It is a proven fact that a retarded circulation indicates an unfavorable prognosis, which ends in an arrest of circulation, i.e., cerebral death. Between these two extremes - normal time of circulation and its arrest - where does the chance to survive lie? When should the neurosurgeon stop his efforts?

According to the little we know from the literature (1, 3, 6, 7, 8) no patient with severe head injury has survived a retarded circulation of more than 6 s. About half of the injured had already died with a slowing down to 5 s. In order to reexamine these reports in the literature and the almost daily decision that has to be made on whether or not to operate, we examined the serial angiograms of 150 patients with severe head injuries and its consecutive symptoms with regard to the speed of flow. Of these 150 cases (3-80 years of age), 79 were extradural and subdural hematomas, 31 intracerebral hematomas, and 40 contusional swelling or edema. With a few exceptions, all hematomas were operated on; 106 patients died.

According to the methods described in the literature, we measured the time of circulation from the moment the contrast medium entered the intracranial part of the carotis artery until the first vein could be seen (GREITZ, 2: the average of arteriovenous flow rate normally is 3.5 ± 0.5 s). The interpreter of the films was quite independent and did not know the clinical course. With the help of the follow-up and medical records, we tried to find a relationship between the course of the disease and the results of measuring the circulation time.

The relation of the prognosis to the retardation in circulation can be clearly demonstrated. Meanwhile, in a normal circulation of 4 s, seven out of nine patients survived, one in two died with a slowing down to 5-6 s, one in three with a slowing down to 7 s, and none survived with a slowing down to 8 s or more (Fig. 1). This coincides with what we know from the literature (Fig. 2). Half of the patients with a slowing of the circulation time to 7 s or more had already died within 2 days of angiography (Fig. 3).

---

[1] This paper includes parts of the M.D. thesis of C. RIECK.

If the initial time of circulation was retarded to 8 s, the unfavorable prognosis could not be influenced, either by operation or by a maximum of intensive care. This was not even possible when a postoperative angiographic control showed a slight improvement in the retarded circulation, as we were able to demonstrate in a few cases. This seems to be an important fact which we believe we have substantiated with these observations.

In summary, we may say that a retardation of circulation of 8 s or more indicates irreparable cerebral damage, which in no case - with or without operation - can be survived. As early as 1972, the late Dr. H. KRAUSS (4), neurosurgeon from Vienna, when asked by an interviewer if he would operate on an identified extradural hematoma with a circulatory slowing to 8 s answered: "... no, there is no sense in it, but with 6 s one is obliged to operate ..." Nothing can be added to this, not even today.

References

1. FREITAG, G., FREITAG, J., KRUMBHOLZ, S., KALISKI, D., WILLENBERG, E.: Relation zwischen zerebraler Blutzirkulationsverlangsamung und Überlebenschance bei gedecktem Schädel-Hirntrauma. Zentralbl. Chir. 100, 210-213 (1975)
2. GREITZ, A.: A radiologic study of the brain circulation by rapid serial angiography of the carotid artery. Acta Radiol. Suppl. 40 (Stockh.) (1956)
3. GRUNERT, V., KRENN, J., KUTSCHA-LISSBERG, E., VALENCAK, E.: Le pronostic des contusions cérébrales. Neurochirurgie 15, 275-281 (1969)
4. KRAUSS, H.: Zerebrale Durchblutungszeit und Überlebensprognose. In: Die Bestimmung des Todeszeitpunktes. KRÖSEL, W., SCHERZER, E. (eds.). Wien: Wilhelm Maudrich 1973
5. LOEW, F., WÜSTNER, S.: Diagnose, Behandlung und Prognose traumatischer Hämatome des Schädelinnern. Wien: Springer 1960
6. SALAH, S., VALENCAK, E.: KUTSCHA-LISSBERG, E., GRUNERT, V.: Dans quelle mesure l'angiographie est-elle un paramètre de la mort cérébrale? Neurochirurgie 18, 49-52 (1972)
7. SCHAPS, P., WEBER, K.: Die Berücksichtigung der Hirn-Kreislauf-Zeit bei akutem schwerem Schädel-Hirn-Trauma. Z. Aerztl. Fortbild. (Jena) 70, 695-698 (1976)
8. SCIALFA, G., CRISTI, G.F.: Prognostic value of cerebral angiography in non-surgical cases of traumatic coma. J. Neurosurg. Sci. 17, 202-204 (1973)
9. TÖNNIS, W., SCHIEFER, W.: Zirkulationsstörungen des Gehirns im Serienangiogramm. Berlin-Heidelberg-New York: Springer 1959

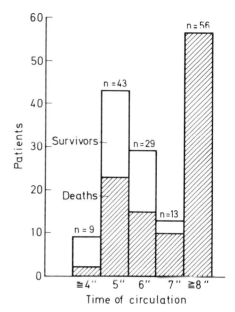

Fig. 1. Change of survival in relation to the speed of flow (our own patients: 150 cases)

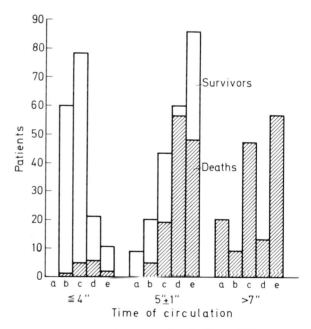

Fig. 2. Chance of survival in relation to the speed of flow (literature and our own patients: 503 cases)
References: a GRUNERT et al., b FREITAG et al., c SCIALFA et al., d SALAH et al., e VOGELSANG et al.

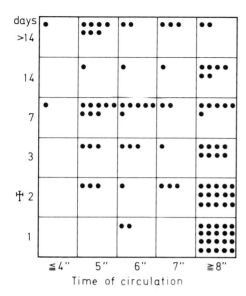

Fig. 3. Clinical death in relation to the speed of flow (our own patients: 106 cases)

Miniaturized Methods of Monitoring Intracranial Pressure in Craniocerebral Trauma Before and After Operation

M. GAAB, O. E. KNOBLICH, K. DIETRICH, and P. GRUSS

Introduction

One of the essential problems in brain injuries is the early recognition, diagnostic clarification, and precise treatment of post-traumatic increases in intracranial pressure (1, 4, 7). A continuous monitoring of intracranial pressure (ICP) after severe craniocerebral trauma allows ominous rises in ICP to be recognized appreciably earlier than by clinical observation of the patient (4, 9). Intracranial hematomas or a traumatic brain edema can thus be clarified diagnostically in time and treated accurately with simultaneous control of the result.

The methods previously available for monitoring ICP are not yet fully satisfactory (8, 9, and our own experience). Measurement of the ventricular pressure with catheters is technically not always possible (ventricular collapse at high pressure, blocked catheters). Ventricular puncture itself constitutes a brain injury. For the duration of measurement, there exists an increasingly appreciable risk of infection of the CSF pathways (10). Measurements of subdural fluid pressure (e.g., with the subdural screw (9)) likewise entail danger of infection and at high ICP with a compressed subarachnoid space are unreliable. The pressure transducers so far obtainable (2, 5) for measurement of epidural pressure are very large. Their epidural implantation necessitates a sterile burhole operation. Since the skin cannot be closed over these transducers, there is danger of infection and of skin necrosis. In vivo calibration is not possible and the systems are expensive.
We have, therefore, tested and developed miniaturized methods in the last 2 years (3). The pressure transducers should be appropriately small (9), technically reliable in zero point constancy and calibration and of good frequency resolution. They should involve little invasion in implantation, be capable of being employed for weeks, be capable of being calibrated enclosed in vivo, and also be cheap.

Methods

In neurosurgical patients, a distinction must be made between measurement of ICP after operation (trepanation) and measurement of ICP in nonoperated patients. In the first case, the pressure transducer can be implanted during operation (which should not thereby be prolonged or complicated). After the end of measurement, it must be possible to remove the receptor without renewed surgical intervention. In the second case, the pressure transducer should be placed in position with a low-risk intervention which is as small as possible, does not require surgical facilities, and can be performed directly in the intensive care unit. For both kinds of application, we use various strain-gauge transducers with the same electronic characteristics (nominal sensitivity 5 µV/V/mm Hg). The transducers can be sterilized in fluids (e.g., Alhydex) or with gas (normal ethylene oxide method) and can be connected to the same measuring chain. Any fullbridge measuring instrument with an alternating voltage supply to the bridge of a maximum of 7.5 V is suitable for this.

1. ICP Monotoring After Neurosurgical Operation

Here, a miniature pressure transducer[1] in the form of a thin flexible catheter is employed (Fig. 1a). The transducer (white tip) is 6 mm long, 4 mm wide, and 1.5 mm thick. The flattened pear shape prevents rotation around the long axis. The cable attached is shielded, coated with silicon rubber, and flexible. Application is in the manner of a drainage tube (Fig. 1b): the transducer is simply inserted epidurally, subdurally, or even intracerebrally (e.g., into a resection cavity) or into the ventricle. In epidural measurements, the side of the pressure transducer membrane (Fig. 1a) is oriented toward the dura. The cable is then led out like a catheter through the wound or a lateral stab incision. The measuring instrument is then calibrated and connected on the ward.

There are two possibilities available for in vivo calibration. In both, there is a small calibration balloon in front of the pressure-transducer membrane which is connected with a thin capillary tube in the cable. A second capillary is connected to the pressure compensation chamber behind the receptor membrane (pressure-difference transducer). In the one version, only the balloon is connected with the hypodermic insertion at the plug (Fig. 1a). By pressure-controlled (e.g., mercury calibrated manometer) air filling of the balloon, the implanted pressure transducer can be calibrated from outside, and the zero point determined indirectly (according to (5)). In the other version, the calibration balloon and pressure compensation chamber are connected together with the hypodermic insertion. The pressure is compensated by filling with air (about 0.1-0.5 ml at will), enabling the zero point to be directly controlled and corrected. After the end of measurement, the transducers are simply drawn out like a drainage tube.

2. Pressure Monitoring in Non-Operated Patients

For this purpose, we experimentally developed our own pressure transducer and a coplanar application technique (3). An appropriately miniaturized pressure transducer is now commercially available[2]. We further improved the application system clinically (Fig. 3). Through the miniaturization, a drillhole of merely 5 mm diameter is necessary. A stab incision is sufficient for this ("percutaneous" application); a small guiding funnel is introduced to avoid further skin contact (for instruments, see Fig. 2b). The small coaxial drill we constructed ourselves (3) permits an adjustment of the distance between the inner and outer drill corresponding to the thread length of the adaptor holder (Fig. 3). This distance determines the depth of the 5 mm boring since the drill decouples on reaching the dura. Since the thread length of the screwed-in adaptor now agrees with the 5 mm drill depth independently of the bone thickness (self-cutting fine thread), the pressure transducer placed in the adaptor holder is now automatically located coplanar to the dura. After removing the guiding funnel, the skin over the miniature transducer is closed completely tension-free, with one to one stitches. Only the thin cable is led through the skin to the measuring instrument. An in vivo calibration with balloon as described above can also be obtained with this pressure transducer.

---

1 Manufactured by Gaeltec Ltd., Scotland (type ICTb).
2 Manufactured by Gaeltic Ltd., Scotland (type 3 AE/special).

Results and Discussion

In our clinic, there are presently five pressure transducers available for postoperative and two for percutaneous application. The transducers were tested for zero point and gain stability in a water bath at $20°-40°$ C and 20 mm Hg pressure for 48 h. The zero point drift was a maximum of 2 mm Hg/24 h, which thus roughly correspond to the data of the manufacturers. Only after immersion in water (saturation of the silicon rubber coat) does a drift of about 10 mm Hg occur in the first 60 min and only in the catheter model. Transducers with an in vivo calibration facility should, therefore, be employed (readjustment about 1-2 h after the implantation). This in vivo adjustment of the zero point can be performed with an accuracy of ± 2 mm Hg. Since the in vivo drift measured up to now is a maximum of about 2 mm Hg/24 h and the gain adjustment does not alter, the accuracy of measurement is ± 4 mm Hg even with measurement over weeks with daily zero point control. A better result is usually attained.

1. Postoperative Measurements

Even rapid frequencies, e.g., the characteristic pulse curve (Fig. 4a), are reproduced well. In the 52 cases to date, the brain pressures were monitored for an average of 3.5 days (max. 12 days). The simplicity of implantation makes it applicable in any trepanation. Complications, in particular infections, have not been observed up to now. Thus far, comparison measurements with the subdural or ventricular pressure (five cases) revealed a good agreement of values taking into account height differences of the recording points, e.g., caused by different positions of the head. Technical failures up to now have been caused exclusively by exogenous damage to the transducers (e.g., pulling out by the patient).

2. Percutaneous Measurements

In contrast to the postoperative implantation, the technique requires some practice. Adaptor holder and drill must first be precisely co-ordinated with each other on a portion of skull. However, the adjustment then remains constant for all adaptors of the same thread length, and in the cases examined to date, a reproducible coplanar implantation without further correction was possible. The least screw-in depth of the thread (= least bone thickness) for stable implantation is about 2 mm. With a mean duration of measurement of 3 days (max. so far 8 days), there have been no complications and also no infection or skin necrosis. Figure 4b shows an example of measurement. Monitoring of intracranial pressure thus not only enables a developing intracranial space-occupying lesion to be recognized but is also a sensitive indicator for alterations in respiration or circulation. The low-risk, low-trauma implantation also suggests an application in neurologic patients (e.g., monitoring and control of therapy in stroke).

Summary

Two miniaturized methods for long-term monitoring of intracranial pressure are described. For measurement after trepanations, a miniature pressure transducer in the form of a catheter (transducer in the tip) is inserted like a drainage at operation epidurally, subdurally, or even intraventricularly. An in vivo calibration from outside permits measurement for several weeks. The transducer is easily extracted after the measurement. An equally small pressure transducer can be implanted percutaneously with a special technique directly in the intensive care unit for monitoring of nonoperated patients. A 5-mm drill hole of constant depth is applied with a self-decoupling special coaxial drill. The transducer put in with an adaptor holder is thus automatically located epidurally coplanar to the dura. The skin is closed free of tension. Complications, especially infections, have not occured up to now.

References

1. BECKER, D.P., MILLER, J.D., YOUNG, H.F., WARD, J.D., ADAMS, W.E.: The critical importance of ICP monitoring in head injury. In: Intracranial Pressure III. BEKS, J.W.F., BOSCH, D.A., BROCK, M. (eds.), pp. 97-100. Berlin-Heidelberg-New York: Springer 1976
2. BEKS, J.W.F., JOURNEE, H.L., ALBARDA, S., FLANDERIJN, H.: The significance of ICP-monitoring in the post-operative period. In: Intracranial Pressure III. BEKS, J.W.F., BOSCH, D.A., BROCK, M. (eds.), pp. 251-254. Berlin-Heidelberg-New York: Springer 1976
3. DIETRICH, K., GAAB, M., KNOBLICH, O.E., SCHUPP, J., OTT, B.: A new miniaturized system for monitoring the epidural pressure in children and adults. Neuropädiatrie $\underline{8}$, 21-28 (1977)
4. GOBIET, W.: Monitoring of intracranial pressure in patients with severe head injury. Neurochirurgia (Stutt.) $\underline{20}$, 35-47 (1977)
5. GOBIET, W., SCHUMACHER, W.: System zur intracraniellen Druckmessung. Hellige data sheet, Freiburg (1977)
6. GOBIET, W., BOCK, W.J., LIESEGANG, J., GROTE, W.: Experience with an intracranial pressure transducer readjustable in vivo. Technical note. J. Neurosurg. $\underline{39}$, 272-276 (1974)
7. GURDJIAN, E.S., THOMAS, L.M.: Surgical management of the patient with head injury. Clin. Neurosurg. $\underline{12}$, 56-74 (1964)
8. LANNER, G.: Neue Methoden und Erkenntnisse der Hirndruckmessung. Acta Chir. Aust. (Suppl.) $\underline{21}$, 1-19 (1976)
9. McGRAW, C.P.: Continuous intracranial pressure monitoring: Review of techniques and presentation of method. Surg. Neurol. $\underline{6}$, 149-155 (1976)
10. SUNDBÄRG, G., KJÄLLQUIST, A., LUNDBERG, N., PONTEN, U.: Complications due to prolonged ventricular fluid pressure recording in clinical practice. In: Intracranial Pressure. BROCK, M., DIETZ, H. (eds.), pp. 348-352. Berlin-Heidelberg-New York: Springer 1972

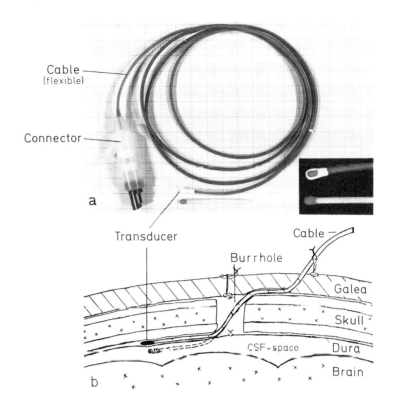

Fig. 1. Pressure transducer for implantation after trepanation
a The miniature pressure transducer sits in the white tip (*inset picture*: membrane side with calibration balloon). The shielded cable is flexible and coated with silicon rubber. Size comparison with a match
b Schematic representation of the possibilities of implantation (in the manner of a drain)

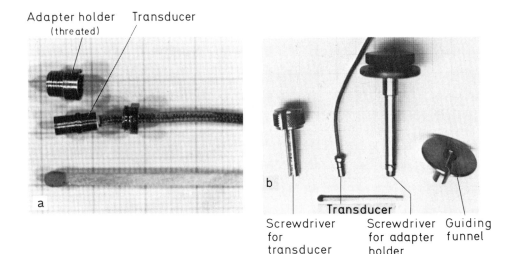

Fig. 2. Pressure-measuring system for percutaneous application in nonoperated patient
a Pressure transducer (silicon-coated metal membrane) with adaptor holder and reverse screw mounted on the cable
b Application instruments for implantation in a miniature drill hole (cf. Fig. 3). Size comparison with a match

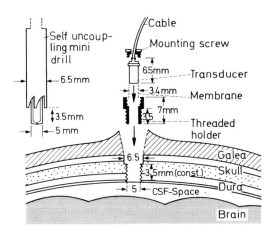

Fig. 3. Scheme of percutaneous application through a 5 mm drill hole. A constant depth of 5 mm is achieved with a special coaxial drill which couples on dural contact. After screwing in an adaptor with appropriate thread length (self-cutting), the pressure transducer is automatically placed epidurally coplanar to the dura

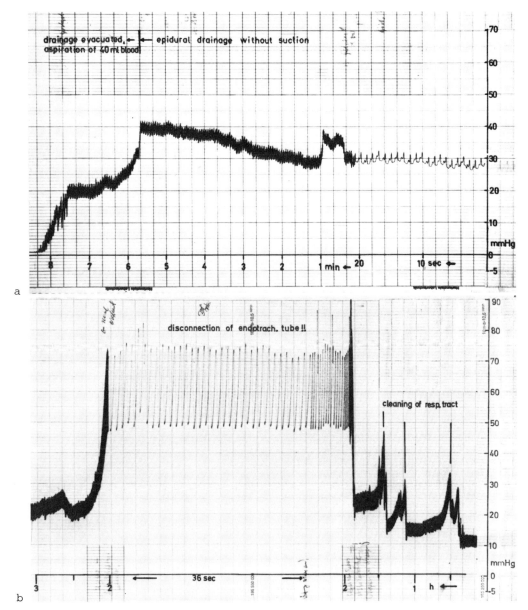

Fig. 4. Examples of measurements
<u>a</u> With pressure transducer in catheter form: extra dural bleeding after an operation on a temporal lobe contusion with disturbed drainage. Demonstration and control of treatment by measurement of epidural pressure
<u>b</u> After percutaneous application: nonoperated patient with primary brain stem damage. Four days pressure measurements: this demonstrates a disturbance of the controlled artificial respiration of the patient by measuring epidural pressure

Classification and Prognosis

Interactions Between Factors Determining Prognosis in Populations of Patients With Severe Head Injury

R. BRAAKMAN[1]

In the last decade, various classifications of coma by levels have been published. A summary of these classifications was given by FROWEIN in 1976 (1). In these classifications of coma an example of which is given in Table 1, the assumption is that different aspects of behavior indicating depth of coma and thus of prognostic significance always occur together. A strict and invariable relation is assumed between abnormalities in these features. The question remains whether this assumption is right or wrong.

Data Bank

In a transatlantic study on comatose patients, the neurosurgical centers of the University of Glasgow and Rotterdam, the Los Angeles County Hospital, and the Neurologic Department of the University of Groningen have built up a data bank of 1000 comatose head injury patients. Included are those patients who do not open their eyes, give no verbal response, and do not obey commands for at least 6 consecutive hours. Of these patients, 70 features are scored on admission, in the first 24 h after onset of coma, after 2-3 days, etc. The patients are followed up for at least 2 years. The outcome is classified in five clearly defined categories (death, persistent vegetative state, severe disability, moderate disability, and good recovery) (2). This outcome is related to the state of the patient in the first weeks.

Table 1. Example of a coma classification in levels as produced by various participants in a symposium on coma grading in 1976. There are various other examples in the literature with sometimes quite differing opinions of the response in a certain feature with similar coma levels

	Coma level			
	1	2	3	4
Motor pattern	Localizing	Flexion	Extension	None
Pupil reaction	+	+	+	-
Eye movement	+	+	Impaired	Absent
Apnea periodic respiration	-	-	-	+
Corneal reflex	+	+	+	-
Speech	-	-	-	-

---

[1] On behalf of the authors of Severe Head Injury in Three Countries (4).

Statistical analysis of the data available in this data bank has identified a limited number of features determining prognosis, whereas the other features are superfluous. Nine of the most important are presented in Table 2. On the basis of information regarding these features obtained in the first few days after the accident, it is possible to predict in each individual patient the probability of a certain outcome on this five point scale. This can be done by computer or nowadays even by calculation on a simple pocket calculator. The prediction has reached an unexpectedly high degree of reliability (a prediction is considered to be reliable if $p > .97$).

In order to monitor the depth of coma, TEASDALE and JENNETT (5) developed a scale in 1974 which was originally called the Glasgow coma scale, but for which we now prefer the name "responsiveness scale" (Table 3). Three aspects of responsiveness are assessed: eye opening, motor response, and verbal response. It is interesting to note that eye opening to which we attach great significance and which was included by FROWEIN in his definition of coma (1) - is not included in most other classifications. On this scale, each response is given a number: high for normal and low for impaired responses. By adding up these numbers, a total responsiveness *score* can be obtained which can vary from 3 to 15.

Table 2. Nine of the most important prognostic features in comatose patients with severe head injury

Best motor response
Total score responsiveness
Eye movements
Pupil reactions
Age
Presence of hematoma
Apnea
Motor pattern
Change (deterioration)

Table 3. Glasgow "coma" or responsiveness scale

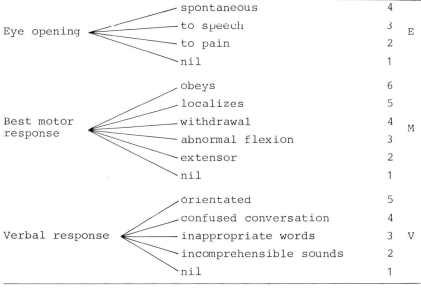

Interactions

In the distribution of the interactions between the three aspects of the responsiveness scale, a number of patterns are noticed which occur often, e.g., the combination $E_1M_4V_1$. However, the relation between the three scores varies considerably and may be different on successive days. The mean improvement curves of the three aspects are not parallel after onset of coma and are also different for those patients who survive compared with those who die. This means that the interaction between eye opening, motor pattern, and speech is not a fixed one, as suggested by classifications with three or four levels, and is time dependent. The variation in interaction between these three aspects and other prognostic factors like eye movement and pupil reactions has been indicated by JENNETT and TEASDALE (3). Some of their results are presented in Tables 4 and 5.

One of the statisticians of our group (Mr. A. Skene, London) investigated the interaction of two "epoch-independent" factors: age and the presence or absence of a hematoma. In our data bank of 1000 patients, he showed that the simplest model which adequately explained the results obtained was the pattern in which hematoma does not appear to have a straightforward effect on outcome except through age. This means that, given a person of a certain age, the presence or absence of a hematoma does not matter. Only in the group of people between 5 and 24 years of age does the presence of a hematoma seem to have a seperate and then adverse effect on outcome. He also established an interrelation between various factors which - according to clinicians - have something to do with the extent of brain damage and prognosis, like responsiveness total score, eye movements, and pupils. The influence of age on outcome is direct and not through relationship with these three factors. These three factors contribute to outcome directly and separately, but within a given level of eye indication and outcome, total score and pupils seem to be independent. This means that the prognostic value of these three indications together (i.e., a certain level in a classification of coma in levels) is less than the sum of the prognostic significance of each individuel indication. Or in other words, if one of the three is missing, less accurate prediction of outcome is possible. If, in order to determine prognosis, coma classifications in levels are used, the maximum effect of the information available is not obtained.

Table 4. Interaction between pupil reaction and responsiveness score

EMV sum	% with nonreacting pupils
3-5	56% of 153
6-7	20% of 164
8-15	9% of 216

Table 5. Interaction between eye movement and responsiveness score. The grading of eye movements is obtained by combining spontaneous eye movements, oculocephalic, and vestibulo-ocular responses

EMV sum	n	Nil	Bad	Impaired	Intact
3-5	120	23%	24%	19%	34%
6-7	135	7%	6%	20%	67%
8-15	182	0.5%	0%	4%	95.5%

Discussion

The interactions between the various features determining prognosis in comatose head injury patients are variable, time dependent, and not yet sufficiently understood. A few abnormal responses are so consistently associated with each other as to make it appropriate to define a certain level of outcome by the occurrence together of several abnormalities as is done in classifications of coma by levels. It is true that classifications by levels are definitely a step forward compared with designations of unconscious patients in terms: like coma, deep coma, semicoma, stupor, subcome, etc. However, overall classifications by levels do not cover all patients; a larger number of patients are in between two levels. So these overall classifications form an intermediate stage and should be abondoned again as soon as more is known about the interactions of other prognostic factors. This moment is - with the use of large data banks like the present one - not far off. Then, monitoring of comatose patients should preferably be performed by assessing several features *separately*, as this permits - with the use of advanced statistical techniques - more confident, accurate, and reliable predictions.

References

1. FROWEIN, R.A.: Classification of coma. Acta Neurochir. (Wien) 34, 5-10 (1976)
2. JENNETT, B., BOND, M.: Assessment of outcome after severe brain damage. A practical scale. Lancet 1975; 480-484
3. JENNETT, B., TEASDALE, G.: Aspects of coma after severe head injury. Lancet 1977; 878-881
4. JENNETT, B., TEASDALE, G., GALBRAITH, S., PICKARD, J., GRANT, H., BRAAKMAN, R., AVEZAAT, C., MAAS, A., MINDERHOUD, J., VECHT, C.J., HEIDEN, J., SMALL, R., CATON, W., KURZE, T.: Severe head injury in three countries. J. Neurol. Neurosurg. Psychiatry 40, 291-298 (1977)
5. TEASDALE, G., JENNETT, B.: Assessment of coma and impaired consciousness. A practical scale. Lancet 1974 ii; 81-85

Limits to Classification and Prognosis of Severe Head Injury

R. A. Frowein, H. W. Steinmann, K. auf der Haar, D. Terhaag, and A. Karimi-Nejad

Based on the efforts originally made by TÖNNIS and LOEW (16) and continued by a great number of authors to establish a prognostic classification of brain damage BUES (4) classified four grades of seriousness which were simplified by LOEW and HERRMANN (13). According to this classification, a first assessment of the seriousness of brain damage can be made from both the type and the duration of the disturbances of brain function. Other classifications have been based on the same factors, as can be seen from the summarized report by MÜLLER (14). BRAAKMANN (1) was able to show that a certain prognosis can be established by certain symptoms or combinations of symptoms in relation to the time elapsed after trauma (cf. 10). Furthermore, the development of intensive therapy has shown that besides type and duration of functional disturbances it is also the *age* of the patient which is of prognostic importance. This can be seen from statistics on mortality, especially the excellent studies by CARLSSON et al. (5), GOUTELLE and MOURET (9), and many others. This third factor, that of age, has not so far been sufficiently considered in the various prognosis schemes, with the possible exception of the one drawn up by OVERGAARD (15). The questions are, what symptoms allow a prognostic classification, in what way, until what time, and at what age.

Syndromes With Acute Prognostic Significance

To allow a prognostic evaluation of the different kinds of syndromes, two groups of patients will be dealt with:
1. Patients who were brought to the clinic by helicopter immediately after trauma (Fig. 1).
2. Seriously injured patients with long-lasting unconsciousness, of more than 48 h duration (Fig. 2).

Of a group of 50 patients transported from the accident site to the clinic by helicopter as quickly as possible, only such patients survived (dotted line) who during the time between accident and admission to the clinic and the following 1-2 h did not suffer from any disturbances or - if any - just slight clouding of consciousness, unconsciousness with or without anisocoria, pareses, or paroxysm or, at the worst, extensor rigidity. However, all those patients died - and many soon after the accident or transport - who showed or developed loss of extremity reactions or dilated and fixed pupils with or without respiratory disturbances lasting for more than 1 h even after intubation and circulatory regulation.

These observations are in accordance with analyses done on 180 patients who had been unconscious for more than 48 h and whose further progress can be evaluated by the appearance and disappearance of different syndromes in the time diagram (Fig. 2). It is obvious that the surviving patients developed pareses, anisocoria, and even extensor rigidity - especially children (triangle) and adolescents (square) (PIA and BUES, 4) - which, however, disappeared by the end of the period of unconsciousness. In the acute stage, the surviving patients did not develop a long-term absence of reaction of their extremities and fixed pupils

for more than 4 h. If there was no extremity reaction and/or the pupils
were fixed and dilated for a longer period, the brain damage suffered
was so serious that the patient did not survive, even if intensive therapy was applied for several days. Therefore, these seem to be the only
symptoms already suggesting an unfavorable prognosis in the acute stage
during the first 24 h. They do not depend on the age of the patient.
Any other kinds of symptoms do not allow a prognosis at this time. This
confirms the common clinical experience that, apart from vegetative
disorder and EEG changes, a few neurologic symptoms are sufficient to
assess the extent of disturbances of brain function in the initial
stage, e.g., disturbance of consciousness, extensor rigidity, dilated
and fixed pupils or complete loss of tone, central respiratory failure.
GERSTENBRAND (8) and BRICOLO (2) also mentioned the importance of
disturbances of eye movement. For this reason, these criteria were incorporated into the Brussels Suggestions on Coma Classification by
BRIHAYE et al. (3a).

Significance of Coma Duration and Age

The leading symptom of severe brain damage is unconsciousness in its
strict meaning, in Oxford defined as "coma," excluding the different
forms of clouding of consciousness (6). This gives rise to the question
of the prognostic significance of the duration of unconsciousness and
the age. Previous studies on 875 cases (with more than 24 h of unconsciousness) have provided results on what duration of unconsciousness
was survived by how many out of 355 patients. This was shown on a
summation curve for each decade. The 5% limit of these courses can be
considered an important marginal value for clinical vital prognosis:
if it is exceeded, the chance for survival drops below 5%. This is the
case with patients over 60 years of age with unconsciousness of more
than 5 days, with patients 50-30 years of age after 12 days, with patients 20-30 years of age after 15 days, and with patients 10-20 years
of age after 20 days, which is four times the value allowed for those
over 60 years of age.

If these values for the chances of survival in each decade are related
to the duration of unconsciousness, we obtain a 95% range for vital
prognosis with respect to age under our present means of diagnosis and
treatment (Fig. 3). It can easily be seen that with long-lasting unconsciousness survival chances of younger children decrease quickly.
This fact will be discussed later by LANGE-COSACK (11) and LANGER and
TERHAAG (12). Maximum values for complete recovery are markedly lower
(dotted line) than the 5% limit of prognosis for survival.

It remains to be seen whether these prognosis values provide a sufficient basis to be considered as marginal values for intensive therapy,
e.g., assisted respiration. These observations are based on 596 patients
of varying ages surviving an unconsciousness of more than 24 h. In the
last 10 years, 26 out of these surviving patients had suffered unconsciousness (horizontal line) that was longer than the 5% marginal value
attributed to their individual age (Table 1). In former times, the
duration of unconsciousness of each patient was simply added up, even
if it was interrupted by clouded consciousness (interrupted line);
nowadays, we consider the end of the first phase of unconsciousness
more significant.

With regard to the age, the number of patients surviving is quite
consistent, i.e., two to four survivals per decade, but eight in the
case of children up to the age of 10. Fourteen of the cases are closed
brain injuries, 12 of them intracranial hematomas. (The three patients

Table 1. Survivors with unconsciousness longer than the 5% limit

No.	Name of patient	Age	Year of treatment	Unconsciousness Time after trauma (days)	Total days	Kind of cerebral trauma Closed/open	Hematoma
26	L.M. 1249/75	71	1975	Secondary 1st-3rd; 4th-7th	7		Subdural, subacute
25	F.D. 218/74	64	1974	Secondary 1st-6th; 8th-10th	6		Intracerebral, subacute
24	Z.A. 372/76	61	1976	Secondary 2nd-9th	7		Intracerebral, subacute
23	W.J. 20946/70	58	1970	Secondary 2nd-12th	11		Subdural, subacute
22	G.I. 876/73	53	1973	Secondary 1st-11th	11		Subdural, acute
21	Z.J. 850/72	51	1972	Acute/ secondary 1st-5th; 8th-11th; 13th-14th	9		Epidural, acute
20	M.W. 17384/67	42	1967	Primary 1st-14th	14	Closed	
19	Z.L. 959/73	40	1973	Primary 1st-13th	13		Subdural, acute
18	G.H. 1133/76	37	1976	Primary 1st-17th	17		Epidural, subdural, acute
17	W.W. 933/72	33	1972	Primary 1st-12th; 19th-22th	14	Closed	
16	W.M. 708/72	31	1972	Acute/ secondary 1st-15th	15		Epidural, subacute
15	K.R. 14451/64	30	1964	Acute 1st-24th	24	Closed	
14	K.T. 20337/69	26	1969	Primary 1st-17th	17	Closed	

Fully-fit	Slightly limited I	Moderate limited II	Unfit	Follow-up time Years	Remarks
			+	2	Before trauma: anti-coagulants. Now: hemiparesis, confined to bed.
	+			1	Hypertension, cardiac insufficiency. Looks after household and herself.
			+	1	Pensioner in good condition.
			+		Hypertension. Nursing home.
			+	0,4	Long-term intubation: stridor. At home: pulmonary embolism, acute exitus after 4 months.
		+		5	
			+	2	In need of care.
	+			4	Alcohol abuse. Epileptic seizures.
		+		1	Alcohol abuse, debility, schizophrenia.
			+	2	Intensive rehabilitation wheel-chair.
		+		1	Crouzon's disease, worktests without success.
		+		13	Associated injuries: contusion pneumonia, fractures of femur.
+				2	After 3 months return to his work. Degree of disablement 20%.

Table 1. Survivors with unconsciousness longer than the 5% limit

No.	Name of patient	Age	Year of treatment	Unconsciousness Time after trauma (days)	Total days	Kind of cerebral trauma Closed/open	Hematoma
13	R.L. 19367/68	23	1968	Primary 1st-29th	29	Closed	
12	N.M. 118/71	20	1971	Primary 1st-17th	17		Epidural, acute
11	K.H. 19248/68	19	1968	Primary 1st-24th	24	Open	
10	S.H. 17306/67	11	1967	Primary 1st-30th	30	Closed	
9	F.A. 20433/69	11	1969	Primary 1st-18th	18		Intracerebral, acute
8	K.F. 13460/64	6	1964	Primary 1st-19th	19	Closed	
7	H.W. 911/72	5	1972	Primary 1st-19th	19	Closed	
6	M.A. 31/75	5	1975	Primary 1st-20th	20		Subdural, acute
5	L.HP. 391/71	5	1971	Primary 1st-20th	20	Closed	
4	R.B. 864/71	4	1971	Primary 1st-5th; 6th-17th	17	Closed	
3	R.E. 17490/67	4	1967	Primary 1st-9th; 10th-22nd	22	Closed	
2	K.A. 286/76	3	1976	Primary 1st-20th	20		Subdural, acute
1	S.M. 1155/72	3	1972	Primary 1st-14th; 17th-23rd	20	Closed	

Follow-up working capacity				Follow-up time Years	Remarks
Fully-fit	Slightly limited I	Moderate limited II	Unfit		
			+	1	Associated injuries: contusion pneumonia, fractures of the leg. After 1 year she died suddenly.
	+			2	Trouble with the economic studies.
			+	5	Sheltered workshop.
	+			10	Finished nonclassical secondary school, epileptic seizures.
		+		7	Sheltered workshop.
		+		10	School for mental disabled. Hemiparesis.
		+		4	School for mental disabled. Hemiparesis.
			+	0,3	Long-term intubation: stidor. After 3 months sudden death.
			+	2	Severe tetraplegia, in need of care, stereotaxic-Operation.
	+			2	Slight disturbance of the right hand.
	+			0,9	
			+	1	Staying in rehabilitation treatment.
	+			5	Promoted in 2nd class of elementary school.

over 50 mentioned before (1975), with exceedingly long period of unconsciousness, suffered from spontaneous, nontraumatic, subdural hematomas.) Follow-up of these surviving patients showed only one case that regained full fitness for work, 19 patients remained considerably disabled, ten patients remained completely disabled or had to be in hospital; three of these patients died from sequelae later on.

To check the neurologic representation, the syndrome time diagrams of the 26 surviving patients with extremely longlasting unconsciousness have been examined in the light of the Brussels Coma Classification and separately for the most important age groups taking the 5% limit into consideration for each of them. According to the explanation already given, of these 26 patients, one has encountered not only the symptoms of coma I and II but also coma III; the last one, accompanied by extensor rigidity, more often occured in the younger than in the older patients.

There are few short-term intervals with marked muscular hypotonia but no long-term ones with fixed dilated pupils. As was to be expected, EEG frequency analyses according to TÖNNIES's method showed a δ-θ dominance. Dominant frequencies with these surviving patients soon increased and - in most cases - did not remain below the θ-level any longer. Vegetative behavior showed relatively stable vital values in some cases even earlier but did not remain constant. For this reason, clinical recognition of those 26 surviving cases with extremely long periods of unconsciousness is not possible at a glance. Neurologically, they only distinguish themselves from a part of those 88 lethal cases with equally long-lasting unconsciousness who died mainly from bronchopulmonary changes or embolism ($\underline{8}$), tracheostenosis ($\underline{2}$), or renal insufficiency ($\underline{6}$). Only those cases can be recognized early as being unfavorable where the patients show a coma IV, in which they remain and, at the same time, where their EEG shows an increasingly shorter sequence of δ-phases leading to a dominance of sub-δ ones and/or a decreasing tension. There were only very few cases of α-comas.

Summary (Fig. 4)

We have *not* discussed:
1. *Slight* brain injuries with only short unconsciousness of up to 2 h.
2. *Moderately severe* brain injuries with unconsciousness of up to 24 h and clouded consciousness.

Serious cases of brain injuries with unconsciousness of more than 24 h showed wide differences according to the age of the patient. Prognosis for survival of patients in coma stages I-III becomes minimal and drops below 5% if unconsciousness has lasted for 5-20 days, depending on the age of the individual patient. No definite prognosis can be made in cases with shorter periods of unconsciousness. Limits for either restricted or complete recovery are below the 5% mark of vital prognosis.

Cases of acute brain damage with coma IV lasting for several hours have an unfavorable prognosis. The syndrome of brain death was not discussed here. Figure 4 shows the symptomatic importance of type and duration of brain function disturbances in relation to the age in cases of serious brain damage with long-lasting unconsciousness. As far as we can judge from our limited experience, the number of patients surviving in cases of extremely long unconsciousness has not increased particularly, and the period of unconsciousness that can be survived has not become any longer.

It seems that the average time of unconsciousness which patients were able to survive has been reduced by the improvement in intensive therapy measures. For this reason, it is of special interest to observe the trend prevailing in other clinics. If these observations are confirmed, all these analyses will lead to a clarification and definition of the groups of patients involved and the limits set for clinically based prognoses for recovery. This should provide guidelines regarding how long highly intensive therapy should be continued.

References

1. BRAAKMAN, R.: See this Volume, pp. 12-15
2. BRICOLO, A., RIZZUTO, N.: Diagnostic criteria for brainstem traumatic lesions. J. Neurosurg. Sci. 20, 17-32 (1976)
3. BRIHAYE, J.: See this Volume, pp. 54-55
3a. BRIHAYE, J., FROWEIN, R.A. LINDGREN, S. LOEW, F., STROOBANDI, G.: Report on the Meeting of the W.F.N.S. Neurotraumatology Comittee, Brussels, 19-23 September 1976. Acta Neurochir. 40, 181-186 (1978)
4. BUES, E.: Längsschnittuntersuchungen und Klassifizierung gedeckter Hirntraumen. Acta Neurochir. (Wien) 12, 702-716 (1965)
5. CARLSSON, C.A., v. ESSEN, C., LÖFGREN, J.: Factors effecting the clinical course of patients with severe head injuries. J. Neurosurg. 29, 242 (1968)
6. FROWEIN, R.A.: Classification of Coma. Acta Neurochir. (Wien) 34, 5-10 (1976)
7. FROWEIN, R.A., TERHAAG, D., AUF DER HAAR, K.: Früh-Prognose akuter Hirnschädigungen. Acta Traumatologie 5, 203-211, 291-298 (1975)
8. GERSTENBRAND, F.: Das traumatische apallische Syndrom. Wien: Springer 1967
9. GOUTELLE, A., MOURET, Ph.: Le pronostic des traumatismes crâniens. Acta Psychiatr. Belg. 70, 445-482 (1970)
10. JENNET, B., TEASDALE, G., BRAAKMAN, R., MINDERHOUD, J., KNILL-JONES, R.: Predicting Outcome in Individual patients after severe Head Injury. Lancet 1976; 1031-1034
11. LANGE-COSACK, H., TEPFER, G.: Das Hirntrauma im Kindes- und Jugendalter. Schriftenreihe Neurologie. Vol. XII. Berlin-Heidelberg-New York: Springer 1973
12. LANGER, M., TERHAAG, D.: See this Volume, pp. 98-100
13. LOEW, F., HERRMANN, H.D.: Die Schädel-Hirn-Verletzungen. In: Handbuch Unfallheilkunde II, 3. Aufl. BÜRKLE DE LA CAMP, H., SCHWAIGER, M. (Hrsg.). Stuttgart: Enke 1966
14. MÜLLER, G.E.: Classification of head injuries. In: Handbook of Clinical Neurology, Vol. XXIII. VINKEN, P.J., BRUYN, G.W. (eds.), pp. 1-22. Amsterdam-Oxford: North Holland, Publishing Company 1975
15. OVERGAARD, J., HOID-HANSEN, O., LAND, A., PEDERSEN, K.K., CHRISTENSEN, S., HAASE, J., HEIN, O., TWEED, W.A.: Prognosis after head injury, based on early clinical examination. Lancet 1973; 631-635
16. TÖNNIS, W., LOEW, F.: Einteilung der gedeckten Hirnschädigungen. Ärztliche Praxis 5, 3 (1953)

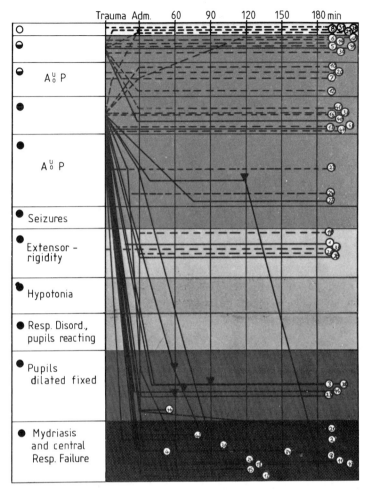

Fig. 1. Cases of 50 patients transported to the clinic by helicopter
--- Survivals
— Nonsurvivals
▼ Time of operation

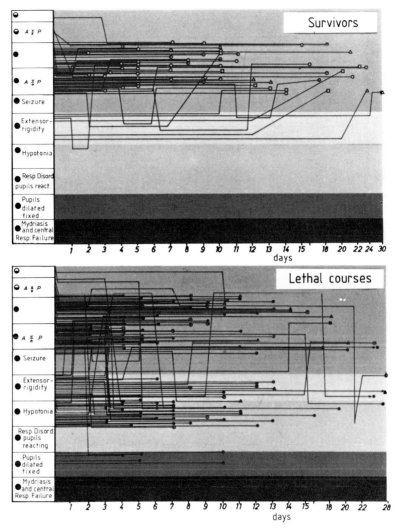

Fig. 2. Serious injuries with unconsciousness of more than 48 h duration (180 cases)

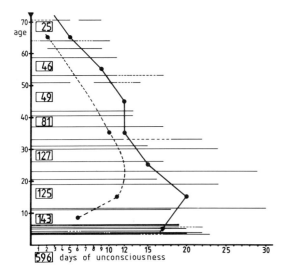

Fig. 3. Limit of 5% for survival after unconsciousness of more than 24 h duration; 26 cases with unconsciousness exceeding the 5% mark
—•— 5% limit of the survivors
--•-- Limit of complete recovery

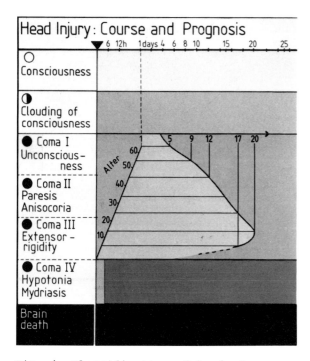

Fig. 4. Classification of brain trauma

Correlations Between Clinical Symptoms and Computerized Tomography Findings in Closed Head Injuries

W. Lanksch, Th. Grumme, and E. Kazner

Up to now, the classification of head injuries has been based on the initial clinical signs and the subsequent progress. The real extent of a traumatic brain lesion cannot be detected exactly by the conventional investigations such as echo ECG, x-rays, or cerebral angiography. Using computerized Tomography (CT), intracranial hemorrhages and contusional lesions can be distinguished. Therefore, a correlation between clinical syndromes and morphologic lesions seems to be possible.

During the past 2.5 years, we have studied 910 patients with head injuries using CT. Extracerebral hematomas and missiles are not taken into consideration here since CT has not essentially improved the diagnosis. We have introduced a grading (3) to classify the different CT findings in contusional lesions.

The first group of severe closed head injuries is characterized by compressed ventricles, absence of cisterns, and a more or less developed periventricular edema in the CT. These findings point to raised intracranial volume as induced by edema not yet visible (2). The contusional lesion type I appears as a well-defined area of low density, corresponding to a localized edema (Fig. 1). The type II lesion is characterized by a more or less expanded edematous area in which small hemorrhages are scattered. More extensive solid or partially confluent hemorrhages can occur (Fig. 2). Contusional lesions of type III appear as intracerebral hemorrhages at the point of impact and at the opposite side (Fig. 3). We have tried to compare CT findings with clinical signs and symptoms of patients with acute head injuries. We were particularly interested in investigating the value of CT in comparison to the clinical criteria in estimating the chances of survival. The correlation between different disturbances of consciousness and CT findings shows an increasing frequency of disturbed consciousness from normal CT to type III lesions. At the same time, the degree of impaired consciousness shows a decreased number of somnolent patients and an increased number of unconscious and comatose patients. The average death rate of patients suffering from diffusely spread edema is 12%, from contusional lesion type I 7%, type II 41%, and type III 70% (Table 1). The overwhelming majority (95%) of the patients belonging to group I were unconscious. In our opinion, this indicates a rise of intracranial pressure.

In 48 unconscious patients, we did not detect any pathologic finding. Therefore, we want to emphasize that CT cannot always detect morphologic lesions. Pupillomotor disturbances can also be related to CT findings in contusional lesions. Type II and III lesions exist with or without mydriasis. In patients showing fixed pupils, we always diagnosed severe traumatic lesions in the CT. In each of the four groups, an increase in the death rate depends on the clinical picture. Out of 30 patients with fixed pupils suffering from contusional lesions of type II and III, not a single one survived (Table 2).

The comparison of CT findings with disturbances of the corticospinal tracts shows that in cases of hemiparesis very often no conclusion can be reached from the CT scan. Comparing the death rates of patients

Table 1. Correlation between disturbance of consciousness and CT findings in 318 contusional lesions; the death rate grows depending on clinical symptoms in each group

	CT	Normal	Diff. edema	Type I	Type II	Type III
Clinical symptoms	Awake	28	3	7	14	2
	Somno-lent	32	20	11 9%	21 9%	9 44%
	Uncon-scious	15	26 8%	10 10%	38 53%	34 70%
	Coma-tose	1	10 50%	1	15 87%	21 86%

Table 2. Mortalities in 318 contusional lesions depending on pupillomotor disturbances and CT findings

	CT	Normal	Diff. edema	Type I	Type II	Type III
Clinical symptoms	Normal		5%	5%	24%	62%
	Mydria-sis		9%	12%	50%	68%
	Fixed pupils		80%		100%	100%

suffering from different contusional lesions with their symptoms of normal, hemiparesis, and bilateral dysfunction of corticospinal tracts, we have found that all patients survived in group I. The mortality increased continuously from type I to type III, and the increase furthermore depends on the clinical picture (Table 3).

We tried to analyze whether the displacement of the midline structure influences the chance of survival. It appears that the location and extent of the lesion as well as brain edema influence the death rate much more than the displacement of the midline structures. In 47% of all contusional lesions midline displacements were absent. In type I lesions, only 17% showed a midline shift. Death in type I lesions is caused exclusively by extracerebral disease. A midline displacement was not present in 40% of all type II lesions, but 22% of the patients died. In the other patients, apart from those suffering from primary or secondary brain stem lesions, we found midline displacements ranging from 3-20 mm. Fatalities increase in relation to the amount of midline shift. A midline displacement of 4-10 mm in patients with type II and III lesions showed a death rate of 59% and 67% respectively; a displacement of 11-20 mm showed a death rate of 93% and 100% for the different type lesions.

In these patients, we analyzed the size of the contusional lesion and the extent of brain edema. We found that lesions up to 2 x 2 cm, without localized or diffuse edema, cannot be considered to be lethal complications. The size of a contusional lesion, apart from those destroying half a hemisphere, cannot be correlated with the death rate. The diffuse brain edema represents a more sensitive factor showing a doubling of the death rate in the two groups of different lesions (Table 4).

Table 3. Death rate of 319 contusional lesions depending on disturbances of the corticospinal tracts and CT findings

	CT	Normal	Diff. edema	Type I	Type II	Type III
Clinical symptoms	Normal		6%		34%	50%
	Hemiparesis			7%	39%	74%
	Bilat. Dysfunctions		25%	54%	94%	96%

Table 4. Death rate of 86 patients in correlation to CT findings (brain edema)

	Brain edema	∅	Localized	Diff. spread out
Size of contusional lesion	cm			
	- 2x2	10	9 ± 2	12 ± 7
	- 5x5	5	16 ± 4	23 ± 13
	5x5			7 ± 6

Seventy percent of all patients suffering from type III lesions died. Nearly half of them showed no midline shift in the CT scan. Only in 10 out of 68 patients did the midline displacement exceed 6 mm. The results were as expected in bilateral type III lesions. The high death rate is caused by extensive cerebral trauma.

Patients suffering from a post-traumatic generalized increase of the intracranial volume usually survived. The compression of the ventricles and the missing cisterns may be due to brain edema not yet visible in an acute stage. The increased volume could also be caused by a post-traumatic vasoparalysis (1).

In conclusion, post-traumatic clinical dysfunctions do not always reveal a corresponding lesion in the CT. The correlation of CT findings and clinical symptoms improves with their severity. Utilizing only the CT findings, it is neither possible to predict the patients outcome nor to decide whether to intervene neurosurgically. A complete diagnosis cannot be based solely on the CT findings.

References

1. LANGFITT, T.W., TANNANBAUM, H.M., KASSEL, N.F.: The etiology of acute brain swelling following experimental head injury. J. Neurosurg. 24, 47 (1966)

2. LANKSCH, W., OETTINGER, W., BAETHMANN, A., KAZNER, E.: CT findings in brain edema compared with direct chemical analysis of tissue samples. In: Dynamics of Brain Edema. POPPINS, H.M., FEINDEL, W. (eds.), p. 283. Berlin-Heidelberg-New York: Springer 1976

3. LANKSCH, W., GRUMME, Th., KAZNER, E.: Schädelhirnverletzungen im Computer Tomogramm. (In press, 1977)

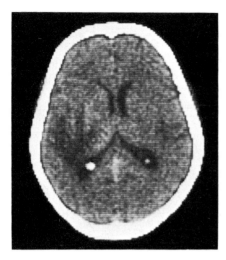 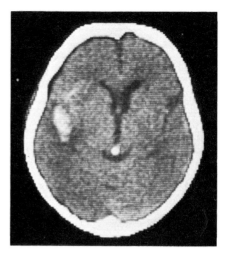

Fig. 1. Contusional lesion type I in the left temporal lobe. (Patient, Gustav S., 59 years, CT No. M 2774)

Fig. 2. Contusional lesion type II in the left temporal lobe. (Patient, Karl, B., 60 years, CT No. M 4411)

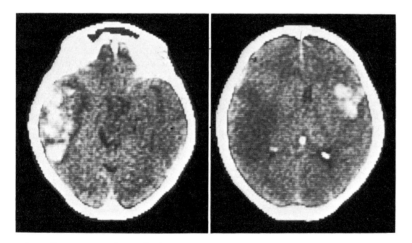

Fig. 3. Contusional lesion type III. Intracerebral hemorrhage in the left temporal lobe and at the opposite site. (Patient, Maria W., 67 years, CT No. M 1316)

Epidemiology, Classifications, and Prognosis of Severe Craniocerebral Injuries: Computer-Assisted Study of 9038 Cases

H. W. PIA, H. ABTAHI, and R. SCHÖNMAYER

This computer-assisted clinical analysis was motivated by the increasing frequency of craniocerebral injuries, as well as by the change of types of injuries sustained and improved diagnostic and therapeutic possibilities. This change in the types of injuries resulted from the different nature of the accidents, accompanying environmental damages, and the increase in the higher age categories. The investigation is based on 9038 cases of craniocerebral injuries, treated 1942-1974 in Giessen. Of these 9038 cases, 1970 cases were treated 1942-1952 in the Department of Surgery, University of Giessen and had been described earlier (PIA, 3-7). We also refer to a computer evaluation of the coded statistical data from 3455 cases originating from the Surgical Clinic during 1960-1974 and from 3793 cases originating from the Neurosurgical Clinic from 1953-1974. The material covers a period of 33 years with a partial exception relating to the years 1953-1960. The cases treated at the Department of Surgery were handled on a consultatory basis with the Department of Neurosurgery. The number of cases admitted increased steadily, predominantly 1942-1952, with an increase from 80 cases yearly to 310 cases yearly. The absolute number of more than 500 cases during the period 1960-1974 shows the further increase and a rising tendency. The striking decrease 1962-1964 cannot be explained.

The comparison of types of injuries shows 20% severe and 80% slight injuries until 1952 (Table 1). Since the Department of Neurosurgery was established, the rate of severe injuries admitted to the Department of Surgery decreased to 10%, whereas the rate of severe head injuries admitted to the Neurosurgic Department increased to 67%. Accordingly, the rate of open cranial injuries and depressed skull fractures, together 20% of all cases, is above average in comparison to the former 3%. A similar increase is shown in the intracranial hematomas with 26% as opposed to 10%. The mortality figures are of limited statistical value because of the different types of injuries, the unknown number of multiple injuries, and other undiscernable facts. However, reliable figures

Table 1. Craniocerebral injuries (Giessen 1942-1974, No. 9038)

	Surgery 1942-1952 No. 1790	Surgery 1960-1974 No. 3455	Neurosurgery 1953-1974 No. 3793	
Slight closed injuries	79	91	33	
Severe closed injuries	16	7	58	
Open craniocerebral injuries	5	2	9	Convexity 3 Basis 6
Fractures	43	13	40	
Impressions	9	-	12.5	
Hematomas	10	3	26	
Epidural Hematomas	3	-	6.4	
Subdural Hematomas	5	-	17.2	
Intracerebral Hematomas	2	-	2.4	

could be obtained for the decrease of mortality in slight head injuries from 2.8% to 1.8% especially in severe closed head injuries from 56% to 37%, and in intracranial hematomas from 84% to 40% (Table 2). Remarkably small or absent is any improved prognosis in open injuries and depressed fractures. The traumatic intracranial hematomas exemplify, in an impressive manner, the diagnostic and therapeutic advances made (Table 3).

Independent of the general increase in the rate of head injuries, we see an increase of traumatic intracranial hematomas from 10%-26%, in different groups, however, 100%-300%. This is not valid in regard to the intracerebral hematomas. Coincidently the percentage of the operated patients rose from 53% to 93%, with the highest increase in the intracerebral hematomas from 42%-85%. These rates particularly show the improvements in diagnosis since the establishment of the Neurosurgical

Table 2. Mortality of craniocerebral injuries (Giessen 1942-1974)

| | Surgery | | | | Neurosurgery | |
| | 1942-1952 | | 1960-1974 | | 1953-1974 | |
	No.	Dead(%)	No.	Dead(%)	No	Dead(%)
Total	1790	11.9	3455	9.7	3793	25.5
Slight injuries	1417	2.8	3085	6	1248	1.8
Severe injuries	373	56	308	34.7	2545	37.1
Open craniocerebral injuries	91	37.3	65	28	349	34.1
					240[a]	15.8[a]
Impression fractures	99	19.1	-	-	447	18.7
Hematomas	186	84	103	47	980	39.6
Epidural Hematomas	58	86	-	-	197	37
Subdural Hematomas	90	82	-	-	653	37
Intracerebral Hematomas	38	87	-	-	89	64

[a]Injuries of the skull basis.

Table 3. Intracranial hematomas (Giessen, No. 1166)

| | Surgery Giessen 1942-1952 | | Neurosurgery Giessen 1952-1974 | |
	No.	%	No.	%
Total	186	10.1	980	25.8
Operation	98	53	909	93
Dead	157	84	386	39,6
Epidural Hematomas	58	3	197	6.3
Operation	34	59	189	95.9
Dead	50	86	72	37
Subdural Hematomas	90	5	653	17.2
Operation	48	53	608	93
Dead	74	82	241	37
Intracerebral Hematomas	38	2.1	89	2.4
Operation	16	42	76	85
Dead	33	87	57	64

Department. Accordingly, the mortality rate shows a fall from 84% to 39.6%. The lowest decrease can be seen in the intracerebral hematomas, i.e., from 87%-64%.

Of the cases discharged from the Department of Neurosurgery, ca. 60% of the epidural hematomas, ca. 55% of the subdural hematomas, and 30% of the intracerebral hematomas were improved. An investigation in 5-year periods since 1955 shows a decrease in mortality from 60%-40%. The mortality rate decreases slightly between 1965 und 1969, but on the whole, there is no notable change. The rate of improvement, on the other hand, increases on the whole and reaches its optimum at 60% during 1965-1969. These results of the treatment of hematomas, particularly the lack of further improvement of mortality rates, were entirely unexpected considering the diagnostic and therapeutic advances. This stimulated a comprehensive investigation of our cases.

Using the extradural hematomas as an example, some factors connected with mortality, clinical course, quality of survival, and treatment will be presented. Of 197 cases, 189 were operated on. The eight unoperated cases were dead on arrival. The autopsies showed the hematoma and accompanying damage. The mortality rate of all cases at 37% and of the operated cases at 34% was remarkably high and showed no notable change in recent years. As expected, there was a distinct influence of age upon mortality, with the highest rates of survival and recovery in childhood and adolescence. In patients aged over 50 years and even in those aged over 30 years, the rate of mortality and severe neurologic defects was higher and that of restitution and slight defects markedly lower than in younger age groups. In patients aged over 60 years complete recovery or recovery with minimal deficits was exceptional. The fact that there were no survivors from the so-called apallic syndrome in patients aged over 60 years needs no further explanation.

The incidence of pulmonary and cardiac complications was high and remained unchanged. In the 4th decade, these complications amounted to 40% and increased in higher age groups. Isolated pulmonary complications appear until the age of 30 years in 3%-4% of the cases, between ages 30 and 50 years in 20%, and thereafter in more than one-third of the cases. The most important clinical and prognostic criteria are the type and pattern of central dysregulation, i.e., the presence or absence of decerebration, the origin, progress, and level of unconsciousness.

The prognosis as regards recovery and lasting damage is unequivocal. Only 7% of the patients with signs of brain stem involvement recovered completely with no neurologic deficit on discharge, whereas among patients without mesencephalic signs, this figure was 36%. Surprisingly, the mortality rate was not influenced by the absence or presence of signs of brain stem involvement. Regarding the types of disturbances of unconsciousness, the mortality rate is highest in patients admitted unconscious at 40%, lower in patients with secondary unconsciousness at 30%, and lowest in patients without loss of consciousness at 7%. Similar agreement can be found in the rates when related to the recovery and persistence of neurologic deficits. The most important morphologic criterion for the prognosis is the existence of isolated hematoma or combined cerebral lesions, whereas the location of the hematoma plays a lesser role. Nowadays, this information can be easily obtained from computerized tomography.

Out of 82 patients with isolated hematomas, 22% died and 50% recovered completely, whereas out of 92 patients with combined lesions, 50% died and only 11% recovered. Statistical analysis of the influence of the timing of the operation upon mortality pointed to the severity of the injury as the only important factor. Among the patients operated on within the first 12 h, 40% died, the mortality rate decreasing among patients operated within the next 12 h and 24 h. Mortality rates of 50%, 30%, and 10% in patients with primary loss of unconsciousness, secondary coma, and those without loss of consciousness are almost identical for patients operated within the first 6 or in the following 6 h after the injury. This indicates that the severity of the cerebral damage plays a more important role than the timing of the operation.

Summary

The analysis of 9038 patients with craniocerebral injuries admitted to the Departments of Surgery and Neurosurgery in Giessen over the period of more than 30 years provided data concerning the epidemiology, classification, and prognosis of these cases. It was revealed that the prognosis for patients with traumatic hematomas has not changed during the last 20 years. The possibilities and limitations of computer-assisted analysis of coded information retrieved from observation charts were presented. It was confirmed that the age, severity, and grade of injury are the decisive clinical criteria in determining the prognosis. The study provides data which point out the limited possibilities of successful treatment in this type of patient in a neurosurgical department which covers a large area.

JAMIESON and YELLAND (1) reported a mortality of 15.6% among 167 patients with epidural hematomas, treated in the years 1956-1967 in Brisbane. In our series, the mortality rate is twice as high. Considerable effort is necessary if improvement in the early diagnosis is to be achieved and avoidance of delay in referral and transport over long distances.

For the present time, we must still recommend that burr holes should be made at the site determined by external injury marks in the hospital to which the patient was first admitted, if any secondary deterioration of the level of consciousness occurs. Transporting the patient to the neurosurgic center or another hospital for angiography cannot be justified.

References

1. JAMIESON, K.G., YELLAND, J.D.N.: Extradural haematoma. Report of 167 cases. J. Neurosurg. 29, 13-23 (1968)
2. LOEW, F., WÜSTNER, S.: Diagnose, Behandlung und Prognose der traumatischen Hämatome des Schädelinnern. Wien: Springer 1960
3. PIA, H.W.: Indikation zu chirurgischem Eingreifen bei Schädel-Hirnverletzungen unter besonderer Berücksichtigung der Verkehrsunfälle. Langenbecks Arch. Chir. 279, 178-180 (1954)
4. PIA, H.W.: Klinik und Behandlung der schweren gedeckten Hirnverletzungen. Langenbecks Arch. Chir. 280, 623-634 (1955)
5. PIA, H.W.: Therapeutische Maßnahmen bei gedeckten Schädel-Hirnverletzungen. Chirurg 27, 415-420 (1956)
6. PIA, H.W.: Die Bewußtseinsstörungen bei Hirnverletzungen. Langenbecks Arch. Chir. 281, 652-661 (1956)
7. PIA, H.W.: Fehler und Gefahren bei der Diagnose und Behandlung gedeckter Hirnverletzungen. Langenbecks Arch. Chir. 298, 110-120 (1961)

8. TÖNNIS, W., FROWEIN, R.A., LOEW, F., GROTE, W., HEMMER, R., KLUG, W., FINKEMEYER, H.: Organisation der Behandlung schwerer Schädel-Hirn-Verletzungen. Stuttgart: Georg Thieme 1968

Using the Frequency Analysis of the EEG for Prognosis in Severe Brain Injuries

W. I. STEUDEL and J. KRÜGER

Introduction

The EEG examination is of great importance for judging brain injuries (15). EEG follow-up in the first days and weeks after the trauma are considered to be of great value (6). In cases of disturbances of consciousness, the EEG examination is as necessary as the assessment of the neurologic status is and provides additional information for classifying the state of unconsciousness and for prognosis (6, 8, 11, 13). Favorable prognostic signs which can be seen in the EEG are sleep patterns in posttraumatic coma (1, 5) and a progressive increase in EEG responses to photic stimulation (16), paroxysmal focal discharges, but without clinical manifestations (6, 17), or a burst suppression pattern signify a bad prognosis (16).

Over the last decade, due to the introduction of computer analysis of the EEG, a new era of EEG application started (7). Based on the frequency analysis (18), this method is suited for calculating disturbances of background activities (12). We examined 20 selected adults with brain injuries who were unconscious for at least 72 h. On the basis of frequency-analyzed EEGs of the first 9 postoperative days, criteria for prognosis are given.

Material and Methods

1. Patients

Twenty patients (17 male and 3 female) aged 18-73 years (mean age: 41.5 years) were all in coma for at least 72 h - no verbal contact even on painful stimulation - (stage II or III according to FISCHGOLD and MATHIS, 1956 (8)). The following brain injuries led to these disturbances of consciousness: eight extradural, five subdural, and five intracerebral hematomas, one depressed fracture, and one contusion not operated on. Nine patients had operations on the right side and ten on the left. For all patients, the treatment was the same, i.e. reduction of edema, prevention of infection, balance of electrolyte status and nutrition. All patients were nasally intubated while in coma. In seven cases, focal seizures occured (focal discharges were only seen twice in the EEG) which were treated with hydantoins and barbiturates.

2. EEG

Patients were electroencephalographically and neurologically examined on the 3rd, 6th, 12th, 15th, and 18th postoperative days. Platinum needle electrodes were placed in the frontal, occipital, and temporal regions. The EEG was recorded together with heart and breathing activities on an Alvar EEG machine and stored on magnetic type (JOHN and REILHOFER 8k60, München) under oscillographic control. Further details are described elsewhere (10) (Figs. 1a and 3a).

3. EEG Spectral Analysis

By fast Fourier transformation, power density spectra of the EEG were computed off-line on a processor (AEG-Telefunken, BIO 16, program ESAP). Main analysis parameters are: frequency resolution: 0.25 Hz, sample length: 4 s (14). One average spectrum was computed from 30 samples (i.e., from 120 s of EEG). The following were calculated from all the bipolar derivations: absolute and percentage power of the common frequency bands, total power, θ-α ratio, cross spectra, and coherence functions. For this study, only the two occipital derivations could be used because they are usually free from disturbing biologic artifacts like muscle activity and eye movements.

Results

In 17 of the 20 cases, a prognosis was made after 9 days based on the spectral analysis which was in agreement with the clinical picture observed 6 months later. Ten patients survived, seven died. The criteria used were mainly the absolute and percentage power of the common frequency bands. According to these two groups, significant differences can be established:

1. *Absolute and percentage power of the common frequency bands in the survivors* (Figs. 1 and 2)
   On the 3rd day, δ-activity predominated in all patients (mean value: 64.4%). The output in the θ-range was lower and in general no longer relevant in the α-range (mean value: 6.85%). During the follow-ups until the 9th day, there was an increase in the absolute and percentage power in the α- and θ-range (Fig. 2). The δ-range was different. The mean value shows a slight increase.

2. *Absolute and percentage power of the common frequency bands in the deaths* (Figs. 3 and 4)
   The δ-activity also predominated in these patients (mean value on the 3rd day: 78.6%), while the output in the α-range was very low (mean value: 4.3%). In the patients who died, the α- and θ-range increased until the 6th day but decreased remarkably until the 9th day (Fig. 2). The δ-range increased until the 9th day. In general, the patients died in the 2nd postoperative week.

In three cases, the correct prognosis could not be established. A poor prognosis was expected in these cases; however, these patients survived. The postoperative course was complicated twice by seizure and once by a bleeding. Two case histories are selected:

Case 1

This 40-year-old patient fell on a stairway and suffered a large left parietal depressed fracture and several lacerations on his left side. After the elevation of the depressed fracture, the patient remained in coma. The hemothorax was first treated conservatively and later removed by operation. On the 3rd postoperative day, focal seizures occurred, which responded to treatment with large doses of barbiturates. The patient deteriorated until the 9th day. Recovery was apparent only after 14 days. After 6 months rehabilitation, little progress had been made.

Case 2

This 35-year-old patient was found in the street after a brawl. He suffered from a left temporal intracerebral hematoma which was removed. On the 3rd postoperative day, further bleeding occurred, which was again removed. After this complication, consciousness was regained very slowly. The patient responded to stimulation after 3 weeks. In addition, the patient suffered from tuberculosis of the lungs. Six months after the trauma, a slight psychosyndrome remained.

Cross-Spectra and Coherence Functions

For the calculation of the cross-spectra and coherences in the θ- and α-range, a minimal power is necessary. Only in five cases did the spectral analysis show sufficient power. Therefore, these criteria were not taken into account.

Discussion

In 17 out of 20 cases of post-traumatic coma, spectral analysis after 9 days permitted a prognosis to be made which was supported by the clinical examination 6 months later. In three cases - which were complicated by focal seizures and a rebleeding - in spite of an unfavorable prognosis based on spectral analysis, the patient recovered. This agrees with observations of CARONNA and PLUM (4) that the EEG shows the irreversible brain damage even though a recovery is possible. This is especially pronounced in patients with barbiturate poisoning. In these three cases, the period of observation (9 days) after the operation is obviously too short. This prognostic tool can only be used with caution for patients on barbiturate medication because of seizures. No significant difference in the age of the patient who survived (mean age: 40 years) and those who died (mean age: 44 years) could be observed. The recovery from post-traumatic coma is known to correlate with the age of the patient. The number of cases was too small to demonstrate this relationship (3).

A further statistical treatment was not possible because there were not enough cases. The correct prognosis in comatose patients based on EEG is in the range of 80%-99% (2, 4). Head trauma tends to result in highly individualistic syndromes (16) and is often affected by complications. Therefore, it is necessary to examine a great number of patients to show the significance of frequency analysis for prognosis. After amplification of the EEG signals, additional criteria, such as the coherence functions, can be obtained which might add to the prognostic value of this method.

Summary

Twenty adults with severe brain injuries were neurologically and electroencephalographically examined every 3 days, from the 3rd to the 18th postoperative day. In 17 of the 20 cases a prognosis could be made after 9 days based on the spectral analysis of the EEG which was in agreement with the clinical picture observed 6 months later. Ten patients survived and seven died. According to these two groups, significant differences can be established: an increase in the absolute and percentage power in the α-range in the survivals and a decrease in the α-range in the deaths. In three cases which were complicated by focal seizures and a rebleeding, the correct prognosis could not be established.

References

1. BERGAMASCO, B.L., BERGAMINI, L., DORIGUZZI, T.: Clinical value of the sleep electroencephalographic patterns in post-traumatic coma. Acta Neurol. Scand. 44, 495-511 (1968)
2. BINNIE, C.D., LLOYD, D.S., SCOTT, D.F., MARGERISON, J.H.: Electroencephaolographic prediction of fatal anoxic brain damage after resuscitation from cardiac arrest. Br. Med. J. 1970/IV, 265-268
3. CARLSSON, C.A., VON ESSEN, C., LÖFGREN, J.: Factors affecting the clinical course of patients with severe head injuries. J. Neurosurg. 29, 242-251 (1968)
4. CORONNA, J.J., PLUM, F.: Prognosis and medical coma. In: Head Injuries. MCLAURIN, R.L. (ed.), pp. 3-9. New York: Grune & Stratton 1976
5. CHATRIAN, G.E., WHITE, J., DALY, D.: EEG patterns resembling those of sleep in certain comatose states after injuries to the head. EEG. Clin. Neurophysiol. 15, 272-280 (1963)
6. COURJON, J.R., NAQUET, R., BAURAND, C. et al.: Valeur diagnostique et prognostique de l'EEG dans les suites immédiates des traumatismes craniens. Rev. EEG. Neurophysiol. 1, 133-150 (1971)
7. DOLCE, G., KÜNKEL, H. (eds.): CEAN. Computerized EEG Analysis. Stuttgart: Fischer 1975
8. FISCHGOLD, H., MATHIS, P.: Obnubilations, comas and stupeurs. EEG Clin. Neurophysiol. (Suppl.) 11, (1959)
9. GERSTENBRAND, F., LACKNER, F., LÜCKING, C.H.: Neurologischer Untersuchungsbogen zur Überwachung akuter traumatischer Hirnschäden. Z. Prakt. Anästh. 6, 437-447 (1971)
10. KRÜGER, J., STEUDEL, W.I., SCHÄFER, M., DOLCE, G.: Cliniconeurological and computer-analysed EEG investigations of patients in coma following operation for cerebral trauma. Adv. Neurosurg. 4, 230-236 (1977)
11. KUBICKI, St., HAAS, J.: Elektro-klinische Korrelation bei Komata unterschiedlicher Genese. Aktuel. Neurol. 2, 103-112 (1975)
12. KÜNKEL, H.: Die Spektralanalyse des EEG. Z. EEG-EMG 3, 15-14 (1972)
13. PLUM, F., POSNER, J.B.: Diagnosis of Stupor and Coma, 2nd ed. New York: Davis 1975
14. SPEHR, W.: EEG spectral analysis in laboratory routine work: The biosignalprocessor BIO 16-1. In: Quantitative Analysis of the EEG. MATEJCEK, M., SCHENK, G.K. (eds.), pp. 497-508. 2nd Symp. of the study group for EEG methodology. Jogny sur Vevey: Switzerland 1975
15. STEINMANN, H.W.: EEG und Hirntrauma. Stuttgart: Thieme 1959
16. STOCKARD, J.J., BICKFORD, R.G., AUNG, M.H.: The electroencephalogram in traumatic brain injury. In: Handbook of Clinical Neurology, Vol. XXIII. VINKEN, P.J., BRUYN, G.W. (eds.), pp. 317-367, Amsterdam: Elsevier 1975
17. VIGOUROUX, R., NAQUET, R., BAURAND, C., et al.: Evolution electroradio-clinique de comas graves prolongés post-traumatiques. Rev. Neurol. (Paris) 110, 72-81 (1964)
18. WELCH, P.D.: The use of the fast Fourier transform for the estimation of power spectra: A method based on time averaging over short, modified periodograms. IEEE Trans. Audio Electroacustics Vol. Au - 15 2, 70-73 (1969)

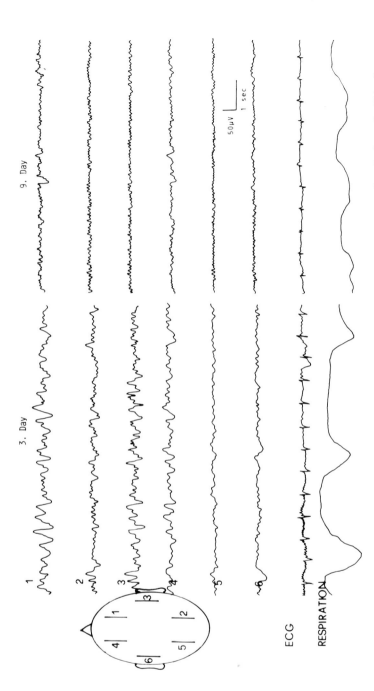

Fig.1. *a* Polygraphic recording of a patient who survived, made on the 3rd and 9th days after the operation of an extradural hematoma on the left side

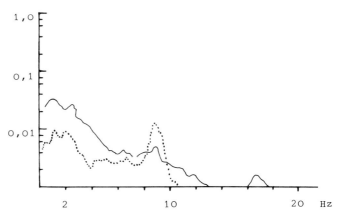

Fig. 1. *b* Autospectra from the left occipital channel of the same patient (x-axis frequency (Hz), y-axis log intensity). ——— 3rd day, ······ 9th day

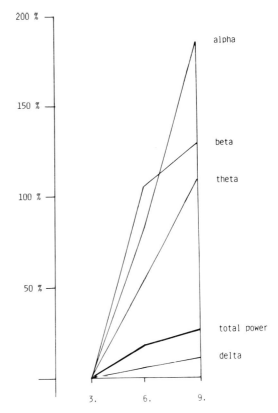

Fig. 2. Percentage change of the absolute power (mean values) on the 6th and 9th postoperative days as compared to the 3rd day in the ten *survivors*

Electroencephalographic (EEG) Differentation of the Apallic Syndrome in Severe Craniocerebral Injuries

H.-E. Nau and W. J. Bock

Introduction

For defining the degree and prognosis of severe craniocerebral injuries, we not only need ancillary investigations, such as axial computerized tomography and angiography which provide information on the morphologic situation, but also measurements of the intracranial pressure and especially electroencephalography which reflect the current functional situation (20) of the patient's brain. The latter is important for recognizing sequelae (32) and offers prognostic hints (2, 14, 33). Only a few reports deal with trauma in the child (22, 25, 34). Literature on severe trauma in children is still rare which is why we tried to do long-term EEG studies and thus to differentiate severe craniocerebral injuries by means of EEG.

Patients

From 1970-1977, we treated 328 craniocerebral injuries in children. Thirty of these (16 females and 14 males) had undergone long-term EEG recordings and eight of these had an apallic syndrome. Among them we found three girls and five boys. Their average age was 7.4 years, whereas patients without an apallic syndrome had an average age of 9.1 years. Two patients in each group died. EEGs were taken, using silver needle electrodes. In the first patients we examined, we recorded daily EEGs. Having some experience, we did the first examination as early as possible after trauma, the second some days later, and then once a week, when the clinical situation did not change.

Results

1. Clinical Observations

In the patients with apallic syndrome, we found one depressed fracture, in the others two depressed fractures, two fractures of the base, and three fractures of the convexity. Intracerebral hematomas were observed in two nonapallic patients. Twelve of these showed lateralized neurologic signs, whereas none of the apallic patients showed any. Extension mechanisms were found in all apallic children but only in nine nonapallic ones. Unconsciousness lasted in apallic children for ca. 41 days on the average, whereas patients without apallic syndrome were only unconscious for about 10.5 days.

2. EEG Alterations in Severe Craniocerebral Injuries Without Apallic Syndrome (Table 1, Fig. 1)

In the acute stage, the EEG changes consisted of a severe generalized slowing. Frequencies were from the δ and slow θ-range (2-5 Ci/s). Sometimes, fast waves of 10-20 Ci/s were superimposed. In this stage, no focally marked alterations could be seen. In four patients only, we found lateralized changes which correspond to x-ray findings or to

Table 1. EEG observations in different stages of severe craniocerebral injuries

Severe craniocerebral injuries		EEG disturbances				Observations
		sub-δ	Activity δ	θ	>θ	
Non-apallic	Early stage		+	(+)		Focal or lateralized alterations seldom Superimposed fast activities sometimes
	Remission			+	(+)	Focal abnormalities frequent Contrecoup seldom Transitory depression of amplitudes seldom
Apallic	Initial complex	+	(+)			High voltage (~200 uV) Asynchrony, desorganization No lateralized alterations Superimposed fast activites sometimes
	Fully developed stage		+	(+)		Amplitude reduction beginning Lateralized or focal activites sometimes
	Remission			+	(+)	Flat EEG (20 uV)

the neurologic examination. As time went on clinical and EEG disturbances which correlated very well decreased, i.e., δ- and θ-waves progressively disappeared and the higher frequencies, charateristic for the age of the patient, began to assert themselves. In this stage, focal abnormalities were more frequent. In nine patients, we found marked focal slowing in some later EEG recordings and in only two patients with one recording a transitory slowing. A real contrecoup was observed once. In two cases, there was a transitory depression of amplitudes.

3. *EEG Alterations in Apallic Children* (Table 1, Fig. 2)

In these patients we were able to find three different EEG pictures which correspond to different clinical stages. In the "initial symptom complex", a generalized slow, especially highvoltage polymorphic sub-δ and δ-activity was to be seen. Asynchrony and disorganization was impressive. Sometimes, faster activities were superimposed. No focus could be found in any case. In the "fully developed stage" of apallic syndrome, δ-activity dominated, with frequencies from 2-4 Ci/s and a simultaneous reduction in amplitude. At this stage, we found some transitory hemispheric slowing.

After this stage, θ-activity increased and the slow δ-waves disappeared completely. Amplitudes became flatter and flatter, which is characteristic for remission. In those cases with an unfavorable course, we saw a recovery of EEG changes without changes in the clinical symptoms.

4. *Particular Observations*

In patients with severe generalized slowing of the EEG, one cannot differentiate any phases of cerebral or electric periodic activity. But such periodic activities can be found, especially in improvement of unconsciousness. The EEG can completely change within a few seconds. As far as we can tell from observations in some patients, the phases of faster activity being more characteristic for the age become longer and longer, until a normal sleep-waking rhythm is consolidated.

Discussion

Observations of EEG alterations in severe craniocerebral injuries are very rare. A very comprehensive study was made by LANGE-COSACK and TEPFER (25). Their results are similar to ours: More boys are injured than girls, a fact which is confirmed by numerous authors like WEINMANN (35). Boys are hurt more severely as a rule. BRANDESKY (5) found that the younger the patient, the better the prognosis. A fatal course may develop from any clinical situation because a lot of complications and preexisting features are important in influencing the course of events (17, 23). Usually, clinical data and pictures correspond to EEG changes (3, 39). In general, our results of EEG disturbances and changes resemble those which GERSTENBRAND (16) has seen in adults. It is reasonable that the more marked the slowing in the EEG is, the less a focal slowing can be distinguished (13). That is why our patients without an apallic syndrome had more focal abnormalities than those with one, but this difference disappeared in the stage of remission. In most cases, there was a marked general slowing to be found in the temporal regions (15). This can be explained by traumatic mechanisms and the structure of the temporal lobes.

The most marked difference in these groups of severe trauma with and without apallic syndromes, however, is the different frequency range (0.5-2 Ci/s and 2-5 Ci/s, respectively) and a relatively clear picture in the one instance or a great desynchronization, hemispheric discordance, and polymorphy of the high voltage waves in the other. Any explanation of EEG alterations, especially of those described, has not yet been given. A possibility for doing so seems to be in the location of the lesion. Slow δ-wave activity can be seen in raised intracranial pressure (12) in deep cerebral lesions (9), or in local edema around a tumor (20). This means that δ-activity is of quite a different origin. In severe head injuries, some mechanisms are possible at the same time. The δ-activity seen immediately after trauma may express the dysfunction of activating systems in the lower brain stem, whereas EEG changes seen some days after trauma (24) could be due to brain swelling, which correspond to pathologic (1) and experimental observations (28). The damage or transient functional disorder of these deep activating structures (26, 27) may be the reason why those EEGs cannot be influenced by any stimuli (31 et al.). The hypothesis that in cases of apallic syndrome deep lesions must exist is confirmed by the great desynchronization of waves, for EEG-synchronizing mechanisms are present in the reticular formation (8, 18). Coma has often been compared with stages of sleep and some authors think sleep recordings to be of more prognostic value (4, 7, 10). EEG changes seem to us to express a recovery of deep brain structures. At this stage, stimuli can influence the EEG.

In some patients, we could find fast frequencies of the β-range which were described by OTTOMO (30), JONES et al. (19), and WESTMORELAND et al. (36) in lesions and circulatory disturbances of the pons. Sometimes, disturbances of cranial nerves pointed to lesions of the pons, but further experimental oberservations and correlation with computerized axial tomography is necessary. Recently, we found rhythmic 12-14 Ci/s activity and bursts of δ-waves, which was regarded as characteristic for deep lesions and a special form of "coma vigil" by COURJON (11). BRENNER et al. (6) described episodic low amplitude and relatively isoelectric EEG patterns in patients with nontraumatic coma with grave prognostic implications. Even 14 and 6 Ci/s positive bursts, resembling ours had been seen in coma cases of hepatic origin by YAMADA et al. (38) and in a case with a penetrating wound of the brain by WYLER and CHATRIAN (37). In summary we can say that the EEG, especially long-term recordings, is a very valuable investigation in severe trauma (21) and also for differentiation of the apallic syndrome (29). The different electric pictures are caused by different disturbances of deep brain structures, and the recovery of those can be shown by characteristic clinical and EEG pictures. Also, experimental work with animal EEGs and computerized tomography correlations can clarify the complicated functional disturbances.

Summary

For defining the extent and the prognosis of severe craniocerebral injuries, we not only need ancillary investigations, such as axial computerized tomography and angiography which provide information about the morphologic situation, but also measurements of the intracranial pressure and especially electroencephalography which reflect the current functional situation. Therefore, we have tried to define the apallic syndrome by doing long-term EEG recordings in children.

In severe craniocerebral injury, severe generalized slowing is dominant with frequencies of about 3 Ci/s, but in cases with the apallic syndrome, a desynchronized high voltage sub-δ/δ-activity is characteristic. Certain clinical stages correlate with certain EEG patterns. Typical seizure potentials were absent in the acute stage. In extensor spasms, no pathognomonic electric patterns could be found. EEG seems to be a valuable method in the differentiation of the apallic syndrome in severe craniocerebral injury.

References

1. ADEBAHR, G., FROMM, H.: Schäden am Hirnstamm bei Hirndruck infolge Schädel-Hirntraumas. Beitr. Gerichtl. Med. 26, 78-83 (1969)
2. ALVISI, C., PAGLIANI, G., VALENTINI, G.: Rilievi sulla patologia, la clinica ed il trattamento di 1679 traumi del capo nella infanzia Riv. Neurol. 39, 254-64 (1969)
3. ANZIMIROV, V.L., GASANOV, J.K., KUMIN, V.A.: Correlation between the circulation of the hemispheres and brain stem regions, and bioelectrical activity in cranio-cerebral injuries (rus). Vopr. Neirokhir. 2, 11-18 (1976)
4. BERGAMASCO, B., BERGAMININ, L., DORIGUZZI, T.: Clinical value of the sleep electroencephalographic patterns in post-traumatic coma. Acta Neurol. Scand. 44, 495-511 (1968)
5. BRANDESKY, G.: Severe head injuries in children: treatment and long-range outlook. Clin. Pediatr. (Phila.) 4, 141-6 (1965)
6. BRENNER, R.P., SCHWARTZMAN, R.J., RICHEY, E.T.: Prognostic significance of episodic low amplitude or relatively isoelectric EEG patterns. Dis. Nerv. Syst. 36 (10), 582-7 (1975)
7. BRICOLO, A., GENTILOMO, A., ROSADINI, B., ROSSI, G.F.: Long-lasting post-traumatic unconsciousness. A study based on nocturnal EEG and polygraphic recording. Acta Neurol. Scand. 44, 513-32 (1968)
8. BUENO, J.R., BOST, K., HIMWICH, H.E.: Lower brain-stem EEG synchronizing mechanisms in the rabbit. Electroencephalog. Clin. Neurophysiol. 24, 25-34 (1968)
9. BUSCH, E.A.: Brain stem contusions: differential diagnosis, therapy, and prognosis. Clin. Neurosurg. 9, 18-33 (1963)
10. BUTENUTH, J., KUBICKI, St.: Klinisch-elektroenzephalographische Schlafbeobachtungen im apallischen Syndrom. Z. EEG-EMG 6, 185-8 (1975)
11. COURJON, J.: Das EEG beim frischen Schädelhirntrauma. In: Beiträge zur Neurochirurgie, Vol. XIV, S. 108-122. Leipzig: Johann Ambrosius Barth 1967
12. DAWSON, R.E., WEBSTER, J.E., GUARDJIAN, E.S.: Serial electroencephalography in acute head injuries. J. Neurosurg. 8, 613-30 (1951)
13. DUMERMUTH, G.: Elektroencephalographie im Kindesalter. Stuttgart: Georg Thieme 1976
14. ENGE, S.: Elektroenzephalographische Untersuchungen in der akuten Phase bei frischen geschlossenen Schädelhirntraumen. Wien. Med. Wochenschr. 116, 417-22 (1966)
15. FÜNFGELD, E.W., RABACHE, C., GASTAUT, H.: Vergleichende hirnelektrische Untersuchungen bei Schädeltraumen - Erfahrungen an einem größeren, unausgelesenen Krankengut. Zentralbl. Neurochir. 17 (5), 326-342 (1957)

16. GERSTENBRAND, F.: Das traumatische apallische Syndrom. Wien-New York: Springer 1967
17. GUTTERMANN, P., SHENKIN, H.: Prognostic features in recovery from traumatic decerebration. J. Neurosurg. 32, 330-5 (1970)
18. HASCKE, W., KLINBERG, D.: In: Neurobiologie. BIESOLD, D., MATTHIES, H. (Hrsg.). Stuttgart-New York: Gustav Fischer 1977
19. JONES, B.N., BINNIE, C.D., FUNG, D., HAMBLIN, J.J.: Reversible coma with an EEG pattern normally associated with wakefulness. Electroencephalog. Clin. Neurophysiol. 33, 107-9 (1972)
20. JUNG, R.: Das Elektroencephalogramm (EEG). In: Handbuch der inneren Medizin, 4. Aufl. Bd. V/1. v. BERMANN, G., FREY, W., SCHWIECK, H. (Hrsg.). Berlin-Göttingen-Heidelberg: Springer 1953
21. KELLAWAY, P.: Head injury in children. Electroencephalog. Clin. Neurophysiol. 7, 497-498 (1955)
22. KOUFEN, H.: Systematische EEG-Längsschnittuntersuchungen in der akuten Phase des kindlichen Schädel-Hirntraumas. Z. EEG-EMG 8, 29-35 (1977)
23. KUGLER, J., RIEGER, H.: Abhängigkeit der Traumafolgen von verschiedenen Vorbedingungen. Wien. Med. Wochenschr. 117, 120-3 (1967)
24. LANDAU-FEREY, J., HAZEMAN, P.: "Fausses aggravations" de L'E.E.G. dans les jours qui suivent un traumatisme cranien de l'etant. Rev. Electroencephalogr. Neurophysiol. Clin. 5 (3), 307-12 (1975)
25. LANGE-COSACK, H., TEPFER, G.: Das Hirntrauma im Kindes- und Jugendalter. Berlin-Heidelberg-New York: Springer 1973
26. LINDSLEY, D.B., BOWDON, J.W., MAGOUN, H.W.: Effect upon the EEG of acute injury to the brain stem activating system. Electroencephalog. Clin. Neurophysiol. 1, 475-86 (1949)
27. MORUZZI, G., MAGOUN, H.W.: Brain stem reticular formation and activation of the EEG. Electroencephalog. Clin. Neurophysiol. 1, 455-73 (1949)
28. NAKAMURA, Y., OHYE, C.: Delta wave production in neocortical EEG by acute lesions within thalamus and hypothalamus of the cat. Electroencephalog. Clin. Neurophysiol. 17, 677-84 (1964)
29. NAU, H.-E., BOCK, W.J.: Electroencephalographic investigation of traumatic apallic syndrome in childhood and adolescence. Acta Neurochir. (Wien) (In press)
30. OTTOMO, E.: Beta wave activity in the electroencephalogram in cases of coma due to acute brain stem lesions. J. Neurol. Neurosurg. Psychiatry 29, 383-90 (1966)
31. PAGNI, C.A., GIOVANELLI, M., TOMEI, G., ZAVANONE, M., SIGNORONI, G., CAPPRICI, E.: Long-term results in 62 cases of post-traumatic complete apallic syndrome. Acta Neurochir. 36, 37-45 (1977)
32. RICKHAM, P.P.: Head injuries in childhood. Helv. Chir. Acta 28, 560-575 (1961)
33. SABIN, T.D., MARK, V.H.: Letter: Computerized axial tomography and electroencephalography. J.A.M.A. 236 (2), 138 (1976)
34. SILVERMAN, D.: Electroencephalographic study of acute head injury in children. Neurology (Mineap.) 12, 273-81 (1962)
35. WEINMANN, H.M.: EEG-Veränderungen als Traumafolge beim Kind. Electroencephalog. Clin. Neurophysiol. 20, 534 (1966)

36. WESTMORELAND, B.F., KLASS, D.W., SHARBROUGH, F.W., REAGAN, Th.J.: Alpha-coma. Electroencephalographic, clinical, pathological, and etiological correlations. Arch. Neurol. 32 (11), 713-8 (1975)
37. WYLER, A.R., CHATRIAN, G.E.: Positive bursts (14- und 6-per second positive spikes) in a patient with a penetrating wound of the brain. Electroencephalog. Clin. Neurophysiol. 32, 317-21 (1972)
38. YAMADA, T., TUCKER, R.P., KOOI, K.A.: Fourteen and six c/sec positive bursts in comatose patients. Electroencephalog. Clin. Neurophysiol. 40 (6), 645-53 (1976)
39. YOSHII, N., MATSUMOTO, K., OSHIDA, K., KAZUNO, T., SAWA, T., MIKAMI, K.: Clinico-electroencephalographic study of 3,200 head injury cases - A comparative work between aged, adults, and children. Keio J. Med. 19, 31-46 (1970)

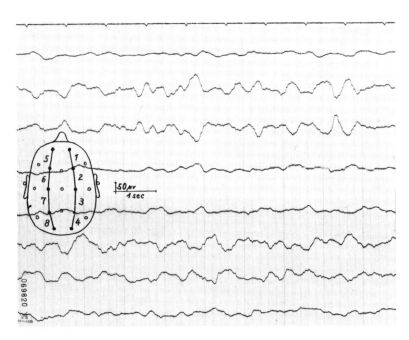

Fig. 1. Typical EEG pattern in a case of severe craniocerebral injury without apallic syndrome

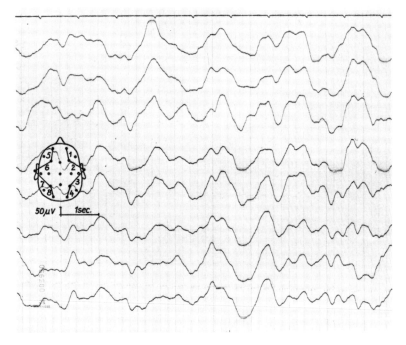

Fig. 2. Typical EEG pattern of patient in the initial stage of an apallic syndrome

Diagnosis of Brain Death by Means of Computerized Tomography
D. KÜHNE and H. ARNOLD

Especially in regard to organ transplantation, an early, certain and safe diagnosis of cerebral death is desirable. Neurologic examination and EEG only allow a statement about the loss of brain function without proving its short-term irreversibility (1, 3). On the other hand, there is no doubt about the diagnosis of brain death, if we have proved an arrest of cerebral circulation, which can normally be done by means of angiography (2) or angioscintigraphy (4). If an organ transplantation is planned, we would usually use one of these means to prove the death of the donor.

We wanted to know in which way computerized tomography could help to establish the arrest of cerebral circulation or any equivalent of it. Normally, the large vessels in the region of the basal cisterns show up after intravenous injection of iodine contrast medium. The circle of Willis, the middle, anterior, and posterior cerebral artery, and the tip of the basilar artery are visible. Impressive is also the increase of filling of the large veins and meningeal structures, e.g., the superior sagittal sinus, the vain of Galen, and the tentorium. An increased density is also to be seen in the very vascular choroid plexus. It may already be visible in the control or Polaroid photograph.

We have measured the change of absorption after rapid intravenous injection of a contrast medium of 65% in the mentioned vascular structures and the white and grey matter. The contrast medium is given in a dose of 1 ml/kg. We examined normal persons and patients who were later angiographically proved to have an arrest of the cerebral circulation and also exhibited the neurologic criteria of brain death (Tables 1 and 2). It is evident that the richly vascular structures show a significantly higher absorption after contrast medium injection in normal cases. In comparison, there are only slight differences in absorption rates in the case of cerebral death: the maximum is 0.9 EMI units and the difference is partly inherent. In cerebral death, the arteries are not to be seen in the basal region after contrast medium injection.

The slight statistically insignificant changes in absorption in the grey and white matter are due to low blood volume in the brain tissue (3%-4%) and to the fact that the contrast medium does not pass the intact blood-brain barrier. With slowly working tomography, the rapid elimination of contrast medium via the kidneys and the extravascular distribution play an important role. The iodine content of the blood decreases during the first 5 min by 20% and by a further 13% during the following 5 min.

Compared with the other methods of contrast medium and isotope angiography, another important advantage of computerized tomography in evaluating clinical brain death, which we have not yet mentioned, is the possibility of getting an impression of the state of the brain and the extent of a possible lesion. In cases of loss of brain function due to brain edema, intoxication, encephalitis, and hypothermia, computerized tomography in combination with contrast medium injection is a mild and comparatively low-risk examination technique, not more endangering than angioscintigraphy. The mode of examination we are using

Table 1. Changes in absorption after i.v. injection of contrast medium (20 normal persons)

	EMI units		
Large cerebral arteries	+ 13.2	−	+ 42.1
Superior sagittal sinus	+ 7.2	−	+ 18.5
Choroid plexus	+ 6.3	−	+ 11.8
White matter	+ 0.3	−	+ 1.1
Grey matter	+ 1.0	−	+ 2.4

Table 2. Changes in absorption after i.v. injection of contrast medium (5 cases of brain death)

	EMI units		
Large cerebral arteries	+ 0.04	−	+ 0.3
Superior sagittal sinus	− 0.4	−	+ 0.1
Choroid plexus	+ 0.07	−	+ 0.7
White matter	− 0.5	−	+ 0.8
Grey matter	+ 0.08	−	+ 0.9

today allows us to diagnose brain death in a very short time, at least to an extent that gives us the indication for angiography. This is important insofar as there is not only a legal contraindication to cerebral angiography in cases of doubt.

A cooperative study would be desirable in order to examine a sufficiently large group of cases of brain death by computerized tomography. Increased introduction of fast scanners, development of automatic subtraction devices, and a biphasic administration of contrast medium which balances the strong decrease during the first 10 min will probably help to improve the information about cerebral circulation, thus providing a method for the diagnosis of brain death. An advantage would be that artifacts such as we know in angiography (5) would not occur, and assessment of the intracranial situation could be made simultaneously.

References

1. ARNOLD, H.: Nervenarzt 47, 529-537 (1976)
2. BÜCHELER, E. et al.: Fortschr. Röntgenstr. 113, 278-281 (1970)
3. KÄUFER, C.: Die Bestimmung des Todes bei irreversiblem Verlust der Hirnfunktionen. Heidelberg: Verlag A. Hüthig 1971
4. MONTZ, R.: Die Sequenzszintigraphie der Hirndurchblutung. Symposium über "Feststellung des Hirntodes", Hamburg 30.8.1974
5. TÄNZER, A.: Die angiographische Diagnostik des dissozierten Hirntodes. Symposium über "Feststellung des Hirntodes", Hamburg 30.8.1974

Classification and Prognosis of Coma: Summary and Conclusion
J. BRIHAYE

Three problems have been dealt with during this session devoted to the classification and outcome of comatose states. The first one is related to the validity of a classification of coma, the second to the various means of grading patients in coma, and the third to the diagnosis of brain death.

Dr. BRAAKMANN feels inclined to think that attempts to scale coma in levels are not worth accepting because he found many inconsistencies in the concurrence of various abnormalities that he has closely examined in a large series of patients; according to him, the individual influence of a series of separate modalities is more informative with regard to prognosis than the creation of a simple overall classification.

For a well-trained clinician, it is correct that dividing comatose states into several levels is not requisite in order to appraise the worsening or the improvement of the patient and to some extent to predict his outcome. But levels have to be looked upon as indicators and not as a strict limit separating patient categories.

In spite of the drawbacks pointed out by Dr. BRAAKMAN, the importance of developing an accurate and generally accepted system of grading coma is obvious for the care of the patient and for the sake of a valid comparison between different groups of patients. During the last conference organized by the neurotraumatology committee of the WFNS in Brussels (September, 1976) (1), it was admitted that a grading system would be useful for a better understanding between people who take care of comatose patients. This preoccupation followed the endeavors made by FROWEIN for a generally accepted meaning of the numerous words used for describing disturbances of consciousness and comatose states. In my opinion, a scale of coma cannot be an unquestioned system; it has to remain a clinical device for a quick and valid appraisal of the patient's state.

With regard to the various means for grading states of coma, I would like once more to emphasize the great value of repeated and frequent clinical examination. The clinical evaluation relies upon symptom groups and at the same time upon laboratory data. Motor reactivity and eye signs (ocular movements and pupil size) are recognized as very valid; glycemia and the degree of brain acidosis are also very predictive and supply valuable and safe information.

Concurring with clinical manifestations and laboratory data, instrumental investigations based either on morphology (radiology, CT scan) or on physiology (EEG, CBF, ICP) are undoubtedly useful but not absolutely necessary. In this respect, STEUDEL and KRÜDER as well as NAU and BOCK have given a fair demonstration of the information provided by the analysis of the EEG. The CT scan, the new arrival, can also supply the clinician with valid information on the extent and multiplicity of brain lesions. When repeated, it also contributes to the prediction of the outcome. On the same line, repeated regional CBF measurements have provided us with information regarding the severity, multiplicity, and evolution of brain lesions.

The prediction of the outcome in comatose patients remains a problem to solve in spite of a careful clinical supervision and complementary investigations.

Whether the patient will survive the injury or not is the first question which we have to answer. I do agree with FROWEIN and his co-workers when they consider the length of coma as one of the best indicators for the prediction of the survival as well as of the severity of sequelae. However we often need the proof of time for the evaluation of the post-traumatic sequelae. Undoubtedly, computer analysis of clinical and laboratory data can be very helpful for the prediction of the outcome, but it is obvious that a machine, however perfect it may be, cannot bring matters to a final decision. The problem of brain death remains debated, and a few months ago, it was still thoroughly being examined in Santiago de Chile by the ad hoc committee of the WFNS. KÖHNE and ARNOLD have just shown that the slow-running blood flow can be appraised on CT scan images which, therefore, can contribute to the diagnosis of brain death.

In fact, with regard to the prediction of brain death and neurologic sequelae, as well as to the scale of comatose states at several levels, the prevalence of the clinical monitoring and of the clinician's experience does not seem questionable, even if complementary investigations are helpful in the management of the patient. Therefore, analysis of large series of patients, as BRAAKMANN and PIA and his collaborators have done, is of great value in giving a better insight into the various problems of craniocerebral injuries.

References

1. Acta Neurochirurgica 40, 181-186 (1978)

Hematomas

Traumatic Intracerebral Hematomas
E. Hamel and A. Karimi-Nejad

Between 1953 and 1976, 150 patients suffering from definite traumatic intracerebral hematoma were operated on in the Neurosurgical University Clinic of Cologne. This was before the era of computerized tomography. The presence of a hematoma was diagnosed exclusively on the basis of angiographic results. In 48% of the cases, a temporal hemorrhage was found, and in 37% a frontal location was stated. Other locations of hematoma were found less frequently (frontotemporal in eight patients, parietal in nine patients, and occipital in six patients). In 92 (61%) of the patients, fractures were noted, which, in 55% of the cases, were found on the same side and, in 40%, on the opposite side. Such attribution was not possible in the case of four patients.

Seriousness of Trauma and Pontine Symptoms

Intracerebral hematomas developed mainly after serious or fairly serious brain trauma, the degree of seriousness being judged by the primary disturbances of consciousness. As can be seen in Table 1, there was an initial unconsciousness in 52% of the cases, which lasted until the time of operation in 41 patients (28%). Fifty-six (39%) patients without primary unconsciousness showed very serious pontine symptoms until the hematoma was verified, either as disturbances of consciousness resembling a transitional stage (cf. WIECK, 4) or clouded consciousness (43 patients), and less frequently as hemiplegia with or without a psychic deficit (13 patients).

As can be seen from Figure 1, however, 13 patients definitely suffering from traumatic hematomas had intervals of 8 h up to 3 weeks with no symptoms at all. In only two patients of 42 and 48 years, suffering from temporal hematomas after slight brain trauma, were the symptomless intervals longer than 48 h. At operation, an intercerebral hematoma was found, which must have been present during the whole interval between trauma and operation. We did not find a fresh hematoma after a symptomless interval in any of the cases, in the sense of delayed apoplexy, according to BOLLINGER (1).

Speed of Development of Hematomas and Their Clinical Course

As can be seen from Figure 2, there were no survivals when clinical manifestation of a hematoma and operation occurred within the first 4 h after trauma. The mortality rate was as high as 80% within 12 h and still 60% within 24 h. The mortality rate was lowest (32%) with patients manifesting a hematoma between the 3rd and the 14th day after trauma.

Table 1. Post-traumatic development of symptoms in 145 cases of traumatic intracerebral hematoma

	Primary and *lasting* unconsciousness	Short primary unconsciousness, interval nearly free of symptoms	No primary unconsciousness but increasing pontine symptoms	No disturbances of consciousness; symptom-free interval
With hemiplegia	7	12	13	
No hemiplegia	34	23	43	13
	41 (28%)	35 (24%)	56 (39%)	13 (9%)

Fig. 1. Post-traumatic development of symptoms with patients suffering from traumatic intracerebral hematomas (with symptomless intervals and no primary unconciousness) (13 patients)

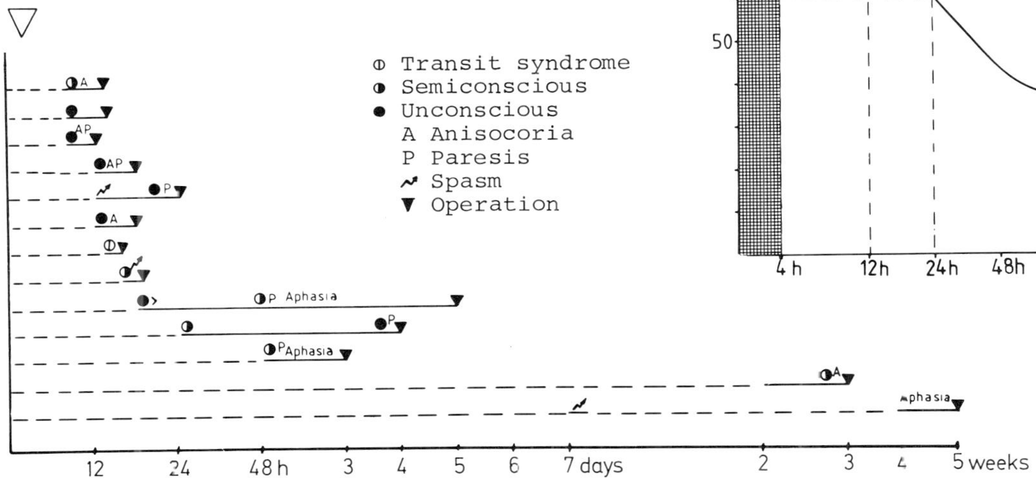

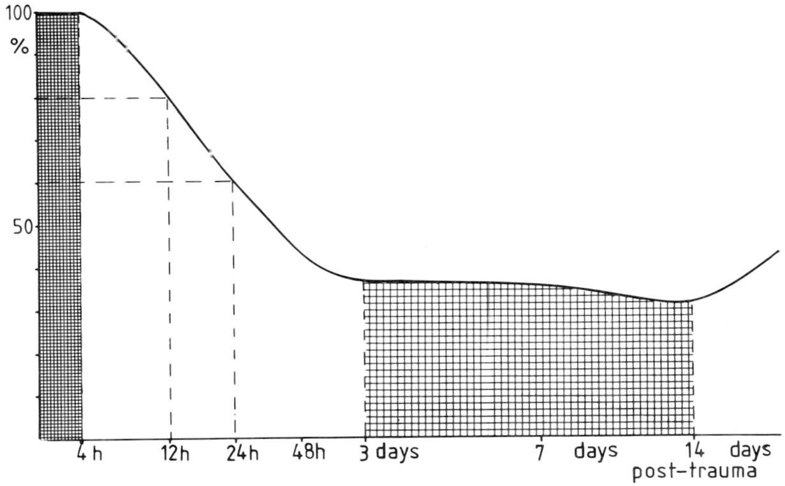

Φ Transit syndrome
⊕ Semiconscious
● Unconscious
A Anisocoria
P Paresis
∼ Spasm
▼ Operation

Fig. 2. Mortality rate in 145 patients with traumatic intracerebral hematomas. No survivals in hematomas developing rapidly within the first 4 h after trauma

According to the macroscopic diagnosis at the first operation, the cases of intracerebral hemorrhage were subdivided into three groups:
1. Hematomas showing inferior cortical contusions without apparent serious contusion of cerebral medulla.
2. Hematomas with marked symptoms of contusion but with the hematoma still being the main cause for the compressing process.
3. Prevalence of contusion with the hematoma being of minor importance.

In accordance with the unfavorable prognosis for rapidely developing hematomas within the first 4 h after trauma, it was mainly contusion hematomas and contusions (Table 2) that were found in this period. Hematomas without contusion which became manifest in this interval were found in patients of more than 60 years of age (four cases), in one patient suffering from previous damage, and also in alcoholics (two cases).

Clinical Symptoms and Results

According to earlier information (2), the results were subdivided into four groups to allow a better survey of their progress:
1. Patients with no neurologic and/or psychic deficit who were fit for work.
2. Patients with slight neurologic and/or psychic disturbances whose fitness for work was slightly impaired.
3. Patients with serious neurologic and/or psychic deficit who remained in need of care.
4. Nonsurviving patients.

As shown in Table 3, mortality was very high (83%) in patients suffering from primary unconsciousness which persisted until the time of operation. If this was combined with the rapid development of a hematoma within the first 12 h, none of the patients survived, even after surgical relief had been given. Patients only survived if the process of development was slow and between 12 and 48 h; this however, was only in patients of less than 30 years of age. In only two cases (the patients being 8 and 23 years of age) was considerable improvement achieved with just a few trivial residual disturbances.

It was only in the case of one patient - a 20-year-old man suffering from an initial 12-h unconsciousness and then regained consciousness, with clinical manifestation of a frontal hematoma after 14 days - that a complete recovery from neurologic and psychic deficit was achieved after primary post-traumatic unconsciousness. Comparable postoperative improvement was only achieved in patients with no primary unconsciousness and slowly increasing disturbances or symptomless intervals (cf. Table 3). In eight out of ten of these cases, the hematoma was localized in the frontal pole. The high mortality rate (62%) of the patients with a symptomless interval is due to the fact that even before operation 8 out of 13 patients were showing symptoms of serious disturbances of brain function due to the hematoma.

Recurring Hemorrhage

Fourteen cases of a recurrence of hemorrhage were verified (seven frontal and seven temporal). The frequency of recurring hemorrhage was independent of the type of operation (osteoplastic or osteoclastic). All patients with such hemorrhages either remained in need of care (six patients) or died (eight patients).

Table 2. Interval between trauma and angiographic demonstration of hematoma, contusion hematoma, and contusions

	4 h	4-12 h	12-24 h	1-3 days	3-7 days	7-14 days	14 days
Hematomas	7	11	24	13	6	9	9
Contusion Hematomas	6	7	16	9	4	4	1
Contusions	6	1	4	4	3	1	
Total	19	19	44	26	13	14	10

Table 3. Results obtained in 145 cases of traumatic intracerebral hematoma in relation to post-traumatic development of symptoms

	Primary and lasting unconsciousness		Short primary unconsciousness, interval nearly free of symptoms		No primary unconsciousness but increasing pontine symptoms		No disturbances of consciousness; symptom-free interval	
No neurologic or psychic deficit (fit over work)	2	5%	1	3%	8	14%	2	15%
Minor neurologic or psychic deficit (fairly fit for work)			5	14%	6	11%	1	8%
Serious neurologic or psychic deficit (in need of care)	5	12%	10	19%	15	27%	2	15%
Deaths	34	83%	19	54%	27	48%	8	62%

Table 4. Results in 145 cases of traumatic intracerebral hematoma, contusion hematoma and contusions

	Hematomas		Contusion hematomas		Contusions		Total	
No neurologic or psychic deficit (fit for work)	7	9%	4	8.5%			11	7%
Minor neurologic or psychic deficit (fairly fit for work)	8	10%	4	8.5%	2	10.5%	14	10%
Serious neurologic or psychic deficit (in need of care)	20	25%	10	21%	2	10.5%	32	22%
Deaths	44	56%	29	62%	15	79%	88	61%

Results

As is shown in Table 4, the rate of mortality with operations performed in 145 cases of traumatic intracerebral hematoma is as high as 61%; 22% of the patients remained in need of permanent care. Considerable improvement of both neurologic and psychic deficits could usually be achieved with younger patients but never when syndromes developed in less than 12 h. Thus, reduction of deficit was achieved with only very minor disturbances remaining in 10% of the cases. Only 11 patients (7%) showed no neurologic or psychic deficits. This was only achieved in one patient older than 40 years of age.

As was to be expected, mortality was higher with contusions (79%) than with hematomas (56%). Surgical treatment of a contusion never led to an improvement of status up to fitness for work. Only 2 out of 19 patients remained with fairly trivial neurologic and psychic deficits. In both of them, carotid angiography showed no hemispheric compression, and the contusion was merely a poor local vascular supply.

Summary

On analyzing the clinical symptoms of 145 patients with definite traumatic intracerebral hematoma, symptomless intervals were observed very rarely. But, in none of the cases did we encounter a fresh hematoma in the sense of traumatic delayed apoplexy. Neither the position of the hematoma nor the kind of operation done showed any relation to the occurrence of recurring hemorrhage. Prognosis was mainly unfavorable when the hematoma became manifest in the first 4 h after trauma. None of the patients suffering from primary unconsciousness persisting until the time of operation survived if a hematoma developed rapidly within 12 h. Surgical treatment of intracerebral hematomas can only lead to satisfying results - both neurologically and socially - if such a hematoma does not develop less than 12 h after trauma. In 17% of the cases, follow-up showed a reduction of disturbances and fitness for work was achieved, mainly with patients under 30 years of age and with a frontal hematoma.

References

1. BOLLINGER, O.: Über traumatische Spätapoplexie. Ein Beitrag zur Lehre von der Hirnerschütterung. (On traumatic delayed Apoplexy. An Contribution to the Studies on Concussion.) In: Internationale Beiträge zur wissenschaftlichen Medizin: Festschrift Rudolf Virchow, Vol. II, S. 457-470. Berlin: Hirschwald 1891
2. KARIMI-NEJAD, A., HAMEL, E., FROWEIN, R.A.: Verlauf der traumatischen intracerebralen Hämatome (The clinical course of traumatic intracerebral Haematomas). (In print)
3. MAYER, E.Th., MEHRAEIN, P., PETERS, G.: Zur Differentialdiagnose der posttraumatischen cerebralen Hämatome (posttraumatische Frühapoplexie) (On the Differential Diagnosis of post-traumatic cerebral Haematomas; Early Post-traumatic Apoplexy). In: BAMMER, G.: Zukunft der Neurologie (The Future of Neurology). Stuttgart: Georg Thieme 1967
4. WIECK, H.H.: Zur Klinik der sogenannten symptomatischen Psychosen (On the clinical manifestations of so-called symptomatic Psychoses) Dtsch. Med. Wochenschr. 81, 1345-1349 (1956)

CT Follow-Up Control of Traumatic Intracerebral Hemorrhage

K. WEIGEL, CHR. B. OSTERTAG, and F. MUNDINGER

The problems regarding the surgical treatment of intracerebral hematoma have been discussed for decades. The CT has made it possible for us to recognize and differentiate intracranial hemorrhage. Not only the site and side of the hemorrhage but also its extent and surroundings can be precisely determined. Traumatic intracerebral hemorrhages are shown in the CT scan as zones of increased density, and they are usually surrounded with a thin less dense border. The density levels of such hematomas lie at 25-35 EMI units; they can be increased to 40 units by means of hemoglobin aggregation. These variations in density compared with normal cerebral tissue provide us not only with the exact location of the intracerebral hemorrhage but also with information about the progress of its resorption in the course of the disease.

Thirty-one of our patients in the last 18 months had traumatic intracerebral hemorrhages, 27 of whom were treated conservatively and four surgically. Of the first group, 23 patients survived, whereas all four of the operated patients died within 4 days of the operation (Table 1). The course of disease in three patients presenting serious initial symptoms after head injury is briefly described. These patients were not operated on although a hematoma was verified by CT.

Case Reports

1. G.R., 30 years old

After a fall from a bicycle, the patient was deeply unconscious and gasping for breath on admission to the Surgical University Clinic. After the vital functions had been secured, a CT scan was performed. This showed an extensive intracerebral hemorrhage in the right frontal region, although without ventricular involvement (Fig. 1a). After intensive care treatment, a control examination 10 days later revealed an extensive zone of reduced density in the area of the original hemorrhage. The original definite shift of approximately 1 cm from right to left had receded considerably (Fig. 1b). In the CT scan 3 months later, a widened ventricular system with rounded contours in all sections was

Table 1. Number of patients with traumatic intracerebral hemorrhage examined by CT scans

	Operated		Nonoperated	
	Alive	Died	Alive	Died
Male	–	4a-d	18	2
Female	–	–	5	2
Total	–	4	23	4

[a] Intraventricular hemorrhage, ventricular puncture.
[b] Right temporal hemorrhage, 1.5 x 2 cm.
[c] Left temporal, paracapsular hemorrhage, 2.5 x 1.5 cm.
[d] Right temporoparietal hemorrhage, 6 x 6 cm.

found with a clearly defined pronounced defect of brain substance in the right frontal region reaching as far as the frontal horn.

2. K.H., 60 years old

After a domestic accident, the patient was admitted to the Surgical Clinic in a comatose state. After appropriate intensive care treatment, a CT scan was performed which revealed a dense lesion in the left frontal region (Fig. 2a). This remained constant in the following days and was surrounded only by a minimal border of edema. A control 3 weeks after the first examination showed a distinct reduction of the left frontal hemorrhage with a decrease in the density and a return in function of the ventricular system (Fig. 2b). Here it can be clearly seen that the initial high density levels of the hematoma decrease with increasing hemoglobin break down. Recent studies by various authors (6, 7) have given reason to correct the notion held until just recently that density reduction is to be equated with the speed of resorption of the hematoma or with the development of an intracerebral cyst. Pathologic examinations in these areas of reduced density, according to the CT scan, showed a completely preserved hematoma clot with greatly increased water storage. The increase of the water content and the reduced hemoglobin molecule concentration are causes of decreased density. These findings and the change of density with the passage of time are consistent with the experiences of the pathologists regarding speed of resorption and disintegration of the hematoma clot. Besides the size of the hematoma, the carabolically efficient, actively resorbing tissue surface nearby is also decisive here (3). A repeat CT scan performed 1.5 months after the onset of the hemorrhage shows a symmetric, in all parts moderately distended ventricular system with rounded contours. In the area of the left frontal white matter, a zone of nonhomogeneous reduced density showed up, which abutted on the left frontal horn. In addition to this, a diffuse cerebral atrophy was starting to develop with markedly expanded subarachnoid spaces (Fig. 2c).

3. K.B., 40 years old

The patient fell from a tree, was responsive for a short time, then became increasingly drowsy, and was in a deep coma when admitted to the Surgical University Clinic. The neurologic state showed a pronounced meningism as well as slight opisthotonus. In the CT scan, a purely intracentricular hemorrhage was shown (Fig. 3a). Three months after conservative treatment, a symmetric generalized moderate dilatation of the ventricular system in middle position was shown in the scan, without distended subarachnoidal or cisternal spaces. There was no evidence of focal damage (Fig. 3b).

Although surgical treatment of all intracerebral hemorrhages has been recommended lately in various studies, with the support of favorable statistics (2, 8), the experiences obtained by means of CT observations on traumatic intracerebral hemorrhage with serious clinical symptoms have allowed to restrict the surgical indications considerably. Surgical intervention is only indicated if clinical deterioration can be established as a result of increasing intracranial pressure.

We consider operation as contraindicated in the case of a brain stem syndrome existing for more than 60 min (5), in the case of a minimal extension of the intracerebral hematoma, as well as in the case of spontaneous improvement of the clinical condition. Here we are in agreement with results of ARANA-INIGUEZ (1), as well as with those of a comprehensive study by the Munich Study Group (4).

At present, the CT scan is the most reliable examination technique by which to differentiate - after an injury-between an intracerebral space-occupying lesion, a ventricular hemorrhage, an extracerebral hemorrhage, and edema. Its speed and dependability, as well as the minimal amount of radiation, make the CT especially suitable for follow-up observation after a brain injury, and it, along with the clinical situation, provides us with exact information as to the time for surgical intervention. The chances of recovery improved even in cases with a problematic initial course. Additional risks such as angiography and brain puncture can be avoided.

Summary

In the last 18 months, 31 patients with traumatic intracerebal hemorrhage have been examined by consecutive CT scans. Twenty-seven were treated conservatively and four surgically. Of the first group, 23 patients survived, whereas all four of the operated patients died within 4 days of operation. The experience gathered up to the present by means of CT observations of traumatic intracerebral hemorrhage have permitted a restriction of the surgical indications. Surgical intervention is only indicated if a clinical deterioration can be established as a result of increasing intracranial pressure.

References

1. ARANA-INIGUEZ, R., WILSON, E., BASTARRICA, E., MEDICI, M.: Cerebral haematoma. Surg. Neurol. 6, 45-52 (1976)
2. BISHARA, S.H.: Intracerebral haemorrhage in closed head injury. Br. J. Surg. 58, 437-441 (1971)
3. KLEIHUES, P.: personal communication
4. LANKSCH, W.: personal communication
5. MARGUTH, F., LANKSCH, W.: Klinische Symptome im Vorfeld des Hirntodes. In: Die Bestimmung des Todeszeitpunktes. KRÖSL, W., SCHERZER, E. (Hrsg.). Wien: W. Maudrich 1973
6. NEW, P.F.J., ARANOW, S.: Attenuation measurements of whole blood and blood fractions in computed tomography. Radiol. 121, 635-640 (1976)
7. NORMAN, D.: Computed tomography in intracerebral haemorrhage.
8. PINEDA, A.: Computed tomography in intracerebral haemorrhage. Surg. Neurol. 8, 55-58 (1977)

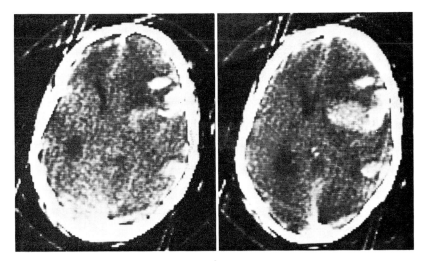

Fig.1. _a_ An extensive intracerebral hemorrhage in the right frontal region

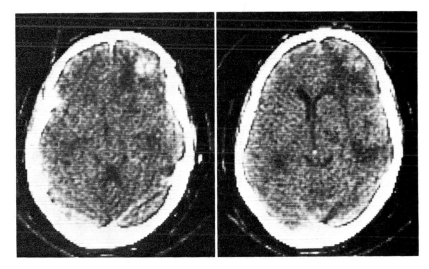

Fig.1. _b_ CT control after 10 days revealed an entensive zone of reduced density in the original area of the hemorrhage

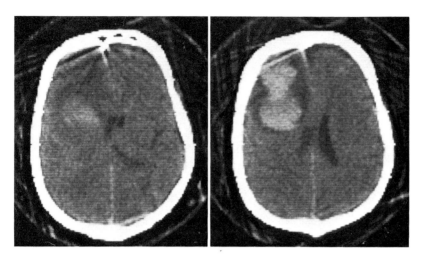

Fig. 2. *a* CT scan showed a dense lesion in the left frontal region

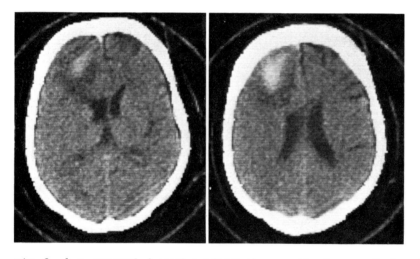

Fig. 2. *b* A control 3 weeks after the accident revealed a distinct reduction of the left frontal hemorrhage

Fig. 3. *b* A follow-up CT scan 3 months after conservative treatment showed a symmetric and generalized moderately distended ventricular system

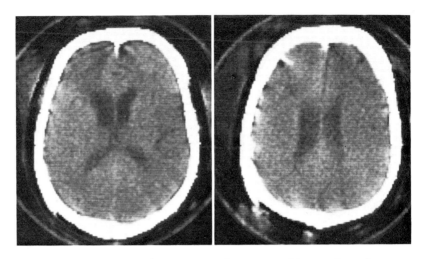

Fig. 2. c A repeated CT scan 1 1/2 months after the first showed a zone of nonhomogeneous reduced density in the left frontal lobe

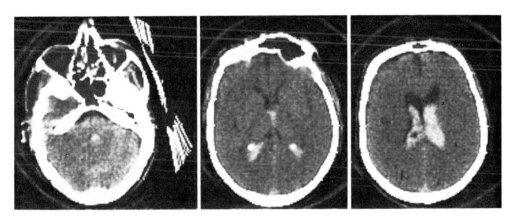

Fig. 3. a CT scan showed a purely intraventricular hemorrhage

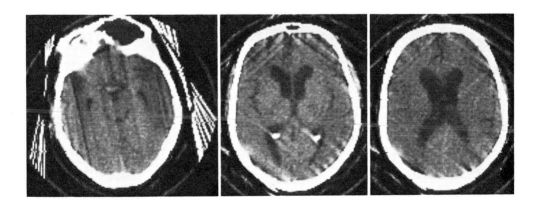

Clinically Nonmanifest Hematomas

H. Huttarsch and G. Cardauns

According to a field study by SCHNELLBÄCHER (4), 80% of all cases of brain damage occuring in the Cologne area are treated in the Neurosurgical Clinic or examined if the presence of a hematoma is suspected. Even so, the number of hematomas that are not verified is unknown, whereas the control exerted on patients treated within the sphere of activity of our clinic is relatively efficient. This is proved by the fact that autopsies on 114 out of 634 of our patients who died from their injuries between 1971 and 1976 were carried out in the Forensic Institute (Table 1). In the remaining cases, prosecution authorities showed no interest in having an autopsy performed.

Comparison of clinical and surgical diagnoses with the results of autopsy showed that in at least 17 of the cases a hematoma was found which had not been previously diagnosed as such. Among these hematomas which were not clinically apparent, there was only one case of an inoperable isolated primary extradural hematoma. Two further cases of extradural hematoma were also combined with an acute subdural one. In eight of the cases, autopsy revealed subdural hematomas and in two of the cases intracerebral hematomas. Autopsy in another five patients showed multiple combined hematomas. Their clinical progress is shown in a time diagram (Fig. 1).

In four cases, there was no chance of either diagnosis or operation. Two of these had cerebral circulatory arrest, and one, because of technical difficulties, insufficient vascular filling; such a frontal intracerebral hematoma would not now be missed by a CT scan. The isolated primary extradural hematoma mentioned above also belongs to this group; this child - who was already moribund - was not admitted to the clinic until 18 h after the accident, after being in two other hospitals. The clinic is interested firstly, in recurrent hemorrhage and secondly in hematomas whose location could not be determined in spite of diagnosis and operation. At autopsy five acute subdural, one chronic subdural and two intracerebral hematomas with epidural, subdural or intracerebral recurrence of hemorrhage were found (Fig. 2).

In nearly two-thirds of the cases examined, it was either because of the acute and swiftly developing clinical process or the advanced stage

Table 1. Survivors, nonsurvivers and number of autopsies among head-injury patients (University Neurosurgical Clinic, Cologne, 1971-1976)

	1529	
Survivors		Nonsurvivors
859		634
		Autopsy
		114
		Massive hematomas
		17

of coma that no further measures could be undertaken. In the other four cases, the situation was as follows. In one case, a control angiography should have been done as well as in two earlier cases, because no marked neurologic improvement was to be seen even after several days; furthermore, the continuing lucidity was misleading, as well as the fact that in another case there were no typical signs of hematoma at angiography, although autopsy revealed an extensive subdural hematoma at the site of the operation. Autopsy of the other five patients revealed multiple hematomas.

In these cases, i.e., three acute subdural hematomas, one intracerebral, and one case of combined extradural and intracerebral hematoma, operation based on the most striking clinical and angiographic findings could not bring about any marked improvement. As a result of the extensive and multiple nature of the injuries, brain damage was too severe to allow any operation to have a successful outcome.

Angiography verification of such combined hematomas was only possible to some extent in one case, which consisted of two hematomas, both of which developed quickly and at different times. In all other cases, it was not possible to differentiat acute combined hematomas by angiography.

According to HAMEL and KARIMI (1), operation on these intracerebral hematomas - even within the first 4 h - would not have been successfull. This fact will have to be borne in mind when considering the location of multiple hematomas and the indications for their surgical treatment.

Summary

Clinical diagnosis and autopsy findings on 114 fatal head injuries seen between 1971 and 1976 have been compared. In at least 17 cases, we found an intracranial hematoma - and among these only one solitary primary extradural one - which had not been previously diagnosed. Rapid deterioration in the clinical state, delays, and technical problems in diagnosis often prevented early treatment or led to inefficient surgical management.

References

1. HAMEL, E., KARIMI-NEJAD, A.: Traumatic intracerebral hematomas. This volume, pp. 56-61
2. KRAULAND, W.: Traumatische intracranielle Blutungen aus path. Sicht. Hefte Unfallheilkunde 78, 213-217 (1964)
3. PENZHOLZ, H.: Blutungen aus klinischer Sicht. Hefte Unfallheilkunde 78, 213 (1964)
4. SCHNELLBÄCHER, M.: Zum Problem der Incidenz von schweren Schädel-Hirn-Verletzungen und sich daraus ergebenden Behandlungsaufgaben. Inaugural-Dissertation, Köln 1975

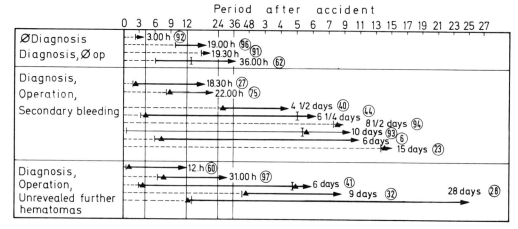

Fig. 1. Time diagram. The clinical course of 17 patients with clinically nonmanifest hematomas
 | Angiography
 I Controlangiography
 ▲ Operation

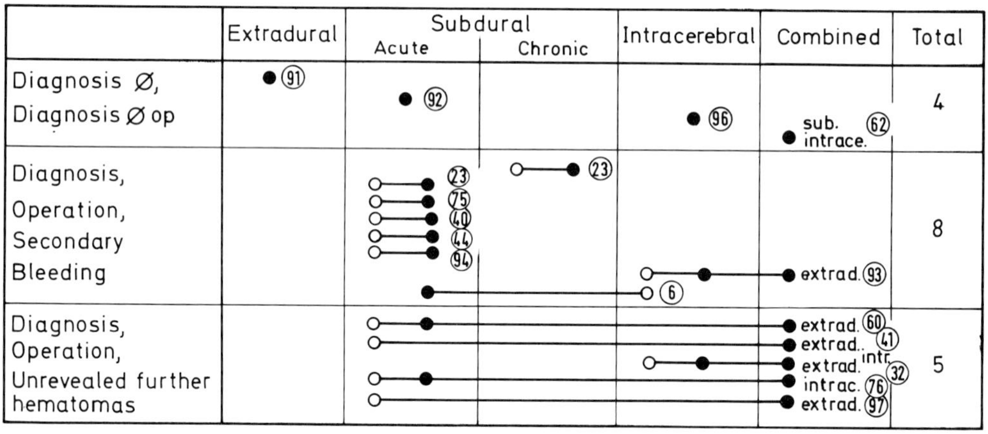

	Extradural	Subdural		Intracerebral	Combined	Total
		Acute	Chronic			
Diagnosis Ø, Diagnosis Ø op	● ⑨⑴	● ⑨⑵		● ⑨⑹	sub. ⑹⑵ ● intrace.	4
Diagnosis, Operation, Secondary Bleeding		○—● ㉓ ○—● ⑺⑸ ○—● ⑷⓪ ○—● ⑷⑷ ○—● ⑼⑷ ● ○—●	○—● ㉓	○—● ⑹	● extrad.⑨⑶	8
Diagnosis, Operation, Unrevealed further hematomas		○—● ○—● ○—● ○—●		○—●	● extrad.⑹⓪ ● extrad..⑷⑴ ● extrad.intr ㉜ ● intrac. ⑺⑹ ● extrad.⑨⑺	5

Fig. 2. Location and character of the clinically nonmanifest intracranial hematomas

Frontobasal Injuries

Head Injuries in Young Motorcyclists
I. SCHÖTER

Fatal motorcylce accidents increase each year (1, 3, 4, 5, 6, 12). In 1975, motorcycle deaths in West Germany totaled 1930 with another 70,709 persons injured (13) (Fig. 1). In 1974, 26% of the victims were killed at an age younger than 18 years and 60% before reaching the age of 25 years (13). It is remarkable that the increasing morbity rate of young and healthy people - much discussed in other countries - (1, 3, 4, 5, 7, 10, 11, 12) is not mentioned in German papers. Motorcycles are supposed to be 12-17 times more dangerous than cars (4, 5, 7). The rate of head injuries in motorcycle accidents ranges from 65%-80% (1, 12). Fatalities and nonreversible neurologic deficits are frequent (1, 2, 3, 8, 10, 12).

Among 537 patients admitted because of motorcycle trauma, we found 162 children and adolescents up to the age of 19 years (30%). Of the victims 89% were drivers or passengers of motorized two-wheeled vehicles, while 11% were injured by motorcyclists. The male sex was predominant (87%). The victims had an average age of 15.7 years with a high incidence of 17-year-old adolescents. Sixty-four percent of the casualities were due to scooter and moped accidents, 34% to motorcycle trauma (Fig. 2). The percentage of severe injuries was equal in the different types of motorized vehicles. One hundred and forty-two of the patients (88%) suffered from head injuries, severe concussion being the most common type of lesion (63%) (Table 1).

Concomitant fractures of the calvarium occurred in 53% and of the visceral cranium in 11%. Severe concussion was accompanied by intracerebral hemorrhage in 19% of the cases. Of the head injuries, 23% were compound injuries. Liquorrhea was present in 56% and meningitis was the consequence in 13% of the cases. One patient developed a brain abscess.

Table 1. Neurosurgic injuries in 162 young motorcyclists

Head injuries	142	88%	Severe concussion	90	63%
			Open injuries	32	23%
			Mild injuries	20	14%
				142	100%
Transverse lesion	5	3%			
Traumatic exeresis of nerve roots	9	5%			
Injuries to peripheral nerves	6	4%			
	162	100%			

Contusions or lacerations were diagnosed at operation in 38% of open injuries. Damaged brain tissue protruded in seven cases and extradural hematomas and intracerebral hemorrhages were encountered in four patients. Only 14% of head injuries were less severe or mild; nevertheless, they were accompanied by cranial fractures in six cases and by long-term changes in EEG in another six. Brain injury was fatal for 37 young patients, 32 of them died from the consequences of severe concussion (Table 2). Concomitant extradural or subdural hematoma was seen in two if these cases. Five persons died after a compound brain injury, one of them from meningitis.

In all fatal cases, the patients remained in a coma for the entire period after the accident. The longest period of survival was 17 days, and the average 3 days. Five patients developed an apallic syndrome. The prognosis of severe concussion is worse than of open brain trauma. Death or an apallic syndrome occurred in 42% of the primary group and in 16% of the later one. Ninety-five patients survived head injury, 56 of them with permanent neurologic deficit. Nonreversible brain damage is obvious in more than 70% of the surviving patients; in another 11% the consequences of long-term changes in EEG have yet to be determined.

The period of unconsciousness seems to be important for later brain function. Weak cerebral function occurred in patients who remained unconscious for an average of 6 days as opposed to 1.6 days in persons with subsequent normal brain function. Only 8% of motorcycle victims recovered completely.

The statistics on the causes of motorcycle trauma reveal that the drivers were to blame for the accidents in 98% of the casualities. Forty percent of the fatalities were the results of travelling at an excessive speed. Nonobservance of traffic regulations and alcohol abuse were the next common causes of accidents (13). As cited by Hunter SHELDON (9), prevention is the only treatment for head injury. Many recommendations have been made:

1. Education of the public, particulalry the young public, concerning frequency and severity of motorcycle trauma (5).
2. Compulsory wearing of crash helmets (1, 2, 3, 4, 5, 6, 8, 10, 11, 12).

Table 2. Consequences of severe head injuries (predominant symptoms)

		Severe concussion		Open Injury		Total	
		90	100%	32	100%	132	100%
Exitus		32	36%	5	16%	37	30%
Permanent deficits	Apallic syndrome	5	6%	–	–	5	4%
	Weak cerebral function	21	23%	9	28%	30	25%
	Fits	3	3%	2	6%	5	4%
	Pareses	9	10%	1	3%	10	8%
	Aphasia	2	2%	–	–	2	2%
	Defect of cranial nerves	2	2%	8	25%	10	8%
Long-term changes in EEG		9	10%	4	13%	13	11%
Complete Recovers		7	8%	3	9%	10	8%

3. Necessity for instruction and specific licensing of all drivers and for all types of cycles (4, 5).
4. Enforcement of speed laws and laws on drinking and driving (12).

However, motorcycling is a "glorious sport" in the opinion of all drivers. In the past, all recommendations were wrecked by public apathy and the prompt reactions from organized cyclists (10).

Summary

Fatal motorcycle accidents in young people increase each year. The histories of 162 victims with an average age of 15.7 years are analyzed. Eighty-eight percent of the patients suffered from head injuries, severe concussion being the most common type of lesion (63%). Brain injury was fatal for 30% of the injured persons. Permanent neurologic deficit occured in 70% of the surviving patients and in 11%, the consequences of trauma are yet to be determined. The period of unconsciousness seems to be important for later brain function. After reviewing the literature, recommendations are made to prevent further casualities.

References

1. BOTHWELL, P.W.: The Problem of Motorcycle Accidents. Practitioner 188, 474-488 (1962)
2. CAIRNS, H., HOLBOURN, H.: Head Injuries in Motor-Cyclists. Br. Med. J. 1943/I, 591-598
3. CLARK, D.W., MORTON, J.H.: The Motorcycle Accident: A Growing Problem. J. Trauma 11, 230-237 (1971)
4. CRACCHIOLO, A., BLAZINA, M., MAC KINNON, D.S.: Motorcycle Injuries to University Students. JAMA 204, 175-176 (1968)
5. DEANER, R.M., FITCHETT, V.H.: Motorcycle Trauma. J. Trauma 15, 678-681 (1975)
6. GUSTILLO, R.B., FOSS, D.L. et al.: Motorcycle Injuries. An Increasing Traffic Problem. Minn. Med. 48, 489-491 (1965)
7. HART, D.N., FRACS, P.W.C., FRACS, W.A.A.: Christchurch Traffic Trauma Survey: Part 2, Victims and Statistics. NZ. Med. J. 81, 543-546 (1975)
8. JAMIESON, K.G., KELLY, D'ARCY: Crash Helmets Reduce Head Injuries. Med. J. Aust. 60 / 2, 806-809 (1973)
9. KEENEY, A.H.: Prevention of Ocular Injuries. Int. Ophthalmol. Clin. 14, 1-10 (1974)
10. KELLEY, A.B.: Motorcycles and Public Apathy. Am. J. Public Health 66, 475-476 (1976)
11. KRAUS, J.F., RIGGINS, R.S., FRANTI, C.E.: Some Epidemiologic Features of Motorcycle Collision Injuries. Am. J. Epidemiol. 102, 99-109 (1975)
12. SMITH, B.H., DEHNER, L.P.: Fatal Motorcycle Accidents of Military Personnel: A Study of 223 Cases. Milit. Med. 134, 1477-1487 (1969)
13. Statistisches Jahrbuch für die BRD. Stuttgart-Berlin-Köln-Mainz: W. Kohlhammer 1976

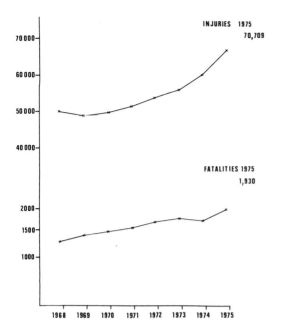

Fig. 1. Motorcycle and motorscooter accidents in West Germany (1968-1975)

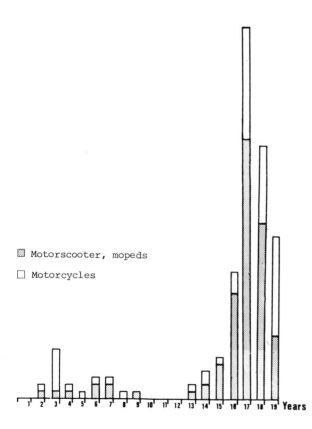

Fig. 2. Accidents with motorized two-wheeled vehicles (age distribution of 162 juveniles)

Safety Helmets and Craniocerebral Injuries

H. E. DIEMATH, B. RICHLING, and G. SORGO[1]

In the last few years, the type of craniocerebral injuries sustained by motorcycle and moped riders seems to have changed. In the past, motorcycle riders used their vehicles mostly as a means of getting to work. Safety helmets were seldom used. With improving economic conditions, two-wheeled motor vehicles were increasingly replaced by automobiles. In recent years, however, there has been another motorcycle and moped boom, but these vehicles are now used more and more for recreation purposes (4).

Due to wider awareness of safety technology and research (1, 2, 5, 8, 9), leather clothing and safety helmets are frequently worn and in some places - Austria for examples - are mandatory for insurance purposes. In Salzburg, in the Department of neurosurgery, numerous case histories have enabled us to confirm the observations of other authors (4, 5, 6). During the years when head protection was generally neglected, the most serious skull injuries were frequently characterized by open depressed fractures of the forehead and crown of the head. These injuries were often accompanied by serious infection of the wounded area and occasionally by extensive damage to parts of the brain. Depending on the functional importance of the site of lesion, e.g., frontal lobes, or the base of these lobes, partial or full recovery of the patients could be expected. Injuries combined with damage to the jaw and orbital areas were occasionally quite serious but not necessarily life threatening.

In recent years, the change to more frequent use of helmets and leather clothing by motorcycle riders has led to a change in the type of motorcycle-related injuries. Open fractures in the frontoparietal area were absent. Instead, however, fractures of the skull base along the posterior fossa and the upper cervical spine were frequently found. These skeletal injuries were accompanied by basal contusions, primary brain stem hemorrhages, and very frequently a distinctive tendency toward generalized brain edema resistant to all treatment (7). The reason for this change in injuries is attributed on the one hand to the high speeds possible with modern vehicles, although riders of lightweight models also sustain the above-mentioned injuries. On the other hand, the use of the customary safety helmet might be one of the reasons for the changes in the type of head injury.

Force hit the bones of the skull within a circumscribed area and the vault of the unprotected skull fractured. By the use of safety helmet, though double walled (9), force is distributed over a larger surface area, therefore diminishing the pressure per cm^2 and leaving the skull intact. In our opinion, the actual energy is only slightly decreased but is transmitted to the atlanto-occipital region and concentrated in a small area. This results in fractures in this area, damage to central parts of the brain, and massive edema. It remains obvious that the protective effect of safety helmets against depressed fractures and

---

[1] We want to thank the Ministerium für Gesundheit und Umweltschutz and the Porsche Konstruktion KG for their generous support of this work.

other skull injuries is irrefutable. It seemed, however, important to us firstly to prove our opinion by experiments and secondly to search for ways of combining the unquestioned protective effects of the helmet with a reduction of the schock wave in order to prevent or diminish the injuries described above.

In cooperation with the research center of Porsche AG, the following experiment was undertaken. A human skull, made to simulate physiologic proportions as authentically as possible, is covered with wet leather and, together with a fluid-filled bladder, is fastened to a hard rubber spinal column of the so-called 50% man/dummy. Sensors which measure the values of acceleration and force are mounted within the skull and in the atlanto-occipital region. On the accelerating sled, this model is projected against a solid barrier, in this case a plexiglass plate. The diversion and recording of force and acceleration values with or without a helmet show the difference in actual force fields in both cases.

Our research at the present time is not yet completed because the technical measuring equipment is very expensive due to the extremely short time intervals and also because the statistical evaluation requires a greater number of tests. Furthermore, it is not only a medical-technical problem, but there are also many details, like weight and material, free movement of the head, and economical viewpoint concerning marketing and product appeal of a newly developed helmet which have to be considered. As there is no doubt as to the safety value of the helmet against trivial and perforating injuries, all our research aims are at showing whether a better distribution and absorption of energy would not heighten the protective effect of the helmet.

Summary

The observation of a change in the pattern of craniocerebral injuries within the last few years has led to the assumption that too great a part of energy is transmitted to the atlanto-occipital region resulting in severe cerebral edema and damage to the central parts of the brain which is resistant to therapeutic measures. This paper reports on the experiments designed to prove this theory and to develop a new helmet, although the protective value of the safety helmet against other injuries is never doubted.

References

1. CHRISTMANN, K., WISCHHUSEN, H.G., EHLER, E., PAN, H.: Untersuchungen über Druckbelastbarkeit und Frakturmechanismus weichteilbedeckter Schädel. Anat. Anz. 139, 274-280 (1976)
2. ELLIS, E.H.: Protective Helmets for Motorcyclists and Car Drivers, Their Design, Function and Evaluation. Technical Aspects of Road Safety. Brüssel: CODITVA 17, 1964
3. FELDKAMP, G., JUNGHANNS, K., PRALL, W.-D.: Motorrad-Boom und Motorrad-Unfälle. Fortschr. Med. 92, 325-329 (1974)
4. FELDKAMP, G., PRALL, W.-D., BÜHLER, G., JUNGHANNS, K.: Unfälle mit motorisierten Zweirädern- Epidemiologie, Klinik, Schutzmöglichkeiten - Eine retrospektive und prospektive Studie. Unfallheilkunde 80, 1-19 (1977)
5. FIALA, E.: Zur Verletzungsmechanik bei Verkehrsunfällen. H. Unfallheilk. 98, 31-52 (1969)

6. KAMIYAMA, S., KÄPPNER, R., SCHMIDT, Gg.: Verletzungskombinationen bei tödlichen Verkehrsunfällen. Mschr. Unfallheilk. 74, 10-30 (1971)

7. RICHLING, B.: Zur Pathomechanik des Sturzhelmes. Wien: Med. Wschr. 127, 313-315 (1977)

8. ZIFFER, D.: Beitrag über die Probleme der mechanischen Widerstandsfähigkeit des menschlichen Körpers und seiner Gewebe. Die Anwendung der Festigkeitsbelastungen auf Konstruktionsfragen von Sturzhelmen und Sicherheitsgurten für Automobilisten. Technical aspects of road safety. Brüssel: CIDITVA 23, 1965

9. ZIFFER, D.: Schutzhelme für Kraftfahrer. Zbl. Verkehrsmed. 3, 72-78 (1967)

Catamneses of Frontobasal Head Injuries
R. A. Pachay

One hundred and nineteen cases of frontobasal injuries operated on in the University Clinic of Cologne were analyzed with respect to their catamnestic results and the time of operation. This is a continuation of our former papers (3, 4, 5).

Time of Operation

In the total number of cases involved (Fig. 1), plastic operations at the anterior base of the skull were performed at extremely different times varying between 1 day up to 18 years after the injury had been suffered. The classic cases of late operation because of CSF fistula and/or meningitis will not be included. But even in patients operated on within the first few days, weeks, or 6 months after the injury, cases of meningitis were observed both at and after the operation. Twenty-one out of 85 of these patients who were operated on died, which means that the repair of the CSF fistula was either too late or technically inadequate. This could be an incentive for considering surgical treatment as early as possible. For this reason, those early operations performed within the first 12 days seem to be of special interest. Figure 2 shows the results obtained, grouped according to survivals and nonsurvivals. Out of a total of 33 patients operated on during the first 12 days, all 12 died, who had been unconscious at the time of operation. However, only one patient, who was conscious and received surgical treatment on the 2nd day died. It should be mentioned that this was a case of combined injuries, including both a renal and a splenic rupture plus pulmonary emphysema. This shows that more frontobasal injuries should not be operated on as long as the patient is unconscious, with the exception of patients, who suffer from space-occupying hematomas.

Despite the fact that they had received early surgical treatment, 7 out of 14 nonsurviving patients developed meningitis in the course of the following 2-4 weeks. This leads to the conclusion that the repair of the CSF fistula must have been technically inadequate under early surgical treatment.

Twenty surviving patients who had received early surgical treatment within the first 12 days, however, did not suffer a relapse of the CSF fistula or develop meningitis. In two cases, however, meningitis developed before the operation on the 4th and 6th days, respectively. In both these cases, there had been no sufficient antibiotic treatment after the accident. This shows that antibiotic prophylaxis is indispensible but should be short-termed to prevent resistance. This data leads to clear conclusions with respect to the time of operation and further requirements. Plastic operation of frontobasal injuries should not be performed on unconscious patients but only on such patients who are either just disorientated or, even better, fully conscious. The operation should be carried out as soon as possible after normalization of brain edema, i.e., after ca. 4-6 days (cf. 1, 2).

Catamnestic Results

Ninety catmneses carried out over several years showed that in the cases of 119 patients operated on, 28% secured a better job than before the time of accident, 37% had a similar job, although seven cases suffered from dysopia, and in four cases, disequilibrium or seizures led to a 45% degree of disablement. This data shows that the results obtained in two-thirds of the patients are either good or at least satisfactory. The same results were presented by DIETZ in 1970 (1).

Twenty-one percent of the patients, however, had to content themselves with inferior employement, and 14% were not able to secure any employment at all. Among the patients with an inferior job, there are six whose degree of disablement is as low as 20% and 13 with a degree of 45%-70%. Together with 13 further patients who are not working at all, there are 26 patients (28%) whose social standard has been considerably impaired. It is only in 7 out of 32 cases that this is due to a marked disturbance in sight, which cannot be influenced and is mainly due to the accident suffered. Five cases with meningitis show the very urgent need for a better timing of the operation and an improvement in the repair.

Seventeen cases suffering from epileptic seizures are especially worth mentioning, since it was in only two cases that the seizures occured before the operation, whereas in eight cases epileptic seizures first occurred more than 2 years after operation. This is striking because former studies on our patients carried out by STEINMANN and OBERTHÜR had shown that 80% of the cases suffering from seizures had epileptic seizures within the first 2 years after closed or open head injuries. For this reason, it is recommended that frontobasal injuries be observed over an especially long period of time and continuous prophylaxis with respect to epileptic seizures should be considered.

References

1. DIETZ, H.: Die fronto-basale Schädel-Hirnverletzung (On Fronto-Basal Brain Injuries). Berlin-Heidelberg-New York: Springer 1970
2. FROWEIN, R.A.: Langenbecks Archiv für klinische Chirurgie. Langenbecks Arch. Chir. 319, 564-565 (1967)
3. KROKER: Die Komplikationen bei fronto-basalen Verletzungen (Complications with Fronto-Basal Injuries) Köln: Thesis 1967
4. THUN: Die nasalen Liquorfisteln, ihre Genese, Diagnostik und Therapie. Dissertation, Köln 1960
5. TÖNNIS, W., FROWEIN, R.A., LOEW, F., GROTE, E., HEMMER, KLUG, N., FINKENMEYER: Organisation der Behandlung schwerer Schädel-Hirn-Verletzungen (On Organising the Treatment of Serious Brain Injuries), pp. 50-57. Stuttgart: Georg Thieme 1968

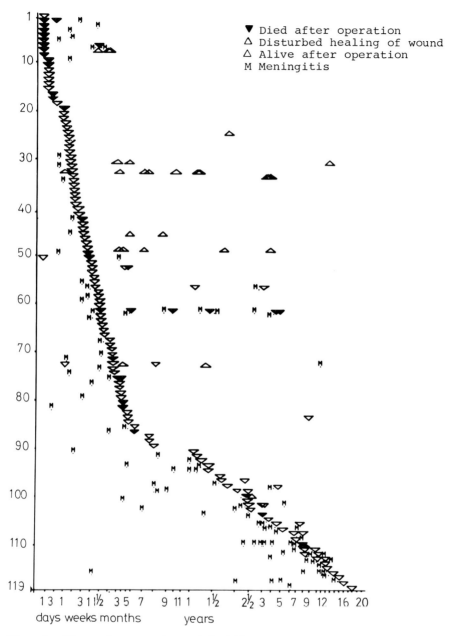

Fig. 1. Time of operation with 119 cases of frontobasal brain injuries

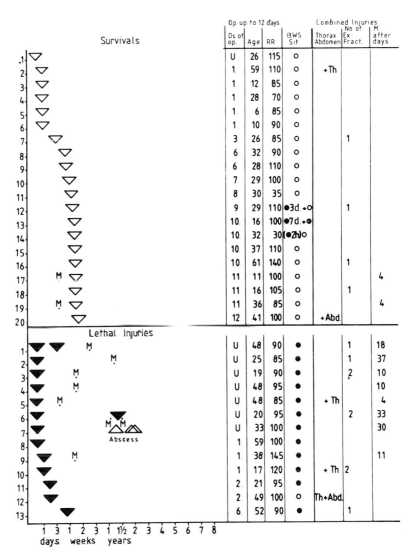

Fig. 2. Early operation of 33 cases of brain injury
BWL State of consciousness
● Unconscious
o Conscious
◐ Clouding of consciousness
M Meningitis

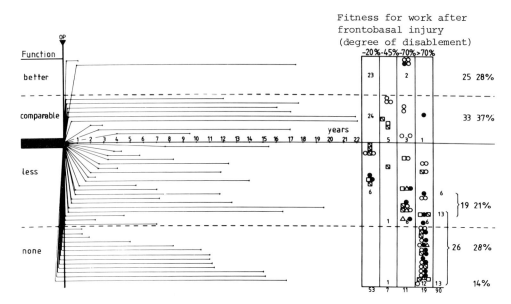

Fig. 3. Catamneses of 90 cases of frontobasal brain injury
o Dysopia
● Attacks
△ Meningitis
◨ Disequilibrium
☐ Weak cerebral function

Prolonged Unconsciousness

Effects of Anti-Parkinsonian Drugs on Behavior and EEG of Comatose Patients[1]

F. MILTNER and J. WICKBOLDT [2]

Introduction

The present interest in catecholamines in cerebral dysfunctions was induced by the various effects that could be elicited by pharmacologic agents known to interfere with aminergic neurotransmission (3, 5, 6, 9, 12). The identification of catecholamines and acetylcholine as transmitters in reticular neurons has led to a more differentiated insight into the functional aspects of NORUZZI and MAGONN's reticular activating system (8, 12).

A few reports have been published about cerebral catecholamine metabolism following head injury in man (3, 13). A clear inverse relationship between the height of the HVA levels and the durations of unconsciousness has been demonstrated (13). Dysfunction of neural systems is reflected by the time course of its reversibility. Therefore, it is of interest to measure both extent and duration of neurologic deficits with noninvasive valid tests.

Up to now, there exist a number of various rational coma classifications which depend on observation and description (10, 11). We prefer the Glasgow coma scale mentioned above (11). More recent investigations propose the evaluation of human cerebral dysfunction with neurophysiologic and neuropharmacological methods (2, 9). This investigation focuses on the relationship between drug-induced bioelectric and behavioral changes in coma and on multimodality-evoked response patterns related to distinct brain stem syndromes.

Methods

Methods obtaining and analysing bioelectric activity from the convexity of the skull and the base in comatose patients have been described elsewhere (9). In 243 comatose patients of both sexes (aged 16-63 years), coma levels were assessed by use of the Glasgow coma scale, in which the degree of coma is determined by the rate of spontaneous eye opening:

---

[1] This investigation was supported by the "Deutsche Forschungsgemeinschaft" (Arbeitsgruppe A I 3).

[2] The authors gratefully acknowledge the competent assistance of M. Stolz.
We thank the following companies for a generous supply of drugs: Hoffmann-La Roche, Merz & Co., Frankfurt/Main, and Knoll AG, Ludwigshafen.

1. Motor responsiveness.
2. Verbal responses.

The clinical course was documented for 14 days and evaluated in relation to the EEG changes obtained. Twenty-four severely injured patients were investigated a total of 102 times during their early phases of intensive care. Clinical diagnosis ranged from brain death, bulbar syndrome to midbrain syndrome. The placement of electrodes was oriented according to the international 10/20 system. We recorded bipolarly from the positions C3-P3, C4-P4, P3-O2, P4-O2, nuchal-suboccipital. Bioelectric activities were amplified and filtered conventionally and fed into a NICOLET 1072 computer. Somatosensory-evoked potentials were recorded in response to electric, supralimitary, and mental nerve stimulation alternately on the right and left side. Visual stimulation was performed using a strobe light flash positioned 0,6 m from the nasion with one pulse per second and fixed intensities. In general, at least 256 responses were averaged to get an adequate signal-to-noise ratio. Sweep durations were varied from 20 ms-400 ms. Results were stored and plotted. Stimulation and recording equipment were mounted on one chart so that it was easily possible to measure at the patient's bed in our intensive care unit.

Results

In general, it can be stated that the spontaneous EEG activity from the cranial convexity and the base changes parallel the patient's clinical course. In agreement with JOUVET (6), we did not register regular circadia rhythmic events in patients persistent in the vegetative state.

1. Drug-Induced Variations

After the rapid intravenous application of L-dopa, amantadine HCl, biperiden tonic arousal reactions occured in 74% of cases. This category of patients showed a marked increase in alertness, which could be recorded in the coma scale (Fig. 1). In 21% of the cases, an alternating EEG pattern occurred. δ-Rhythmus and irregular, low amplituded 6-8 cps traces alternate each other. In addition, applied arousal stimuli triggered a δ-rhytmic reaction. These patients showed slowly increasing coma levels (Fig. 1). It can be stated that under antparkinsonian drugs, clinical assessed coma ranges tend to differ significantly ($p < 0.05$). Especially these coma ranges of severly injured patients who did not respond to pharmacologic stimulation (4) are isolated from the others (Fig. 1).

2. Multimodality-Evoked Responses in Brain Stem Syndromes

Twenty-Four severely head-injured patients were investigated during the early phases of neurosurgical intensive care. In brain death, neither cortical nor nuchal responses to somatosensory stimulation could be obtained (Fig. 2). The bulbar syndrome is characterized by normal nuchal but absent cortical responses to somatosensory stimulation (Fig. 2). Midbrain syndromes showed marked differences in the amplited of the primary responses when results of alternate stimulation sites were compared with each other. As a rule, the lower the coma level, the shorter the cerebral response was. Improvement in coma levels was accompanied by the occurrence of waves belonging to the late primary or even secondary cortical responses.

Discussion

Intact neural systems located in the brain stem reticular core are the functional basis of waking and sleeping (1, 3, 4, 5, 6). More or less reversible dysfunction of these systems cause coma (7, 12, 13). In neurosurgical intensive care units, it is of importance to define a patient's final outcome as early as possible by means of valuable functional tests (2, 9, 10, 11, 13). As a result findings, it is suggested that in addition to EEG monitoring during the early phases of hospitalization, drugs known to influence the reticular activating system should be employed. Long-term assessment of coma levels has proved to be useful for registering spontaneous and druginduced variations. To complete the neurophysiologic assay, multimodality-evoked response studies should be performed. This enables the investigator to obtain further information about the extent of the neurologic deficits and its probable reversibility.

Summary

Following severe head injuries, extended lesions of the mesodiencephalic region often interrupt ascending catecholamine and cholinergic pathways. In 243 comatose patients, coma levels were assessed using the Glasgow coma scale. This clinical evaluation of coma was accompanied by neurophysiologic investigations, which included long-term EEG monitoring, multimodality-evoked response studies, and a neuropharmacologic approach (L-dopa, amantadine HCl and biperiden). Bioelectrical findings were found to be closely correlated with the patients' final outcome.

References

1. DOMINO, E.D., DREN, A.T., YANAMOTO, K.: Pharmacologic evidence for cholinergic mechanism in neocortical and limbic activating systems. In: Structure and Function of the Limbic System. ADEY, W.R., TOKINAZE, T. (eds.), Vol. XXVII, pp. 237-364. Amsterdam-London-New York: Elsevier 1967

2. GREENBERG, R.P., MAYER, A.J., BECKER, D.P.: The prognostic value of evoked potentials in human mechanical head injury. In: Head Injuries. Proceedings of the Second Chicago Symposium on Neural Trauma. MCLAUREN, R.L. (ed.), pp. 81-88. New York-San Francisco-London: Grune & Stratton 1976

3. HARNER, R.N., DORMAN, R.M.: Mechanisms of electroencephalographic and behavioral changes produced by parenteral L-Dopa. Electroencephalog. Clin. Neurophysiol. 27, 672 (1969)

4. HEPPNER, F., ARGYROPOULOS, G., LANNER, G.: Anticholinergische Behandlung des Schädelhirntraumas. Wschr. Unfallheilkunde 76, 341-358 (1973)

5. JONES, B.E., BOBILLIER, P., PIN, C., JOUVET, M.: The effect of lesions of catecholamine-containing neurons upon monoamine content of the brain and EEG and behavioral waking in the cat. Brain Res. 58, 157-177 (1973)

6. JOUVET, M.: The role of monoamines and acetylcholine-containing neurons in the regulation of the sleep-waking cycle. Rev. Physiol. 64, 166-307 (1972)

7. LINDSLEY, D.F. RANF, S.K., FERNANDEZ, F.C., WYRWICKA, W.: Effects of anti-parkinsonian drugs on the motor activity and EEG of cats with subthalamic lesions. Exp. Neurol. 47, 404-418 (1975)

8. MAJ, J., SOWINSKA, H., BARAN, L.: The effect of amantadine on motor activity and catalepsy in rats. Psychopharmacol. 12, 295-307 (1972)
9. MILTNER, F., WICKBOLDT, J.: Arousal Reactions with Unconscious Patients Eliciting by L-Dopa, Amantadine-HCl and Akineton. In: Advances in Neurosurgery, Vol. 4, p. 6. WÜLLENWEBER, R. et al. (eds.). Berlin-Heidelberg-New York: Springer 1977
10. PLUM, F., POSNER, J.B.: Diagnosis of Stupor and Coma, 2nd ed. New York: Davis 1972
11. TEASDALE, G., JENNETT, B.: Assessment and prognosis of coma after head injury. Acta Neurochir. (Wien) 34, 45-55 (1976)
12. UNGERSTEDT, U.: Stereotaxic mapping of monoamine pathways in the rat brain. Acta Physiol. Scand. (Suppl.) 367, 1-48 (1971)
13. VECHT, Ch.J., VAN WOERKOM, Th.C., TEELKEN, A.W., MINDERHOUD, J.M.: On the nature of brain-stem disorders in severe head-injured patients. I. Acta Neurochir. (Wien) 34, 11-21 (1976)
14. WILLIAMSON, P.D., GOFF, W.R., ALLISON, T.: Somatosensory evoked responses in patients with unilateral cerebral lesions. Electroencephalogr. Clin. Neurophysiol. 28, 566-575 (1970)

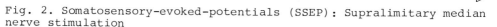

Fig. 2. Somatosensory-evoked-potentials (SSEP): Supralimitary median nerve stimulation
<u>A</u> C3-P3, C4-P4, nuchal and suboccipital points
  1 Bulbar brain syndrome, only nuchal potentials
  2 Brain death no response
<u>B</u> Traces one and three: C3-P3
  Traces two and four: C4-P4
  SSEPs after bilateral alternative median nerve stimulation
  1 Transitionalstage (Bulbar-Midbrain Syndrome)
  2 Midbrain Syndrome
Note: At all lowered amplitudes shortened responses and marked differences in amplitudes of primary response

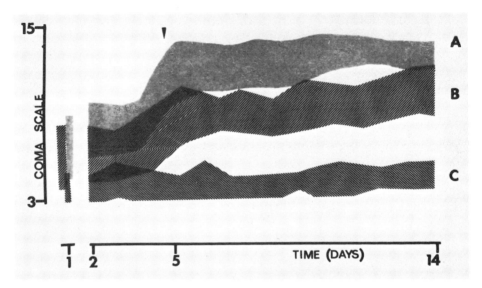

Fig. 1. Assessment and course of coma (Glasgow Coma Scale: range defined by 2 sign variation of 243 patients)
A *First category*: Tonic electroencephalographic arousal reaction following i.v. application of Antiparkinsonian drugs
B *Second category*: Alternative EEG pattern elicited by drug injection
C *Third category*: None-responders
Note: Bioelectrical none-responders remain in a persistent vegetative state (pvs)

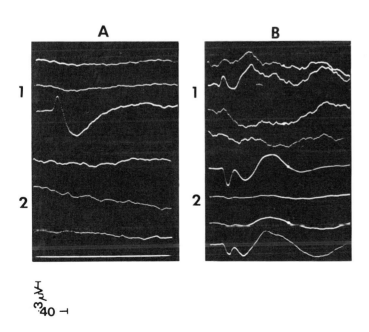

Long-Term Observation of Patients With Closed Head Injuries and a 24 h Period of Unconsciousness

O. LEITHOLF and E. KNECHT

Out of a total of 12,316 patients seen in the years 1974-1976, of whom 2900 had suffered head injuries, we selected 113 patients fulfilling three conditions: 1. a closed head injury, 2. a period of unconsciousness of at least 24 h, and 3. treatment in our clinics at least three times. On the average, the trauma had occurred 5-8 years before the last phase of treatment.

With 71 of these patients, the clinical treatment began between the 1st and the end of the 2nd year following the trauma. We divided the length of unconsciousness into periods ranging from days to weeks; the result was that 22 patients had been unconsciousness between 5 and 10 days and 43 patients between 11 days and several weeks. It was remarkable that of 87 patients under 45 years of age, 53 had been unconscious for more than 5 days.

After having investigated the course of the accidents, we can state that 81% of all injuries were caused by traffic accidents, whereas only 19% were due to accidents at work, at home, or elsewhere. After traffic accidents, the length of unconsciousness was between 11 and 21 days, with 27% at the top of the list.

Statements regarding anterograde or retrograde amnesia were, as had been expected, so uncertain that they could hardly be used in the statistical evaluation. However, most of our patients were believed to have had an amnesia up to 1 day, which was claimed mainly by patients having been unconscious for 5-10 days, whereas those patients having remained unconscious for 11-21 days spoke of an amnesia lasting 2-3 weeks ([3], [4]).

Directly after the trauma, 61 patients suffered a hemiparalysis, 27 of which were moderate and 12 serious. Forty percent of the patients with a moderate hemiparalysis had been unconscious for more than 5 days, in comparison to 84% with serious paralysis. After at least three clinical treatments, these paralyses improved noticeably; they were described as light in 28%, as moderate in 10%, and as serious in only 1% of the patients.

Twelve of our patients had a temporary aphasia which fully subsided within 2 years after the trauma. At the last investigation in our clinics, 14 patients (ten of whom had been unconscious longer than 5 days) still suffered from an aphasia since the trauma.

In our last observation, psychologic deterioration could be determined as moderate secondary loss of brain function in 59% of the patients; 3 having an orbital-frontal brain syndrome had been unconscious for more than 11 days ([3], [4]). Surprisingly high was the number of patients with a high frontal brain syndrome which we saw in 16% of the patients, 59% of whom had been unconscious for a long time.

Concerning the results of the electroencephalograms, one can only say that 50% of the patients with a diffuse abnormality had been unconscious for more than 21 days. A focus at the point of impact existed in 63% of the patients, 58% of whom had remained unconscious for a very long period of time.

In 90%, contrecoup injuries were found mainly in patients with a length of unconsciousness between 5 and 21 days. Ten percent of the patients had abnormalities typical of seizures. After an 8-year observation, the electroencephalograms of about half the patients were still pathologic, especially those having been unconscious for over 3 weeks. Only 22 patients presented seizures. Eight patients showed the first signs of seizures in the 1st year following the trauma already, in 8 other patients between the 1st and the 4th years. A period of latency of more than 4 years existed in six cases. In the last survey, frequent generalized seizures were presented by five patients, all belonging to the group having been unconscious for 5-10 days.

Although a focus could not always be localized, 14% of the patients had a right temporal and 33% a left temporal or frontotemporal focus, a fact sustaining common observations in the literature. Deep brain regions were also affected in more than half of the patients, 45% of whom had been unconscious for 11-21 days.

Last but not least, a word about the social consequences. Of the 113 patients, 63% had resumed working by the end of the 2nd post-traumatic year. At the last clinical treatment, 34% worked full-time at their former place of employement, 30% had new jobs, 6% worked part-time, and 27% of all patients received pensions.

In summary it can be said that in patients with a severe closed head injury a state of unconsciousness lasting one to several *weeks* seems more frequent than unconsciousness for just 1-5 *days*. Particularly often involved in traffic accidents are younger male patients. It seems that a clinical treatment in the second to third rehabilitation stage in the 1st year after the trauma offers especially good prospects of success, since 75% of the patients, in whom a long state of unconsciousness had existed, could resume work after 1-2 years. At the last clinical admission, only 23% were unable to work. We also saw that treatment in the 1st post-traumatic year could usually reduce the initially moderate and severe hemiparalysis to a light paralysis. In only 11% of the patients was there still a moderate paralysis. But even if the first treatments were performed later, the tendencies toward good improvement of the hemiparalyses could be observed. On the other hand, aphasias improved within the first 2 years after the trauma in only half the cases. Psychologic disorders also subsided more slowly than expected. Remarkable here was the high percentage of patients with high frontal personality change, especially with those having been unconscious for a very long period of time.

Noteworthy, however, is that already after 1 year 44%, and at our last observation, 70% of our 113 patients were working again. As expected, we could also prove that the prognosis is unfavorable after a *very* long state of unconsciousness, particularly with respect to reincorporation into working life, since over half of 30 patients receiving full pensions had been unconscious for more than 5 days.

After a long-term observation of a larger number of patients with a serious, closed head injury, we can for the most part confirm the statements made in the literature, especially by FROWEIN (1), PAMPUS, and SEIDENFADEN (2), except for the fact that the majority of our patients could resume working earlier.

Summary

Following an observation over several years of 113 patients who had been unconscious for more than 24 h after a closed head injury, the clinical and social results are discussed and compared to the respective length of unconsciousness. Even after a long state of unconsciousness, hemiparalyses improved well, whereas aphasias improved in only about 50% of the cases. Psychologic disorders lasted a relatively long time. At the last examination, 70% of all patients had resumed working.

References

1. FROWEIN, R.A., AUF DER HAAR, K., TERHAAG, D., KIENZEL, W., WIECK, H.H.: Arbeitsfähigkeit und Abbausyndrome nach Hirntrauma mit langdauernder Bewußtlosigkeit. Monatsschr. Unfallheilk. 71, 233-249 (1968)

2. PAMPUS, I., SEIDENFADEN, I.: Rehabilitation Hirnverletzter. Stuttgart-Berlin-Köln-Mainz: W. Kohlhammer 1974

3. SCHMIEDER, F.: Heilverfahren und Rehabilitation bei Hirnverletzten. Unfallmed. Tagungen der Landesverbände der gewerbl. Berufsgenossenschaften. Heft 3, Unfallmed., Tagung in Baden-Baden, November 1967

4. SCHMIEDER, F.: Möglichkeiten und Mängel in der Rehabilitation Hirngeschädigter. Rehabilitation (Stuttg.) 11, 90-93 (1972)

Late Sequelae of Head Injury in Infancy and Early Childhood, With Special Reference to Child Abuse

B. WIDER, H. LANGE-COSACK, and H. J. SCHLESENER

In follow-up examinations of children who had suffered severe brain injury at a very early age, it became apparent that child abuse was a major cause, both in respect to its incidence, especially in the first 18 months of life, and the severity of permanent neurologic and mental disturbances.

Materials and Methods

All children up to 5 years of age, who had been treated for severe brain injury in the neurosurgical department of the Charlottenburg Clinic between 1962 and 1971 were selected for our study. These included:
1. All compound fractures.
2. Closed injuries accompanied by loss of consciousness lasting more than 1/2 h.
3. Depressed fractures and growing fractures with cerebral contusion.

Minor injuries and chronic subdural hematomas of undetermined origin were not included. Sixty-one children met these criteria, and in 14 cases the cause of brain injury was child abuse. If one compares the incidence of different causes of injury in the various age groups, it is clear that child abuse is more common in the first 2 years of life and that traffic accidents claimed more victims among 3- and 4-year-olds. Falls of all types were rather evenly distributed among all age groups.

We shall report exclusively on the cases of child abuse. In order to widen our survey, we included four cases of severe brain injury caused by child abuse from the period 1972-1974. The age distribution of the 18 injured children can be found in Figure 1. Follow-up material on 12 out of 14 survivors was available.

Results

1. Early Stage

Regarding the *circumstances of injury*, in most cases the *offender* was the father, mainly under the influence of alcohol, usually with passive complicity on the part of the mother. If the offender was the mother, there was frequently evidence of an immature personality and an associated emotional stress situation.

As far as the *mechanism of injury* can be reconstructed, the children were struck on the head, violently shaken, or thrown against hard objects. Children were thrown to the ground or against their cribs; one mother grasped her son by the legs and threw him against the wall. In most cases, there was evidence of *repeated injury*.

In most cases, the *basic immediate lesions* consisted of cerebral contusions, associated with one compound fracture and eight cases of intracranial hemorrhage (five subdural, one extradural, and two intracerebral hematomas). We can only deal briefly with the four *fatalities*. Intracerebral hemorrhage (two subdural and two intracerebral) with the rapid development of a space-occupying lesion was the significant factor in all four cases. Operative decompression took place too late because all four children were brought to the hospital in desparate condition.

With respect to the *initial symptoms* (Table 1), most of the children were deeply comatose at the time of admission and displayed more or less extensive signs of midbrain compression; out of five surgically treated patients, there were four cases of acute subdural or extradural clots and one case of a space-occupying contusion (one further surgical case had a compound depressed fracture elevated). There were no cases of apallic syndrome (post-traumatic stupor or coma vigile).

2. Late Stage

All patients were followed up with neurologic, EEG, radiologic, psychiatric, and psychometric studies for at least 4 and up to 14 years after injury. Age at the time of follow-up examination ranged from 4-19 years.

Regarding *permanent neurologic damage*, only 3 of 12 children demonstrated no neurologic symptoms, and two others showed only moderate deficits. Five children had hemiparases with growth retardation on the affected side and were considerably handicapped as a result. Motor development was arrested entirely in two children; they were unable to walk, stand, or even to sit unassisted as a result of inadequate head control. Both were blind due to optic nerve atropy.

Permanent psychologic disturbances were even more severe than neurologic deficits. Speech and mental development were entirely arrested in the two previously mentioned children, both of whom had been injured at the age of 3 months. Communication was impossible in these two cases. A global reduction of intelligence was the characteristic psychopathologic residual deficit in five other children, two of whom attend a special school for the mentally handicapped and two others a special school for problem learners.

Figure 2 shows the distribution of intelligence quotients (IQ) in ten of the children who were followed. Intelligence could not be tested in the two most severely handicapped patients. Two children had above-average and two others average IQs; the others were conspicuously below average. All of the children demonstrated psychologic abnormalities: partial deficiencies in perceptual and cognitive functions, poor concentration, and behavior abnormalities were observed in the four children with normal IQs. Several patients had secondary neurotic symptoms which cannot be discussed here.

The *severity of psychologic and neurologic deficits* can be correlated *with the duration of the initial loss of consciousness* (Fig. 3). It must be emphasized that in our experience severe permanent damage in older children only occurs when a much longer period of unconsciousness or a traumatic apallic syndrome was observed. With one exception, *EEG results* remained pathologic until the end of the follow-up period, which lasted several years. Seven of the 12 children - including the two most severely handicapped - continued to suffer from *posttraumatic epilepsy*. Eight patients were examined with CT scan and six demonstrated severe pathologic findings such as defects and atrophy of grey or white matter (Fig. 4).

Table 1. Initial symptoms. A severe clinical course was often associated with midbrain compression and brain stem symptoms, which were especially pronounced in the cases with the longest periods of unconsciousness

No. 12	Unconsciousness Group	Duration	Brain stem syndrome	Respir. arrest	Hematoma	Op.	Neuro.	Initial convuls.
1	VI 1 week	8 days	+	+	Acute subdural	+	+	+
2	V 1-5	5 days	+			+	+	+
3		6 days	(+)				+	+
4		5 days	−		Extradural	+	+	+
5		2 days	+					
6	IV 1-24	12 h	(+)		Acute subdural	+	+	+
7		4 h	(+)	(+)			−	−
8		2 h	(+)				+	+
9		1.5 h	−		Acute subdural	+F.P.	+	+
10	II Drowsyness	1 day	−				−	−
11	I No alt. of consciousness, depressed fracture	−					−	−
12	Compound fracture, no alter. of consciousness	−				+	+	−

Discussion

Although the number of cases that we observed is small, we consider it important to point out child abuse as a cause of severe brain injury in infants and to call attention to the severity of its consequences, especially since there are few references in the literature (2, 3, 5, 6, 7).

Since repeated trauma is characteristic of child abuse (1, 4, 12, 13, 14) and a significant number of cases, if not the majority, is undetected, we must pursue all possible means of prevention, which include:
1. Education of the public.
2. Improved medical information about the need for adequate initial diagnostic procedures.
3. Early and prolonged social and psychologic assistance to endangered families (4, 9, 10, 11).

The *following factors* seem to be *decisive causes of the frequency of severe permanent damage*:
1. Extraordinary violence causing the injury.
2. Frequently repeated traumas.
3. The special reaction of the immature brain.
4. Delayed admission to the hospital, which might be attributed to parental fear of discovery of child abuse.

Summary

We reported on follow-up studies of children up to 5 years of age who sustained severe brain injuries caused by child abuse. Four of the 18 patients died of the immediate results of injury. The majority of the survivors displayed considerable permanent psychopathologic and neurologic symptoms which corresponded to the severity of the initial symptoms.

References

1. BAST, H., BERNECKER, A., KASTIEN, I., SCHMITT, G., WOLFF, R. (Arbeitsgruppe Kinderschutz): Gewalt gegen Kinder. Kindesmißhandlungen und ihre Ursachen. rororo-Taschenbuch 6934

2. DZIEDZIC-WITKOWSKA, T., KAMRAI-MAZURKIEWICZ, K.: Zespót bitego dziecka (The battered child syndrome). Polski Tydgodnik Lekarski 31/6, 239-240 (1976)

3. FINK, B.: Das Delikt der körperlichen Kindesmißhandlung. Kriminologische Schriftenreihe 34. Hamburg: Kriminalistik-Verlag 1968

4. HELFER, R.A., KEMPE, C.H.: The Battered Child, 2nd ed. London: University of Chicago Press, Ltd. 1968

5. JAMES, H.E., SCHUT, L.: The Neurosurgeon and the Battered Child. Surg. Neurol. 2, 415 (1977)

6. JACOBI, G., KOCH, H., EMRICH, R., RITZ, A.: Neuropädiatrische und neuro-radiologische Befunde beim schweren Schädel-Hirn-Trauma des Säuglings und jungen Kleinkindes. In: Bücherei des Pädiaters. VIVELL, O., BURMEISTER, W. (eds.). Heft 70, S. 63, Stuttgart: Enke 1973

7. KRAULAND, W.: Über die Zeitbestimmung von Schädelhirnverletzungen. Beitr. z. Gerichtl. Med. 30, 226 (1973)

8. LANGE-COSACK, H., WIDER, B., SCHLESENER, H.-J.: Hirntraumen nach Mißhandlungen im frühen Kindesalter. Festschrift für Prof. Dr. KRAULAND. Berlin: Zentrale Universitätsdruckerei. April 1977

9. LYNCH, M.A.: Child abuse - the critical path. J. of Maternal and Child Health, July 1976

10. LYNCH, M.A., ROBERTS, J., GORDON, M.: Child abuse: early warnings in the maternity hospital. Dev. Med. Child Neurol. Dec. 1976

11. LYNCH, M.A., ROBERTS, J.: Predicting child abuse: signs of bonding failure in the maternity hospital. Br. Med. J. 1, 624-626 (1977)

12. NAU, E.: Das Delikt der Kindesmißhandlung in forensisch-psychiatrischer Sicht. Münch. med. Wochenschr. 106, 972 (1964)

13. NAU, E.: Kindesmißhandlung. Monatsschr. Kinderheilkunde 115, 192 (1967)

14. SCHMITT, Y.D., KEMPE, C.H.: The battered child syndrome. In: Handbook of Clinical Neurology, Vol. 23, p. 60. VINKEN, P.J., BRUYN, G.W. (eds.). Amsterdam: North-Holland publishing Comp. New York: Wiley Interscience Division, John Wiley and Sons, Inc.

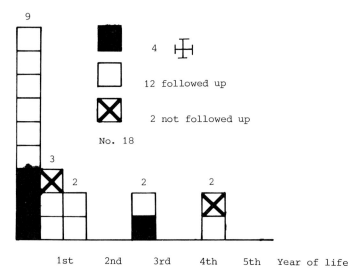

Fig. 1. Age distribution. The incidence of severe brain injury after child abuse in the first 18 months of life should be noted

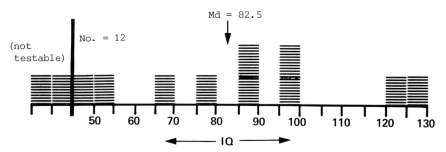

Fig. 2. Distribution of intelligence quotients. The mean value (82.5) is shifted to the left in comparison with the normal population. In the two cases on the left of the ordinate, the handicap was so severe that intelligence could not be tested

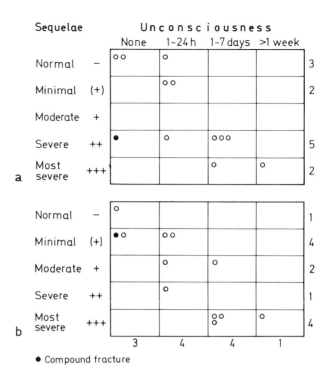

Fig. 3. Severity of permanent neurologic and psychologic symptoms correlated with the duration of the initial loss of consciousness
a Permanent neurologic damage (No. = 12)
b Permanent psychologic damage (No. = 12)

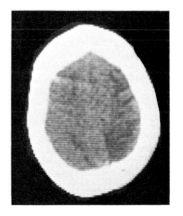

Fig. 4. Computerized tomography (CT scan) shows right-sided cortical atrophy

Follow-Up Studies After Craniocerebral Injury in Children
M. LANGER and D. TERHAAG

FROWEIN (1, 2) has shown that children's mortality in relationship to age is in an exceptional position. In our patients (Fig. 1), the mortality of serious craniocerebral injuries drops from 77% in the group of injured persons older than 60 years of age to 47% in the middle-aged group and to 43% in children up to 10 years of age.

LANGE-COSACK (3) has pointed out that the better average in children does not apply to all age groups. In the patients here, the mortality during the years from 1964-1974 was 46% in the group between 7 and 10 years of age, 33% in the group between 3 and 7 years of age, and 65% in the group between 0 and 3 years of age. However, it should be taken into consideration that the number of children in the youngest group is comparatively small. At the same time, it becomes apparent that the duration of unconsciousness which is *survived* by children is also limited (5). This becomes even more pronounced when the developments in the form of summation graphs of the surviving group are studied (Fig. 2). The 5% survival limit was 11 days in the group of children between 0 and 3 years of age, but it became clearly more favorable for children between 7 and 10 years of age with 16 days and increased to 18 days in children between 3 and 7 years of age. By means of 58 catamnestic examinations within 2 and 20 years after the accident, it became clear that a different grade of recovery is reached in the three age groups depending upon the duration of unconsciousness (4). In the course of these examinations, the post-traumatic neurologic, the psychic syndrome, and the development of fits or electroencephalographic changes were evaluated separately (Fig. 3).

Neurologic symptoms of disturbances such as tonus disturbances, ataxia, or pareses showed improvement only during the first 3-4 years after the trauma. The course of improvement was again the lowest for the youngest group of children up to 3 years of age: three out of five serious symptoms remained; in the 3-7-year-olds, 5 out of 16, and in the group of older children 2 out of 10. It was quite clear that this limited tendency toward improvement within age groups was correlated to the duration of unconsciousness.

The examination of electroencephalographic changes and of the development of organic cerebral disorders (seizures) and of the psychic syndromes - this particularly regarding the possible efficiency at school - resulted in showing, in principle, the same tendencies, although classification was more difficult.

A summary of the neurologic, psychic, and electroencephalographic sequelae (Fig. 4), which have been defined catamnestically, shows that as a rule longer periods of unconsciousness result in a more serious syndrome of neurologic deficiencies. Among 58 children, full recovery after a duration of unconsciousness of more than 24 h was noted only once. Restitution with little or hardly any disturbing symptoms was noted only if the duration of unconsciousness did not exceed 6 days in children between 3 and 5 years of age, in a few cases following an unconsciousness of up to 12 days. Moderate sequelae were found after a duration of up to 17 days of unconsciousness. After longer periods, there always remained serious and very serious deficiency syndromes. In four out of five children of up to 3 years of age, there were always only serious and moderate neurologic, psychic, and electroencephalographic changes to be found, in spite of a duration of follow-up of 3-14 years.

In summary, the above findings show that the smallest children up to the 3rd year of life show not only the worst prognosis for survival but also the most limited chance of recovery. It also shows that in all age groups the duration of unconsciousness after which a good or satisfactory recovery can be expected is on the average, comparatively limited.

References

1. FROWEIN, R.A., TERHAAG, D., AUF DER HAAR, K.: Früh-Prognose akuter Hirnschädigungen. Akt. Traumatologie 5, 203-211, 291-298 (1975)
2. FROWEIN, R.A., STEINMANN, H.W., AUF DER HAAR, K., TERHAAG, D., KARIMI-NEJAD, A.: Limits to classification and prognosis of severe head injury. This volume, pp. 16-26
3. LANGE-COSACK, H., TEPFER, G.: Das Hirntrauma im Kindes- und Jugendalter. Schriftenreihe Neurologie, Vol. XII. Berlin-Heidelber-New York: Springer 1973
4. LANGER, M.: Prognose schwerer Schädel-Hirntraumen bei Kindern bis 10 Jahren. Diss. Köln 1977
5. TERHAAG, D.: Prognosis of severe head and brain injury in childhood. In: Advances in Neurosurgery, Vol. 4. WÜLLENWEBER, R., BROCK, M., HAMER, J., KLINGER, M., SPOERRI, O. (eds.), pp. 191-195. Berlin-Heidelberg-New York: Springer 1977

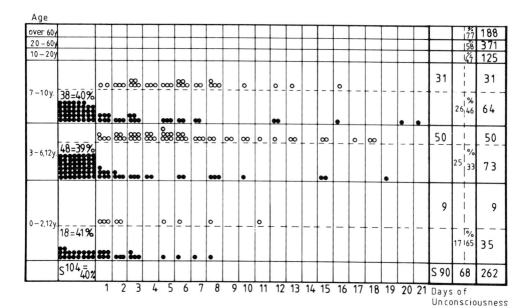

Fig. 1. Distribution of the observed periods of unconsciousnes-longer than 24 h - in 90 surviving and 68 deceased children in the three age groups. Severe craniocerebral injury 262 children up to 10 years, 1964-1974 Cologne
o Survivor
● Nonsurvivor

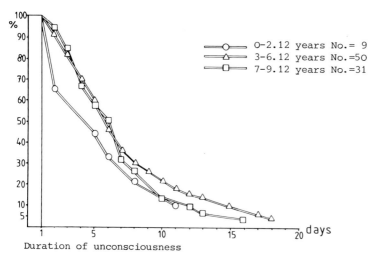

Fig. 2. Summation graphs in percent of the 90 surviving children in the last three age groups, related to the duration of unconsciousness

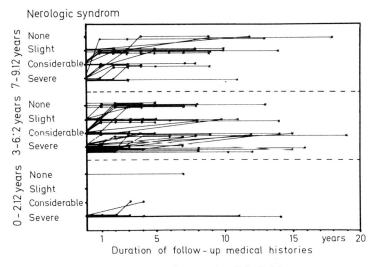

Fig. 3. Progress of the post-traumatic syndrome in 58 follow-ups - 2-20 years after the accident - for the age groups: 0-2.12, 3-6.12, and 7-9.12 years. Course of neurologic syndrome: 90 surviving children, unconsciousness > 24 h
x Time of Examination

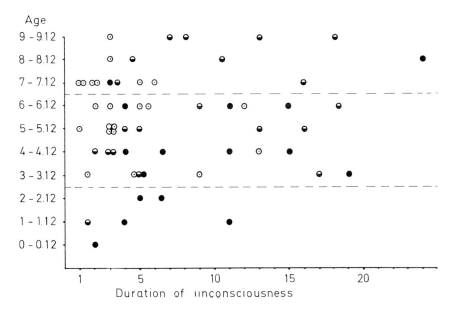

○ None ◉ Slight ◐ Considerable ● Severe   Pathologic dysfunction

Fig. 4. Synopsis of the neurologic, psychopathologic and electroencephalographic disturbances of functions in relation to age at the moment of accident and duration of unconsciousness. 58 follow-up medical histories after craniocerebral injury of children

The "Fall-Asleep-Syndrome" – A Kind of Secondary Disturbance of Consciousness After Head Injury in Children

S. TODOROW and E. HEISS

Secondary clouding or loss of consciousness following a free interval after head injury is usually a sign of dangerous post-traumatic complications, e.g., intracranial hematoma or brain edema. Yet in children after head injury, a benign state may occur which is also characterized by an alteration in consciousness. A child injured in the head who is not unconscious after the trauma even for a short time becomes increasingly tired and drowsy and falls asleep. The child can be awakened only by strong stimuli and only for a short time. Most often, one cannot establish contact with the child; he cries or turns away from the examiner. According to MEALEY (2), this state occurs often and is common enough to be considered a special post-traumatic syndrome.

A case for illustration: A boy, 9 years old, slipped on ice and fell on the back of his head. Just after the trauma, he did not become unconscious and there were no neurologic symptoms. One hour later he complained of increasing headache, nausea, and an invincible need for sleep. He fell asleep deeply and restlessly and could be awakened only with great effort. On admission 2 h after the accident, he could not be aroused and he responded to painful stimuli only by whimpering or mumbling indistinctly and with feeble protracted defense movements. His pupils changed in size and showed anisocoria and slow reaction to light. Babinski's sign was positive on the right leg. There persisted a moderate tachycardia with normal blood pressure. A bruise mark was found over the occiput, but no skull fracture could be found by x-ray examination. There was no displacement of the midline echo. During the following 3 h, the boy remained in this lethargic state, but showed a more and more distinct arousal reaction at reexamination. After a period of 4 h, he was fully awake and orientated, he remembered the accident, and was aware of the time until the onset of the great fatigue. He complained of headache, he looked pale, and his pulse was still labile. Anisocoria and Babinski's sign persisted further, but these signs disappeared the following day. The EEG recorded 1 day after the trauma showed a moderate slowing of basal activity as well as a focal dysrhythmia over the left occipital region. This was no longer present in the record 7 days later.

For this state following head injury in children which is very alarming though benign as to prognosis, PLUM and POSNER (3) used the term "post-traumatic stupor in children;" LANGE-COSACK and TEPFER (1) used the term "Einschlafsyndrom." The incidence rate of this condition following head injury is unknown. In 300 children aged 4-14 years, who were admitted to the department of pediatric surgery at Tübingen University on account of mild head injury in the past 4 years, this state of secondary clouding of consciousness occurred in 24 cases. The "fall-asleep syndrome" ("Einschlafsyndrom"), therefore, does not seem to be rare - it was found in about 8% of children hospitalized because of mild head injury.

Table 1 presents a survey of the cases and symptoms. In all age groups there were more boys than girls according to the relationship of hospitalized children with slight concussion. This relationship may depend on the kind of accident, i.e., falling off a bicycle or falling from a great height. Remarkable is the high incidence of occipital injury.

Table 1. Synopsis of all cases (No. = 24) of "fall-asleep-syndrome"

Age	4- 6 years	No. = 9
	7-10 years	No. = 10
	11-14 years	No. = 5
Trauma (impact)	occipital	No. = 11
	frontal	No. = 8
	not to be localized exactly	No. = 5
Fracture	No. = 3 (all of them occipital)	
Initial unconsciousness	Ø None	
Retrograde Amnesia	Ø None	
Lucid period	15-60 min	No. = 18
	1- 3 h	No. = 6
Duration of fall-asleep state	1-3 h	No. = 15
	3-5 h	No. = 8
	more than 5 h	No. = 1
Neurologic signs	No. = 11	7 with changes of pupils 5 with reflex aberration 3 with pyramided signs 2 with ataxia
Vegetative symptoms	No. = 20	12 with vomiting 14 with tachycardia or unstable pulse or paleness or transpiration
EEG (first record on the 1st to 3rd day after trauma)	Normal:	No. = 8
	Pathologic (becoming normal within 5 days to 6 weeks)	No. = 12

The information about the lack of initial loss of consciousness was confirmed by the patient's report of the circumstances of the accident. The leading sign in all cases was the onset of an invincible fatigue and a sleep-like state within a relatively short time after the head injury, independent of time of day, in three-fourth of the cases within 15-60 min after the accident. All children remained in a sleep-like state less than 5 h, most of them even less than 3 h; in five cases this state was accompanied by moderate motor restlessness. The only case which presented a fall-asleep syndrome lasting longer than 5 h was examined by angiography under anesthesia in this state. Eleven patients showed neurologic signs, and 20 showed symptoms of vegetative disturbances. Usually the children recovered completely on the 2nd day after the injury.

The EEG was recorded in 20 children, the first record on the 1st-3rd day after injury. We are sorry not to have an EEG record during the sleep-like conditions, none is known to us in the literature. In eight cases there was only a slight to moderate slowing of basal activity, in four cases, there were focal occipital changes. The EEG changes disappeared during the 5th day and 6th week after the injury.

The pathophysiologic mechanisms underlying the fall-asleep syndrome or post-traumatic stupor in children are unknown. Clinical signs remind one of conditions following the unconsciousness after brain concussion wherein the patients also suffer from fatique and repeatedly tend to fall into a refreshing sleep. In the fall-asleep syndrome, however, this state occurs belatedly after a free interval after the brain trauma, usually without an initial loss of consciousness. The EEG changes often last several days to weeks and point to a more serious brain injury than could be supposed according to clinical conditions and course.

The fall-asleep syndrome does not cause diagnostic difficulties after the recovery which already occurs in some cases before hospitalization or soon after, although the actual clinical condition of a child with fall-asleep syndrome may worry the examiner in view of the differential diagnosis.

Summary

The state of post-traumatic stupor in children, called the fall-asleep syndrome ("Einschlafsyndrom") in the German literature is presented. The characteristic secondary sleep-like clouding of consciousness following a free interval after a head injury was observed in 24 children. A synopsis of the symptomatology, course, and EEG findings of these cases is presented. The diagnostic difficulties of this prognostically benign syndrome are emphasized.

References

1. LANGE-COSACK, H., TEPFER, G.: Das Hirntrauma im Kindes- und Jugendalter. Berlin-Heidelberg-New York: Springer 1973
2. MEALEY, J.: Pediatric Head Injuries. Springfield (Ill.): Ch. C. Thomas 1968
3. PLUM, F., POSNER, J.B.: The Diagnosis of Stupor and Coma, 2nd ed. Philadelphia: Davis 1972

Memory Sequelae After Severe Head Injuries

A. Violon, J. Demol, and J. Brihaye

Brain damage is very frequently associated with disturbances of memory. In general, the greater the brain damage, the more severe the memory deficit is. Sometimes, mnestic disturbances are so troublesome that they prevent the return to any professional position. Moreover, the deficit in memory is difficult to handle with regard to methods of reeducation. Therefore, it appears necessary to go further into the problem of memory, which is the purpose of the present study.

Thanks to the tests of the 15 words of REY (2) and of the complex picture of REY (1) we have taken two aspects into consideration; evocation and recogition of memory. To make the difference between evocation and recogniton clear, we will recall to mind the test of the 15 words: the examiner reads aloud 15 words, the patient has to repeat them immediately in the order he prefers; this exercise is performed five times consecutively, and the number of words correctly repeated is scored. The result is directly related to the evocation of the words which have been uttered. Then one reads a text in which the 15 words are included, and the patient has to point out the words that he recognizes. This part of the test is related to the recognition phenomenon and the score obtained by the patient depends on the mnestic trace left in his brain.

Forty-one patients were examined with these methods. They had all suffered from a severe head injury and remained in coma for at least 7 days; the longest period of coma was 58 days. Not a single patient was seen by us as a medicolegal case. The age of the patients extended from 3-70 years. One-half of the patients were tested in the course of the 2 years following injury and the other half were tested from 2-7 years after injury. Mnestic disorders were divided into four categories according to the severity of the disturbance, ranging from undisturbed to severe deficiency.

Results

During the 1st month which follows coma, not a single patient had recovered normal memory. In 75% of the cases, the mnestic disturbance is severe and is usually associated with disorientation in space and time. From the 2nd to the 6th month after injury, 23% of the cases had recovered good memory. All these patients were in coma during a period which did not exceed 10 days. From the 7th to the 18th month, more than 50% of the patients progressively recovered their mnestic capacities. In this group, the relationship between the age or the length of coma and the degree of recovery tends to be distinctly less. Two years after injury, 10% of the patients still experienced severe memory disturbances. Figure 1 gives a general view of the evolution of mnestic disorders in time.

This study also confirms previous studies made by our group (3), according to which memory recovers more slowly and less completely than other mental abilities after severe brain damage. In general, it shows that the strategy of active research in evocation is especially inadequate, far more than the ability of recognizing newly learned data. Indeed, in our patients, a few years after injury, 52% have recovered a normal ability for recognition while only 21% have regained normal ability for evocation (Table 1). This ability to recognize learned data means that the information has been stored, even when the active recall remains defective. This observation may lead to the development of a new strategy for the reeducation of patients with post-traumatic mnestic disturbances.

With regard to the social rehabilitation in relation to the memory deficit, we have observed that all patients with severe mnestic disturbances were unable to resume their work while the patients, who had recovered a good mnestic function were working again. However, among the patients who have resumed a position, 50% still have mild mnestic disorders and 20% experience more marked disorders (Table 2). In addition to the mnestic deficit, other neurologic disorders interfere with their professional life. In this respect, 37% of our patients are definitively disabled and unable to work or to study in normal schools, and 11% are doing it with great difficulties.

In conclusion, the present study confirms that memory recovers very slowly after a severe brain injury. It also demonstrates that the process of active recall is particularly affected, far more than the ability for recognition of newly learned data. Finally, it emphasizes the relationship between amnestic disturbances and the possibility of resuming a professional life.

Table 1. Long-term mnestic recovery: evocation and recognition

	Evocation	Recognition
Normal	21%	52%
Disturbed	79%	48%

Table 2. Social life at least 2 years after the injury

Back to work	52%
Definitely unable to work or go to normal schools	37%
Following school with difficulties	11%

References

1. REY, A.: Test de copie d'une figure complexe. Paris: Centre de Psychologie Appliquée 1959
2. REY, A.: L'examen clinique en psychologie. Paris: Presse Universitaire Française 1964
3. VIOLON, A., DE MOL, J.: Etude neuropsychologique de l'évolution à court terme des traumatisés crâniens. Acta Psychiatr. Belg. 74, 176-232 (1974)

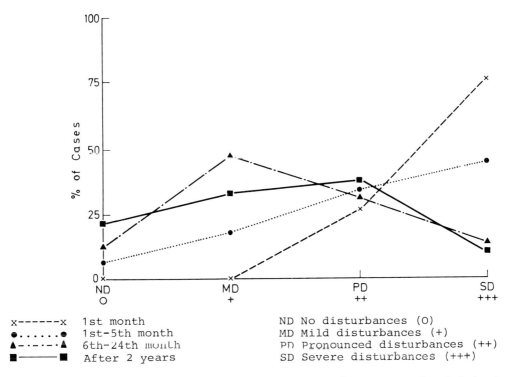

Fig. 1. Development of amnestic disturbances after severe head injuries

Clinical Aspects and Research

Notes on the Development of Interest in North America in Head Injury
J. P. Evans

The purpose of this brief communication is not to present a profound analysis of the problems of the head-injured patient nor to offer a nationalistic survey of North American accomplishments in the field. Rather, I propose to review, in summary fashion, steps taken in the past and being made at present, in the belief that a backward look may throw some light on the future. I trust that the selected bibliography may prove useful for European colleagues. My comments will be limited to the North American experience. Canadian and United States neurologic surgeons share a great deal, and for our present purposes may be looked on as a common group.

It is recognized that the mortality figures utilized throughout this paper are only approximate, but they are valid indices of striking improvement. I have divided my presentation into five phases. The first of these I have called the "descriptive period" which bridges the years between the American Revolutionary War of 1775 and the Spanish-American War at the end of the 19th century. Review of the literature indicates a rough average mortality rate among various armies of the period of 61%.

In phase II, the World War I period, neurologic surgery had come of age. The fundaments of neurologic surgery-anesthesia, asepsis, cerebral localization, and the principles of wound healing were well-established. In the American forces, the genius of Cushing, with his neurologic team concept, made it possible to lower the mortality figures for penetrating cerebral wounds to about 30%.

Phase III, the World War II period, found neurologic surgery well-established in North America. In both Canada and the United States, there was a small but well-defined group of senior and junior fully trained neurologic surgeons to assume direction of field, base, and zone of interior neurosurgic units, leaving skeleton staffs to provide care for civilians. The development of an effective military neurosurgic effort was greatly aided by the fact that, beginning in the 1920s, residency programs in general surgery had been developed. From this large pool of well-trained young surgeons, some 200 were selected, trained in neurosurgic techniques for 3-6 months, and then made available to assist the established neurologic surgeons. In many instances, the younger men found themselves strongly attracted to neurologic surgery, developed great competence, and were extremely effective. Many retained their interest and now comprise an important cadre in the some 2400 certified neurologic surgeons in the United States and Canada.

As the result of the efforts of these men, aided by string support from the Surgeon General's Office and by the devotion of military nurses and corpsmen, a combined effort was made at utilizing fluids, blood, antibiotics, and improved transportation, which reduced head wound mortality to 13%.

But throughout phase III, there was evident an increasingly important civilian input to the understanding of the various factors militating against recovery and restitution of function. Extensive studies were made of pathologic alterations, and a start was made toward better understanding of the vagaries of intracranial pressure changes. Neurosurgeons benefited from the blood fraction studies which produced hemostatic agents, including Gelfoam and of course the Bovie electrocautery, which had been developed in the late 1920s under civilian circumstances and was widely used by military neurosurgeons.

Phase IV may aptly be named "neurosurgery refined." From the military point of view, due to superb spirit, competence, and organization among neurosurgic teams in Korea, the mortality in those cases of penetrating craniocerebral wounds reaching a neurosurgical facility dropped to 7.78%, and the final figures for the Vietnam War promise to be about the same. Rapid triage made possible by a wide use of helicopters enhanced the results.

But recognition should also be given to the developments in the civilian section stimulated by the impact of increasing industrialization and traffic. Through the good offices of the National Institutes of Health and specifically what was then known as the National Institute of Neurologic Disease and Stroke, this increasing interest in civilian head injuries has been drawn together into two Head Injury Conferences. A significant resolution offered at the first conference in 1966 was:

"It is recommended, therefore, that consideration be given to the establishment of several centers devoted to head injury investigation. Such centers should be located in areas where proper clinical material is available, where laboratory facilities may be utilized, where ancillary technics and services may be called upon, and where a high level of interest in problems of head injury already exists. Specialized centers, in conjunction with hospitals with large accident services, would permit prospective studies to develop data concerning the mode of injury, clinical states, treatment, and acute and chronic convalescence. They would also provide opportunity for training general surgeons, urologists, practitioners, and paramedical personnel in the emergency care of head injuries."

As a reflection of the results of this concerted effort, the five areas of primary interest at the second Head Injury Conference in 1975 are exemplified in the chapter headings of the final report:

Prognostic Considerations
Blood Brain Barrier
Respiratory Pathophysiology
Cerebral Microcirculation
Pressure Volume Relationships

These titles are but a scant indication of the vast increase in interest in North America in the neurophysiologic and neurochemical aspects of head injury.

In view of the fact that the head cannot be separated from the body, the development of emergency medical services in the United States is of great importance. Among these efforts have been the work of the

American College of Surgeons' Committee on Trauma functioning actually since 1922, the Committee on Injuries of the American Academy of Orthopedic Surgeons established in 1965, and the efforts of the National Research Council from 1966 onward. As the result of the enhanced interst in roadside trauma, a Federal Department of Transportation has been established, national training programs are being promoted, and prevention of the so-called "second accident" at the site of the injury is being emphasized.

Thus, one can see that no longer is the head injury problem the exclusive but intermittent interest of the military whose accomplishments have been so impressive. Currently, in peacetime, this vast field is subject to intensive investigation which is producing fascinating results that are now appearing in the literature.

What of phase V ? The question is an imposing one, and its final answer probably lies in the decisions of our statesmen. Very probably, we, of the surgical world, both military and civilian, are in the best position to urge upon our leaders the avoidance of that ultimate folly, the nuclear holocaust (Fig. 1).

References

Phase I

BARNES, J.H.: Medical and Surgical History of the Rebellion (1861-1865), Vol. 1, Chap. 1. Washington: Government Printing Office, Second Issue 1875

BORDEN, W.C.: Military Surgery. Washington: Government Printing Office 1905

BROWN, H.: E.: The Medical Department of the United States Army from 1775 to 1873. Washington: Surgeon General's Office 1873

CHISHOLM, J.J.: A Manual of Military Surgery for the Use of Surgeons of the Confederate Army. Richmond (Va.): West & Johnston 1861

DUNCAN, L.C.: Medical Department of the United States Army in the Civilian War. Washington: Surgeon General's Office 1914

SENN, N.: Surgical Aspects of the Spanish-American War. Chicago: American Medical Associated Press 1900

Phase II

CUSHING, H.C.: From a Surgeon's Journal, 1915-1918. Boston: Little Brown & Co. 1936

KEEN, W.W.: The Treatment of War Wounds. Philadelphia: W.B. Saunders 1917

Phase III

HAYS, S.B.: Surgery in World War II, Vol. 1: Neurosurgery. Washington: Office of the Surgeon General 1958

Symposium on Treatment of Trauma in the Armed Forces. Washington: Army Medical Service Graduate School 1952

Phase IV

Head Injury Conference - Proceedings. CAVENESS, W.F., WALKER, A.E. (eds.). Philadelphia: Lippincott 1966

Head Injuries, Second Chicago Symposium on Neural Trauma. McLAURIN, R.W. (ed.). New York: Grune & Stratton 1976

Neurological Surgery of Trauma. MEIROWSKY, A.M. (ed.). Washington: Office of the Surgeon General 1965

ROCKWOOD, C.A. Jr., et al.: History of Emergency Medical Services in the United States. J. Trauma 16, 299-308 (1976)

 or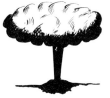

Fig. 1. Phase V: **Further**   HAVOC
the ultimate question   **development**

Schedule for the Care of Extremity Fractures in Patients With Serious Brain Injuries

W. REICHMANN, J. ROSENBERGER, and B. HORTEN

Patients with multiple injuries need the immediate care of a team of anesthesiologists, surgeons, and neurosurgeons, regardless of whether the patient is taken to a surgical or a neurosurgical hospital. A schedule of life-saving measures must be followed. Diagnostics have to be restricted to essential things (Table 1).

A brain injury must be admitted as early as possible, the course of the disease must be controlled. An x-ray survey of thorax and abdomen (pelvis) and x-rays of the skeleton according to clinical findings should be undertaken. If possible, one should perform x-rays of the injured parts of the body in the shock room, including an x-ray of the vertebral column in case of paralysis or if a whiplash injury is assumed. Detailed roentgenologic diagnostics of an extremity, for example, are allowed only if the vital functions are under control. This system has been well-tested. Diagnostic and therapeutic steps are taken according to their priority rating. The early care of extremity fractures offers the best chance for good results - particularly in patients with multiple injuries. Nevertheless, life-threatening injuries of abdomen, brain, and thorax have absolute priority. If the general state of the patient is good enough, medical treatment in different parts of the body can be carried out simultaneously. This demands high quality personnel and medical equipment. As long as the blood circulation can be maintained only by infusions, surgical procedures on extremity fractures are very dangerous. During the first 8 h after the injury, the following measures are necessary if possible: careful positioning, aseptic wound debridement of open fractures, and temporary immobilization by wire extension. Setting and a plaster cast - if necessary temporarily - is possible during the primary period. If the general state does not allow an immediate operation, the measures described reduce such complications as: superinfection, disturbances of local circulation and coagulation, and paralysis due to pressure. Such damages finally lead to an unsatisfactory result.

In seriously brain-damaged patients, conservative therapy leads to an extensive immobilization because the patient is supposed to be inactive for a longer period of time. Unstabilized joints and limbs cannot be trained systematically. For this reason, we prefer the operative treat-

Table 1. Schedule for the treatment of multitraumatized patients with serious craniocerebral injuries

1. Protection of vital functions
2. Special diagnostics
3. Interdisciplinary therapy according to priorities
    a) Craniocerebral injuries
    b) Thoracicoabdominal injuries
    c) Injuries of the extremities
4. Therapeutic procedure
    a) Simultaneous
    b) Serial

ment of fractures in seriously injured people. That method, we believe, has proved effective (Table 2).

Indications for Operative Treatment

1. Open fracture II and III: the risk of infection is extremely high if interfragmentary fixation is not absolute. This may favor a septic process. In the absence of contraindications, we favor an osteosynthesis during the first 8-h-period that allows an early mobilization.

2. We see a special urgency in the care of accompanying blood vessel injuries of the danger of ischemia. Generally, a reconstruction of arteries is justified only after a good osteosynthesis.

3. Multiple fractures: in case of conservative treatment, immobilization of a patient increases with the number of fractures. Because of the severity and duration of the surgical intervention, all precautions to save blood and to shorten the time of operation must be taken, i.e., two teams of surgeons, pneumatic blood block, and the availability of stored blood. Because of the high risk, this treatment should be performed in the secondary phase (after the first 8-h-period until the end of the 2nd week).

4. After the akinetic phase, one must rely upon a hyperkinetic period in the unconscious patient. In this phase, even well-stabilized fractures are highly endangered. This is the reason why the so-called minimal osteosynthesis is not indicated.

5. Long-term unconscious patients demand particularly great efforts on the part of the intensive care unit. This concerns especially very old persons and children. Consequently, the surgeon has to decide on an early osteosynthesis in these groups.

Contraindications for Operative Treatment

1. Poor prognosis quo ad vitam due to brain damage or to shock or to decreased vital functions are a contraindication for any surgical procedure.

2. The treatment of extremity fractures has to be postponed in case of persistent, unclear, or renewed loss of blood due to thoracic or

Table 2. Indications and contraindications for operative therapy

Special indications for osteosynthesis of fractures in patients with multiple injuries and serious craniocerebral injuries
1. Open fractures II and III
2. Blood vessel injuries
3. Multiple fractures
4. Motor restlessness
5. Improvement of intensive care

Contraindications for osteosynthesis
1. Poor prognosis
   a) Craniocerebral injury
   b) Generally
2. Unverified thoracal and abdominal injuries
3. Signs of infection
   a) Extremity wound
   b) Urinary passage, respiratory tract, abdomen

abdominal injuries. Two or three cavity injuries have such a high mortality that the care of extremity fractures must be delayed (Table 3).

3. Infections of open fractures as well as fever from general infections, bronchogenic, or urologic infections may impair the progress of healing dramatically. To prevent a spreading septicemia, an immediate amputation is sometimes needed.

Since 1963, more than 1000 people with multiple injuries have been treated at the University Clinic Cologne-Lindenthal, Department of Surgery. More than 50% had head injuries, in 6% a three-cavity injury was found. The possibility of giving definitive advice for the individual case through general therapy plans seems to be of limited value (Table 4).

In the 10-year statistics shown here, only patients with serious brain damages were considered, i.e., an unconsciousness of at least several

Table 3. Mortality in relation to the degree of multiple injuries

Type of injury	No. of patients	Died	%
Brain extremities	77	17	22
Brain, thorax extremities	54	33	61
Brain, abdomen extremities	9	4	44
Brain, thorax, abdomen extremities	15	14	93
Total	155	68	44

Table 4. Therapy and mortality of 155 patients with multiple trauma and serious craniocerebral injuries and fractures of the extremities (1968-1977)

Therapy	No. of patients	Died	%
Without fracture therapy	23	16	70
Conservative fracture therapy	68	40	59
Operative fracture therapie			
Primarily operated	20	8	40
Early secondary operated	29	3	10
Late secondary operated	15	1	7
Total operative therapy	64	12	19

hours. We were not able to treat 23 patients with extremity injuries within a propitious period. Sixty-eight injured people were treated conservatively; 64 persons were operated on. Twenty persons were operated during the primary phase (first 8-h-period), 29 were operated on during the early secondary phase (after 8 h until the end of the 2nd week), and 15 patients were treated late secondarily (after the end of the 2nd week). Twenty patients primarily operated on suffered mostly from open fractures or limbs endangered by ischemia.

Patients with multiple injuries and serious head injuries present many problems to medical treatment. Good chances are provided by modern techniques; we are, nevertheless, supposed to be modest in our hopes of success.

Angiographic Demonstration of Vascular Injuries Following Head Injury and Its Significance

N. FRECKMANN, K. SARTOR, and K. MATSUMOTO

Since the advent of computerized tomography (CT) in 1973, the importance of cerebral angiography in the evaluation of head trauma has been greatly reduced. Cranial CT very reliably detects intracranial hematomas of recent origin, it also clearly differentiates intracerebral hemorrhage from brain edema (4, 7, 8, 9). The vascular injury, however, which caused the hematoma, can only be demonstrated angiographically, if at all. In certain cases, e.g., where the larger caliber vessels at the base of the brain are injured, angiography provides detailed information not obtainable from CT studies. The same is true for intracranial AV fistulas and aneurysms of traumatic origin (6). In order to classify vascular injuries which could be recognized on the angiograms and find out the relative frequencies of the various types of lesions, we reviewed the head injury cases of a large general hospital.

Material and Methods

The serial cerebral angiograms of 345 patients with head injuries treated at the Allgemeines Krankenhaus Altona, Hamburg (FRG) from July, 1971 until the end of 1976 (5.5 years) were reviewed in conjunction with the patient charts (Table 1).

In most cases, angiography had been performed by direct puncture of the common carotid artery[1]. Rarely, the internal carotid artery had been injected. Furthermore, catheter studies had been done infrequently, mainly due to the emergency character of the majority of the angiographic examinations considered here. In all cases, rapid biplane serial angiography was performed. In many additional series, different projections (i.e., oblique, axial, or subaxial views) were obtained. In addition, series with a slower or faster than normal sequence of film had been employed in certain cases. Occasionally, direct serial magnification and simultaneous single-phase angiotomography had been performed as well. While reviewing the angiograms, we looked carefully for vascular injuries. For better visualization of such lesions, photographic subtractions were made in a larger number of cases. The plain skull films of the patients were also reviewed in order to recognize accompanying fractures or other changes attributable to the trauma.

Table 1. Age and sex distribution

	Total	-15	-25	-35	-45	-55	-65	Over 65 years
Total No. of cases	345	70	71	48	42	34	27	53
Male	253	48	51	38	37	25	14	35
Female	92	22	20	10	5	9	13	18

---

[1] The contrast medium used was Angiografin (Schering).

Results

In 62 cases (18% of 345), lesions of extra- and intracranial vessels were found on the angiograms. In 23 cases (37% of 62), there was more than one lesion in the same patient. Age and sex distribution were not different from the total number of angiographically examined head injury patients shown in Table 1. As other authors did before, we divided the various lesions into *five* groups or types of vascular injury (Fig. 1). The final diagnoses and the distribution of skull fractures in the 62 patients with angiographically demonstrated injuries of extra- and intracranial vessels are shown in Table 2.

Classification and incidence of angiographically verified vascular injuries were as follows:

1. External carotid artery system
    Superficial (extracranial branches: laceration (rupture) and complete disruption of vascular continuity[1]; nine cases, eight *with* visible extravasation of contrast medium
    Deep (intracranial/dural) branches
    Laceration (rupture) and complete disruption of middle meningeal artery or branches; ten cases, nine *with* visible extravasation of contrast medium
    AV fistulas of middle meningeal artery or branches; five cases, in three fistulous communications with middle meningeal veins, in two with diploic veins (Fig. 2)
2. Internal carotid artery system
    Internal carotid artery
    Traumatic occlusion of cervical segment at the atlas/axis level; one case
    Traumatic stenosis of anterior portion of siphon (fracture of sphenoid body); one case
    Dissecting aneurysm of carotid siphon (fracture of petrous bone, additional fracture of sphenoid body?); one case
    Traumatic aneurysms at level of anterior portion of siphon (fractures of sphenoid body and petrous bone); two cases (Fig. 3).
    Traumatic direct carotid artery-cavernous sinus fistulas due to large tear in carotid wall; three cases (Fig. 4)
    Intimal tear of supraclinoid segment (fractures of the skull base in all but four patients); 19 cases (Fig. 5).

Table 2. Clinical diagnoses and distribution of skull fractures in 62 patients with angiographically verified vascular injury

Clinical diagnosis	No. fracture	Fracture of the skull vault	Fracture of the skull bases	Total
Brain contusion	5	4	15	24
Epidural hematoma	-	18	(8)	18
Subdural hematoma	3	4	9	16
Open head injuries gun shot injuries	-	3	1	4

---

[1] Exact differentiation between laceration or rupture of a vessel (*without* break in continuity) and complete disruption is not always possible angiographically as laceration plus thrombosis may mimic complete severing of the vessel.

Dural branches of internal carotid artery
AV fistulas between meningeohypophyseal trunk and basal sinuses;
16 cases (Fig. 3).
Main branches of the internal carotid artery including their
cortical rami
Traumatic occlusion of middle cerebral artery branches; three cases
Laceration (rupture) or disruption of middle artery with extravasation of contrast medium; one case (Fig. 6).
Traumatic aneurysm of insular branch of middle cerebral artery; one case (Fig. 7).
Laceration (rupture) or disruption of terminal cortical branches of anterior or middle cerebral artery, *all* with extravasation of contrast medium; 12 cases
Traumatic aneurysm of cortical branches of anterior or middle cerebral artery branch/frontopolar branch of anterior cerebral artery with fistulous communication to adjacent cortical vein); two cases
3. Veins: laceration of bridging veins with visible extravasation of contrast medium; two cases.

Course of Disease

The patient with the traumatic occlusion of the carotid artery at the atlas/axis level died shortly after admission. In patients with injuries of the extracranial branches of the external carotid artery, the outcome was mainly dependent on the severity of the concomitant trauma to the skull and brain. The course of disease in patients with angiographically verified injuries of intracranial vessels is tabularized in Table 3.

Discussion

The relatively high number of angiographically demonstrated injuries of extra- and intracranial vessels in our material may be explained, at least in part, by the short time interval between trauma and angiography in many of our cases. The Allgemeines Krankenhaus Altona, Hamburg can be reached very rapidly by helicopter or ambulance from almost any point in the area covered by the hospital's neursurgical trauma unit. Also, due to large experience with head trauma, our Department of Radiology produces angiograms of good quality even in emergency situations. Aside

Table 3. Course of disease in cases with injuries of intracranial vessels[1]

Type of injury	Died	PVS	SD	SLD	GR
Meningeal vessels (15) of external carotid artery	9	3	1	1	1
Internal carotid artery (26)	22	3	1	-	-
Meningohypophyseal trunk (16)	11	2	2	-	1
Intracranial branches of internal carotid artery (20)	20	-	-	-	-

Died: lethal outcome in the clinic; PVS: persistent vegetative state;
SD: severe deficits; SLD: slight deficits; GR: good recovery.

[1] The number of 77 vascular injuries in the result of multiple lesions in certain patients.

from injury of the meningeal vessels, trauma to the arteries at the base of the brain was unexpectedly frequent. In these cases, intimal tears of the intracranial carotid segments (19 cases = 30.6% of 62) and lacerations of the meningohypophyseal trunk (6,11) with development of AV fistulous communications to basal sinuses (16 cases = 25.8% of 62) were found most frequently. Both types of vascular injury were very often accompanied by fractures of the base of the skull (2,10) (26 cases = 74% of 35). Angiographically visible trauma to cranial vessels was found much more often in patients with fractures of the base of the skull than in patients who had not sustained any osseous trauma to the head. This shows that generally only very heavy blunt trauma to the head can produce such vascular injury (1,5). Also, there is a direct relationship between the break in bone continuity and laceration or disruption of a vessel in many instances (12). This is particularly true when the damaged vessel is located at the fracture site or at the base of the brain where it is less able to evade bony fragments or the impact of shearing forces.

Considering the final outcome in the 62 cases where injuries of cranial vessels were found angiographically, one may say the following: the more proximal and the deeper within the skull and brain the lesion was located, the worse the final outcome was.

Conclusion

If clinical signs and plain skull films in severe head trauma make the involvement of the base of the skull likely, cerebral angiography is still preferable to CT as the next diagnostic step in many instances. In such cases, angiography, if performed properly, included all necessary projections, often shows both the hematoma *and* the lacerated or disrupted vessel. Clinical signs plus angiographic findings probably yield better criteria for the decision on which therapeutic measures should be taken in a considerable number of cases. The type of vascular injury may be more significant for the prognosis than the intracranial hematoma itself. Active bleeding from a vessel, angiographically manifested as extravasation of contrast material, does not necessarily have a grave prognosis as long as the site of hemorrhage is located peripherally and superficially (1). Massive hemorrhage from larger caliber arteries at the base of the brain is usually very rapidly fatal. This fact may lead the neurosurgeon to the decision not to operate on the patient for the developing hematoma. If CT is performed as the only radiologic procedure, this would lead more often to an active but vain approach in such cases.

Summary

The cerebral angiograms of 345 patients with severe head trauma (1971-1976) were reviewed in conjunction with the charts. Attention was directed chiefly to vascular injuries. An unsuspectedly high number of such lesions were found. Particularly striking was the relative incidence of injuries to arteries and veins/sinuses at the base of the brain. These were very often associated with fractures of the base of the skull and had a grave prognosis. In head injury patients with signs of intracranial hemorrhage *and* involvement of the base of the skull, angiography is probably still preferable to computerized tomography as the major radioloc procedure.

References

1. ALLAN, D.M., WITCOMBE, J.B.: Intracranial extravasation of contrast medium during carotid angiography. Br. J. Radiol. 50, 404-411 (1977)

2. ARCHER, C.R., SUNDARAM, M.: Uncommon sphenoidal fractures and their sequelae. Radiology 122, 157-161 (1977)

3. BERGERON, R.T., RUMBOUGH, C.L.: Skull trauma. In: Radiology of the Skull and Brain. NEWTON, T.H., POTTS, D.G. (eds.), Vol. I/2, pp. 763-818. St. Louis: Mosby 1975

4. DUBLIN, A.B., FRENCH, B.N., RENNICK, J.M.: Computed tomography in head trauma. Radiology 122, 365-369 (1977)

5. GLICKMAN, M.G.: Angiography in head trauma. In: Radiology of the Skull and Brain. NEWTON, T.H., POTTS, D.G. (eds.), Vol II/4, pp. 2598-2658. St. Louis: Mosby 1974

6. HUBER, P.: Angiographie beim Schädel-Hirntrauma. Akt. Neurologie 4, 41-60 (1977)

7. KAZNER, E., LANKSCH, W., STEINHOFF, H., WILSKE, J.: Die axiale Computer-Tomographie des Gehirnschädels - Anwendungsmöglichkeiten und klinische Ergebnisse. Fortschr. Neurol. Psychiat. 43, 487 (1975)

8. KOO, A.H., LaROQUE, R.L.: Evaluation of head trauma by computed tomography. Radiology 123, 345-350 (1977)

9. LANGE, S., GRUMME, Th., MEESE, W., ZUM WINKEL, K.: Das epi- und subdurale Hämatom im Computertomogramm. Fortschr. Röntgenstr. 125/6, 537-540 (1976)

10. MARKWALDNER, H.: Neurochirurgische Komplikationen der Schädelbasisfrakturen. Ther. Umschau 31/9, 621-25 (1974)

11. NEWTON, T.H., HOYT, W.F.: Dural arterivenous shunts in the region of cavernous sinus. Neuroradiology 1, 71-81 (1970)

12. RUMBAUGH, C.L., BERGERON, R.T., KURZE, T.: Intracranial vascular damage associated with skull fractures. Radiology 104, 81-87 (1972)

Fig. 2. AV fistulas between anterior (*upper arrow*) and posterior branch of middle meningeal artery and their corresponding veins; tram-track sign (*lower arrows*)

Fig. 3. Rupture of internal carotid artery with development of small false aneurysm (*anterior arrow*). Also laceration of branches of meningohypophyseal trunk with AV fistula between these and basilar plexus (*posterior arrow*)

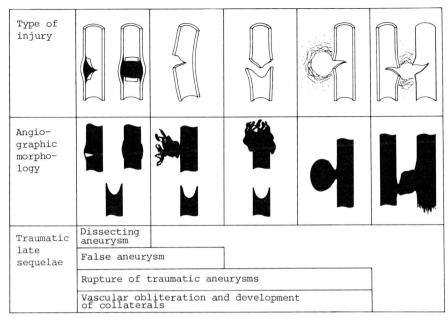

Fig. 1. Type of injury and angiographic morphology (modified after PROST and HAERTEL, 1976)

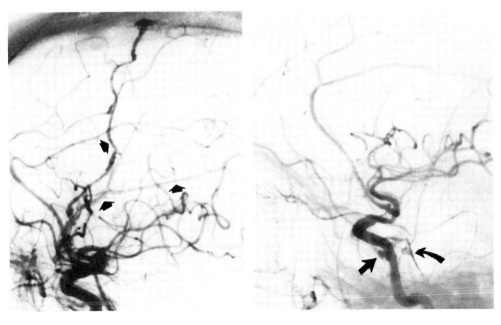

Fig. 2

Fig. 3

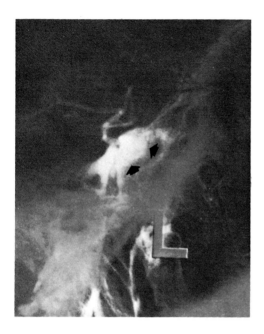

Fig. 4. Rupture of internal carotid artery at the level of siphon; massive contrast filling (*arrows*) of cavernous sinus due to direct carotid-cavernous sinus fistula

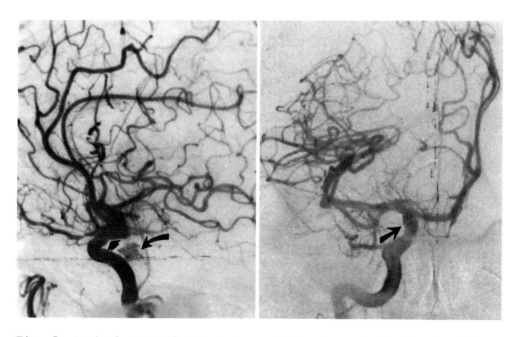

Fig. 5. Intimal tear of internal carotid artery at the level of the supraclinoid segment. *Arrow* points to intimal flap

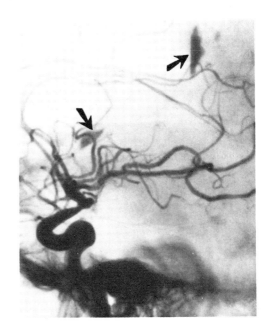

Fig. 6. Extravasation from two cortical branches of middle cerebral artery. *Arrows* point to pools of extravasated contrast medium

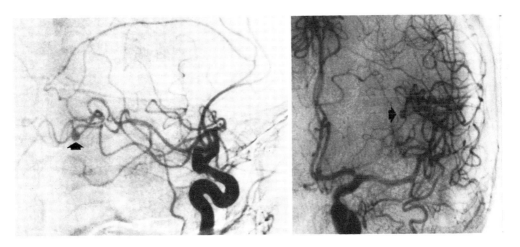

Fig. 7. Rupture of a posterior insular branch of the middle cerebral artery with development of an intracerebral false aneurysm (*arrows*); posteroanterior and lateral projection

Traumatic Aneurysms
A. LAUN

Aneurysms of traumatic origin are uncommon and not well-known. In 1922, MENSCHEL (17) reported on a pathologic description of a false aneurysm of the right vertebral artery. The first clinical case report of a traumatic aneurysm (TRA) of the carotid artery was published by BIRLEY in 1928 (3). Further autopsy reports were published by KRAULAND (15) in 1949 and clinical findings of TRA were discussed by POUYANNE et al. (18) in 1959. The subject was also reviewed by HIRSCH et al. (1962) (13), BURTON et al. (1968) (5), RAIMONDI (1968) (20), RUMBACH (1970) (22), ACOSTA et al. (1972) (1), and BENOIT and WARTZMANN (1973) (2).

This paper reviews the 70 cases published to date in the literature to which three personal observations are added, aneurysms of the middle meningeal artery, the callosomarginal artery, and the arteria gyri angularis. The analysis comprises iatrogenic aneurysms with the exception of TRA of the carotid artery and carotid-cavernous sinus fistulas.

Incidence and Localization

The analysis of the literature revealed 70 cases of TRA. Topographic distribution after adding three personal observations is presented in Table 1. With the exception of a few cases, TRA of the middle meningeal

Table 1. Traumatic and iatrogenic cerebral aneurysms (No. = 73)

Traumatic aneurysms			
Middle meningeal artery			20
Intracerebral arteries			45
Anterior choroideal artery		1	
Anterior cerebral artery		13	
A_1 segment	2		
A_2 segment	3		
Peripheral branches	8		
Middle cerebral artery		29	
Main branch	1		
Main junction	1		
Peripheral branches	27		
Posterior cerebral artery		1	
Peripheral branch	1		
Vertebral artery		1	
Iatrogenic aneurysms			8
Anterior cerebral artery		4	
Middle cerebral artery		4	
			73

artery were localized in the temporal area (Fig. 1, Table 2). Out of 20 cases, 14 were combined with epidural and the remaining six with subdural or combined hematomas. Eighty percent of these aneurysms were associated with skull fractures.

TRA of the cerebral arteries were reported in 45 instances (Tables 1 and 3). Most commonly, they are located on the cortical branches of the middle cerebral artery (Fig. 3); they are found far less frequently on the branches of the anterior cerebral artery (Fig. 2). Cases of aneurysms localized at the central branches of the cerebral arteries are exceptional. TRA of the anterior cerebral artery were more often associated with open head injuries (eight cases) than with closed ones (five cases). This contrasts with aneurysms of the middle cerebral artery branches. Among the latter, closed head injuries were present in 24 cases and open head injuries in five. Only in 2 out of 13 cases of the anterior cerebral artery aneurysms was there no fracture. Among 29 cases of aneurysms of branches of the middle cerebral artery, there was no skull fracture visible in 16 cases. Accompanying hematomas are the rule. They are usually subdural, less frequently intracerebral or combined. In many cases, cerebral contusion was found particularly in cases of TRA of deeper branches of cerebral arteries. Iatrogenic aneurysms occur, as suspected, at the site of the operative trauma (Table 4).

Pathogenesis

Iatrogenic aneurysms were described after surgery for brain tumor, brain puncture for access to the ventricles, puncture of bilateral subdural hematomas, leucotomy, and puncture for brain abscess.

All the aneurysms of the middle meningeal artery developed after closed craniocerebral injuries. In his anatomopathologic study, HASSLER (12) described defects of the wall of middle meningeal artery in its intracranial course. Because of a close relationship of the artery to the dura, direct distortion and laceration of the vascular wall can occur at the time of injury leading to the development of an aneurysmal sac. It is interesting to notice that no fracture was found in four cases, and in two further cases, the skull fracture was at a site distant to the false aneurysm. In these two cases, direct laceration of the arte-

Table 2. Traumatic aneurysms of the middle meningeal artery (No. = 20)

Hematoma	N	Fracture		Localization		
		+	-	Frontal	Temp.	Occ.
Epidural	14	11	3	-	12	2
Unilateral epidural and bilateral subdural	1	1	-	-	1	-
Subdural	2	1	1	1[a]	1[b]	-
Subdural and intracerebral	2	2	-	-	2[a]	-
Intracerebral	1	1	-	-	1	-
	20	16	4	1	17	2

[a] Two aneurysms without relation to the fracture.
[b] Angiographic evidence of development of aneurysm.

Table 3. Traumatic aneurysms of intracerebral arteries

	No.	Open	Injury missile + penetr. inj.	Closed	Fracture +	Fracture -	Hematoma Epi.	Hematoma Sub.	Hematoma Intr.	Comb.	Laceration
Anterior cerebral artery	13	4	4	5	11	2	-	2	1	1	8
A₁	2	-	1	1	2	-	-	-	-	-	1
A₂	3	1	1	1	3	-	-	-	1	-	2
Frontopol. art.	2	-	1	1	1	1	-	-	-	1 sub.+epi.	1
Pericallosa art.	4	2	1	1	3	1	-	1	-	-	3
Callosomarg. art.	1	1	-	-	1	-	-	-	-	-	1
Cortical branches	1	-	-	1	1	-	-	1	-	-	-
Middle cerebral artery	29	1	4	24	13	16	-	17	5	4	7
Main branch	2	-	1	1	2	-	-	-	-	1 sub.+intr.	2
Cortical branches	27	1	3	23	11	16	-	17	5	1 sub.+epi. / 2 sub.+intr.	5

Table 4. Iatrogenic intracerebral aneurysms (No. = 8)

	Branch	Operation	Onset
Anterior cerebral artery	A₁	Aneurysm of the ACOA	22 days
	FPoA	Orbital roof meningeoma	12 months
	A₂/FPoA	Frontal glioma	12 days
	PCAA	Leukotomy	4 weeks
Middle cerebral artery	Main branch	Meniongeoma of the orbital roof	17 days
	Post. temp. artery	Brain abscess	?
	Art. gyri angul	Ventr. punction for Pudenz drainage	15 days
	Cortical branch	Punction for bilateral subdural hydroma	?

rial wall was postulated. Aneurysms of the middle meningeal artery were combined with epidural subacute or chronic hematomas in 75% of the cases. Isolated subdural hematomas were found in two cases.

According to BURTON et al. (5) TRA of the cortical branches develop because of:
1. Direct injury to the arterial wall in cases of perforating or open head injuries.
2. Indirect injury of the artery in cases of closed head injuries.

This opinion was supported by the experimental findings of WHITE et al. (26), who was able to produce experimental defects in the vascular wall by injecting iso- and hypertonic solutions or hyaluronidase into the arterial wall in dogs. At the site of the defect produced in the vascular wall, saccular aneurysms originated in the course of the experiment. In patients who sustained a perforating brain injury, the aneurysms were found in the vicinity of the injury canal (1, 6, 8, 11, 14). In some cases of open head injury, bone fragments (1, 23) or missiles were found in the immediate vicinity of the aneurysms.

More difficult to understand is the development of TRA in cases of closed head injuries. DRAKE (9) and VANCE (25) described arterial and venous communicating and bridging vessels and cortical arteries which are adherent to the arachnoid membrane and dura mater. Rotatory movements of the brain (19) during the head injury can easily cause rupture or partial injury to the vascular wall. Depending upon the local situation, the false aneurysm develops instead of a hematoma.

Histology

Histologic exmaination was performed in 11 out of 20 cases of aneurysms of the middle meningeal artery. In all the cases where false aneurysms were found, the wall of the aneurysm consisted of blood clot and layers of fibrin. Histologic examination was performed in approximately 40% of all the other aneurysms reported. In four cases, true aneurysms were found (7, 10, 21, 23), in the remaining ones, the histologic picture corresponded to that of a false aneurysm, which proves its traumatic origin of course.

Diagnosis

In 19% of the cases, the development of an aneurysm was demonstrated by repeated angiography. This includes four cases of iatrogenic lesions. The diagnosis, therefore, has to be based upon clinical observations. TRA usually rupture in the 2nd or 3rd week after the trauma. The subarachnoid, subdural, or intracerebral bleeding produces rapid clinical deterioration which leads to angiographic examination and the operative treatment. True traumatic aneurysms possess a very solid wall and may rupture after several years (7, 23). Spontaneous thrombosis demonstrated angiographically was reported in five cases (2, 4, 22, 24). It may result in a rapid improvement in the clinical course (BRENNER) (4).

Therapy

Fifty patients were operated upon. Of this number, ten patients died (20%). Out of 23 patients who were not operated upon, 13 died (57%). In six cases, the diagnosis was made at autopsy (15, 16, 17, 23). BURTON (5) reported an overall mortality of almost 55%. The mortality of the series analyzed is 33%. In spite of considerable difficulties in the diagnosis, early angiography is indicated in cases of unexplained deteriation of the clinical state and should be followed by immediate operation.

Summary

The review of the literature to which three personal cases of false traumatic aneurysms are added is presented. The review comprises eight cases of iatrogenic aneurysms. Localization of the aneurysms and diagnostic and therapeutic problems are discussed. The relatively unfavorable prognosis so far can be improved by early angiography and computerized tomography with simultaneous demonstration of aneurysm and hematoma.

References

1. ACOSTA, C., WILLIAMS, Ph.E., Jr., CLARK, K.: Traumatic aneurysms of the cerebral vessels. J. Neurosurg. 36, 531-536 (1972)

2. BENOIT, B.G., WORTZMAN, G.: Traumatic cerebral aneurysms. Clinical features and natural history. J. Neurol. Neurosurg. Psychiatry 36, 127-138 (1973)

3. BIRLEY, J.L.: Traumatic aneurysm of the intracranial portion of the internal carotid artery. Brain 51, 184-208 (1928)

4. BRENNER, H.: Frontale Schädelspaltung mit traumatischem Aneurysma der Arteria pericallosa. Acta Neurochir. (Wien) 10, 145-152 (1962)

5. BURTON, Ch., VELASCO, F., DORMAN, J.: Traumatic aneurysm of a peripheral cerebral artery. J. Neurosurg. 28, 468-474 (1968)

6. CHADDUK, W.M.: Traumatic cerebral aneurysm due to speargun injury. J. Neurosurg. 31, 77-79 (1969)

7. COURVILLE, C.B.: Traumatic aneurysm of an intracranial artery. Bull. Los Angeles Neurol. Soc. 25, 48-54 (1960)

8. CRESSMAN, M.R., HAYES, G.J.: Traumatic aneurysm of the anterior chorioidal artery. J. Neurosurg. 24, 102-104 (1966)

9. DRAKE, Ch. G.: Subdural hematoma from arterial rupture. J. Neurosurg. 18, 597-601 (1961)

10. EICHLER, A., STORY, J.L., BENNETT, D.E., GALO, M.V.: Traumatic aneurysm of a cerebral artery. J. Neurosurg. 31, 72-76 (1969)

11. FERRY, D.J., KEMPE, L.G.: False aneurysm secondary to penetration of the brain through orbito facial wounds. Report of two cases. J. Neurosurg. 36, 503-506 (1972)

12. HASSLER, O.: Medical defects in the meningeal arteries. J. Neurosurg. 19, 337-340 (1962)

13. HIRSCH, J.F., DAVID, M., SACHS, M.: Les anévrysmes artériels traumatiques intracraniens. Neurochirurgie 8, 189-201 (1962)

14. KLUG, N.: Besonderheiten perforierender Schädelhirnverletzungen unter Friedensverhältnissen. Inaugural-Dissertation, Heidelberg 1968

15. KRAULAND, W.: Zur Entstehung traumatischer Aneurysmen der Schlagadern am Hirngrund. Schweiz. Z. Pathol. Bakteriol. 12, 113-127 (1949)

16. KRAULAND, W.: Verletzungen der Schlagaderzweige an der Mantelfläche des Großhirns durch stumpfe Gewalt ohne Schädelbruch als Quelle tödlicher subduraler Blutungen. Dtsch. Z. Nervenheilk. 175, 54-65 (1956)

17. MENSCHEL: Ärzte Sachverst. Ztg. 1922, o. 13, zit. nach KRAULAND 1949: Traum. Aneurysma der Art. vertebr. re.

18. POUYANNE, H., LEMAN, P., GOT, M., GOUAZE, A.: Anévrysme artériel traumatique de la méningée moyenne gauche. Neurochirurgie 5, 311-315 (1959)

19. PUDENZ, R.H., SHELDEN, C.H.: The lucite calvarium - A method for direct observation of the brain. J. Neurosurg. 3, 487-505 (1946)

20. RAIMONDI, A.J.: Intracranial false aneurysms. Neurochirurgia (Stuttg.) 11, 219-233 (1968)

21. RASKIND, R.: An intracranial arterial aneurysm associated with a recurrent meningeoma. J. Neurosurg. 23, 622-625 (1965)

22. RUMBAUGH, C.L., et al.: Traumatic aneurysms of cortical cerebral arteries. Radiology 96, 49-54 (1970)

23. SCHMID, K.O.: Zur Morphologie der posttraumatischen Anosmie und des intracerebralen posttraumatischen Aneurysmas. Fallbericht einer traumatischen Spätapoplexie. Virchows Arch. (Pathol. Anat.) 334, 67-78 (1961)

24. SCHUGK, P., VAPALAHTI, M., TROUPP, H.: Lokalisierte intrakranielle Gefäßschädigungen bei Schädel-Hirn-Trauma. Acta Neurochir. (Wien) 22, 327-337 (1970)

25. VANCE, B.M.: Ruptures of surface blood vessels on cerebral hemispheres as a cause of subdural hemorrhage. Arch. Surg. 61, 992-1006 (1950)

26. WHITE, J.C., SAYRE, G.P., WHISNANT, J.P.: Experimental destruction of the media for the production of intracranial arterial aneurysms. J. Neurosurg. 18, 741-745 (1961)

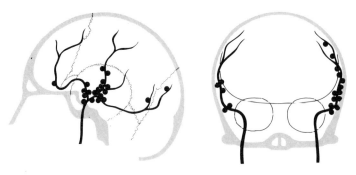

Fig. 1. Localization of traumatic aneurysms of the middle meningeal artery

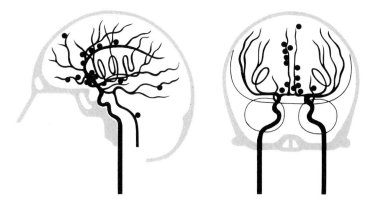

Fig. 2. Localization of traumatic aneurysms of intracerebral arteries with exception of the middle cerebral artery

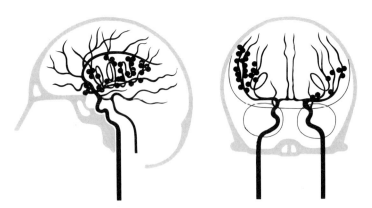

Fig. 3. Localization of traumatic aneurysms of the middle cerebral artery

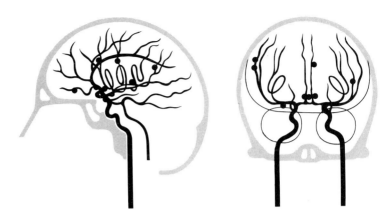

Fig. 4. Localization of iatrogenic intracerebral aneurysms

The Prognostic Value of Biochemical Data From Blood and CSF: Analysis in Patients With Severe Head Injury

L. AUER, E. MARTH, W. PETEK, H. HOLZER, and G. GELL

Introduction

The prognosis of outcome and survival chances for severely head-injured patients has been for many years a challenging problem for neurosurgeons. Extent, localization, and further development of traumatic brain lesions are often difficult to judge, preventing us from making a definite prognosis. The problem has become even greater by the increasing possibilities of intensive care and treatment of brain edema (1, 15, 16, 18, 19, 23, 27, 35), the first becoming a problem of medical economics in hopeless cases, the second creating an additional number of patients with traumatic apallic syndrome (persistent vegetative state) (17, 31). The attempt to find laboratory values of prognostic relevance should be seen in this light, although it is evident that decisive therapeutic steps will never be made dependent only on changes of such humoral factors.

Selection of Patients and Methods

A total of one hundred patients were divided into three groups according to the results of investigations, such as the clinical picture, EEG, CT scan, carotid angiography, etc. One group included patients lacking severe damage to the brain, these serve as a control group. The second group consists of patients with severe head injury who survived the trauma and the third group consists of those who did not survive the acute stage.

Blood samples were taken daily for the determination of serum proteins (2, 3), urea, uric acid, creatinine, platelets, fibrinogen, thromboplastin time, partial thromboplastin time, plasma thrombin time, platelet aggregation tests, and other routine investigations. Special globulins, such as α-1-antitrypsin, α-2-macrogolbulin (α-2-M), and haptoglobulin, were determined according to the radial immunodiffusion method (M-partigen test, Behring). From patients with an external ventricular drainage (1), ventricular CSF probes were withdrawn daily for the estimation of protein and hemoglobin content, polyacrylamide gel electrophoresis, and protease activity using TAME and/or BAPA as substrates (4).

Results

Electrophoretic determination of single plasma proteins showed doubling of the α-2-globulins during the first 10 days after a severe injury, when mean values of a series of 48 patients were calculated (2). An increase in α-globulins had already been described earlier (13); α-1-globulins were also increased, but to a less marked degree. At first, observations without statistical analysis seemed to indicate that α-1-antitrypsin is not responsible for this increase in α-1-globulins. In view of the other most important protease inhibitor in the blood, i.e., α-2-M, this was also found not to cause an increase in its fraction. On the contrary, it was decreased down to 40% of the normal

values in patients with extensive brain tissue lesions, thus indicating
a certain prognostic value. Moreover, haptoglobulin could be shown
to cause a significant increase in α-2-globulins and to increase up to
the sevenfold of normal (6) (Fig. 1). Interestingly, there was a very
good correlation with the extent of tissue lesions, but not with the
survival chances.

The most striking correlation between laboratory value changes and survival chances was seen in serum urea measurements. Here, nonsurvivors
had significantly (p = 0.1) higher values than survivors with a clear
threshold at 100 mg% (Fig. 2). None of the patients with urea levels
above this threshold survived the acute stage following a severe head
injury. These changes often run parallel with sodium retention (13, 26)
which is also a poor prognostic sign (28, 29).

Single values over 300 mg% were seen in nonsurvivors. Uric acid and
creatinine demonstrated a behavior dissociated from urea, showing later
and less marked increases. This fact, however, allows some conclusion
on the nature of urea increase, which appears rather to derive from
shock and central dysregulation as a sign of a hypercatabolic state than
from primary renal insufficiency (7, 25). This assumption receives
further support from measurements of urine urea which can increase up
to 90 g pro day and creatinine clearance values, which remain normal
for several days after injury (14, 28, 29).

Platelets and fibrinogen were found to be further prognostic indicators,
the first being significantly lower, the second higher in nonsurvivors
than in survivors (8). However, these data do not correlate with the
occurrence of disseminated intravascular coagulation which is an extremely rare event (8, 39). Serum proteinase activity is a possible,
but not a regular poor prognostic sign (4). Ventricular CSF proteins
are a much better indicator when investigated with the polyacrylamide
gel electrophoresis method. Here, our first observations showed a series
of bands that do not appear normally but occur in severely injured patients and remain or even worsen in nonsurvivors, whereas it normalizes
within a week or so in the survivors (Fig. 3). The molecular weight of
these bands lies between 16,000 and 60,000.

Discussion and Conclusion

This short review on our present state of laboratory value investigations shows that there are several factors which clearly indicate a bad
prognosis, poor survival chances, or extensive tissue lesions. The
aim of these investigations should not be to discuss the possible origin
of these changes, which has been done elsewhere (2-8), but to put
forth the question of whether there exists the possibility to form,
sooner or later, a network of factors for early differentiation of
those patients with no survival chances from those with a fair prognosis. Among such factors, persistently high intracranial pressure
(9, 20, 27, 32, 38) and several laboratory values such as blood and
CSF lactate (21, 22, 33, 35) have been mentioned in the literature.
Another attempt that fits into this concept is the "coma scale" from
the Glasgow group, which aims to detect different patterns of clinical
signs in patients with different survival chances (30). It is to be
hoped that evaluation of further laboratory values and other data compared with the aid of a computerized schedule will show us in the next
years whether it is possible to find a "no-chance pattern."

Summary

A description of a series of biochemical factors from the blood and ventricular CSF in order is given to determine the prognostic value in patients with a severe head injury. One of the most striking plasma factors indicating poor survival chances turned out to be the urea level, whereas the extent of tissue damage is reflected by the serum haptoglobulin level.

References

1. AUER, L., OBERBAUER, R., TRITTHART, H.: Externe Ventrikeldrainage - ein neuer Aspekt zur operativen Behandlung des Schädelhirntraumas Neurochirurgia 20, 48-55 (1977)

2. AUER, L., PETEK, W.: Serum globulin changes in patients with craniocerebral trauma. J. Neurol. Neurosurg. Psychiatry 39, 1076-1080 (1976)

3. AUER, L., PETEK, W.: Serumproteinveränderungen bei Patienten mit Schädelhirntrauma - Vergleich zwischen Alpha-2- und Alpha-2-M-Globulinabweichungen. Acta Neurochir. 33, 301-309 (1976)

4. AUER, L., MARTH, E.: Proteolytische Enzymaktivität im Liquor cerebrospinalis nach Schädelhirntrauma. Vorläufige Mitteilung.

5. AUER, L., PETEK, W.: Serum-Alpha-2-M-Globulinveränderungen bei Patienten mit Schädelhirntrauma. Acta Chir. Austriaca. (In press)

6. AUER, L., PETEK, W.: Serum haptoglobulin changes in patients with severe isolated head injury. Acta Neurochir. (In press)

7. AUER, L., HOLZER, H., TRITTHART, H., GELL, G.: Azotemia in severe head injury - central dysregulation of renal failure? Acta Neurochir. (In press)

8. AUER, L.: Disturbances of the coagulatory system in patients with severe cerebral trauma. Acta Neurochir. (In press)

9. AUER, L., TRITTHART, H., EKHART, E.: Therapeutical consequences of simultaneous ICP and blood pressure measurement in patients with severe head injury. Proc. 6th Int. Congr. Neurol. Surg. Exc. Med. 418, 115-116 (1977)

10. AUER, L., WENDT, P., HUBER, P., BLÜMEL, G.: Untersuchungen über proteolytische Enzymaktivität nach experimentellem Schädelhirntrauma. Neue Aspekte Trasylol-Therapie 7, 229-239 (1975)

11. BARRETT, A.J.: Inhibitors of lysosomal proteinases. In: Proteinase Inhibitors. FRITZ, H., TSCHESCHE, H., GREENE, L.J., TRUSCHEIT, E. (eds.), pp. 574-580. Berlin-Heidelberg-New York: Springer 1974

12. BARRETT, A.J., STARKEY, P.M., MUNN, E.A.: The unique nature of interaction of alpha-2-macroglobulin with proteases. In: Proteinase Inhibitors. FRITZ, H., TSCHESCHE, H., GREENE, L.J., TRUSCHEIT, E. (eds.), pp. 72-77. Berlin-Heidelberg-New York: Springer 1974

13. BRILMAYER, H., FROWEIN, R.A.: Eiweiß- und Elektrolytveränderungen im Blut und Urin während des akuten Stadiums nach Schädelhirnverletzungen und nach Hirnoperationen. Langenbecks Arch. Chir. 294, 205-216 (19607

14. BUCHNER, H.: Eiweißstoffwechsel und Trauma. Langenbecks Arch. Chir. 283, 361-370 (1956)

15. FAUPEL, G., REULEN, H.J., MÜLLER, D., SCHÜRMANN, K.: Double blind study on the effects of steroids on severe closed head injury. In: Dynamics of Brain Edema. PAPPIUS, H.M., FEINDEL, W. (eds.), pp. 337-358. Berlin-Heidelberg-New York: Springer 1976
16. FROWEIN, R.A., KARIMI-NEJAD, A., RICHARD, K.B.: Influence of ventilation and hyperventilation on brain edema and intracranial pressure. In: Advances in Neurosurgery, Vol. 1. SCHÜRMANN, K., BROCK, M., REULEN, H.J., VOTH, D. (eds.), pp. 114-127. Berlin-Heidelberg-New York: Springer 1973
17. GERSTENBRAND, F.: Das traumatische apallische Syndrom. Wien: Springer 1967
18. GOBIET, W.: The influence of various doses of dexamethasone on intracranial pressure in patients with severe head injury. In: Dynamics of Brain Edema. PAPPIUS, H.M., FEINDEL, W. (eds.), pp. 351-356. Berlin-Heidelberg-New York: Springer 1976
19. GOBIET, W.: Monitoring of intracranial pressure in patients with severe head injury. Neurochirurgia 20, 35-47 (1977)
20. GOBIET, W., BOCK, W.J., LIESEGANG, J., GROTE, W.: Intracranial pressure, hemodynamics and metabolic disorders in patients with severe head injury. In: Advances in Neurosurgery, Vol. 1. SCHÜRMANN, K., BROCK, M., REULEN, H.J., VOTH, D. (eds.), pp. 68-72. Berlin-Heidelberg-New York: Springer 1973
21. HAUSDÖRFER, J., HELLER, W., OLDENKOTT, P., STOLZ, I.C.: Alternations of metabolism in brain edema following head injury. In: Advances in Neurosurgery, Vol. 1. SCHÜRMANN, K., BROCK, M., REULEN, H.J., VOTH, D. (eds.), pp. 34-41. Berlin-Heidelberg-New York: Springer 1973
22. HELLER, W., OLDENKOTT, P.: Enzymdiagnostik bei traumatisch bedingten Hirnerkrankungen. Acte Neurochir. 20, 299-308 (1969)
23. HEPPNER, F., DIEMATH, H.E.: Klinische Erfahrungen mit der anticholinergischen Behandlung des gedeckten Schädelhirntraumas. Mschr. Unfallheilk. 61, 11-20 (1958)
24. HEPPNER, F., LANNER, G., AUER, L.: Die Behandlung des traumatischen Hirnödems. Wien. Med. Wschr. 126, 105-109 (1976)
25. HIGGINS, G. et. al.: Metabolic disorders in head injury. Lancet 9, 61-67 (1954)
26. HOFMEISTER, L., SCHAEFER, H.: Wasser-, Elektrolyt- und Eiweißhaushalt beim Schädelhirntrauma. Med. Klin. 43, 1959-1961 (1959)
27. HOLBACH, K.: Verbesserte Reversibilität des traumatischen Mittelhirnsyndroms bei Anwendung der hyperbaren Oxygenierung. Acta Neurochir. 30, 247-258 (1974)
28. HOLZER, H., AUER, L., TRITTHART, H., EKHART, E.: Akutes Nierenversagen und Hyperkatabolie nach Schädelhirntrauma. Paper given at the 2nd Donausymposion for Nephrology, Budapest, 26th-28th September, 1977
29. HOLZER, H., AUER, L., TRITTHART, H., EKHART, E.: Hypertabolie und Nierenversagen nach schwerem Schädelhirntrauma. 1977 (In preparation)
30. JENNETT, B., BOND, M.: Assessment of outcome after severe brain damage. Lancet 2, 480-485 (1975)
31. JENNETT, B., PLUM, F.: Persistent vegetative state after brain damage. Lancet 1, 734-737 (1972)

32. LUNDBERG, N., TROUPP, H., LORIN, H.: Continous recording of the ventricular fluid pressure in patients with severe acute traumatic brain injury. J. Neurosurg. 22, 581-590 (1965)
33. McLAURIN, R.L.: Liquorlaktat bei Hirntraumen. Med. Trib. 5, 1 (1974)
34. RABOW, L., HEBBE, B., LIEDEN, G.: Enzyme analysis for evaluating acute head injury. Acta Chir. Scand. 137, 305-309 (1971)
35. SCHUBERT, F., WALLENFANG, T., REULEN, H.J., SCHÜRMANN, K.: The influence of ventilatory changes in CSF-lactate and CSF L/P-ratio. In: Advances in Neurosurgery, Vol. 1. SCHÜRMANN, K., BROCK, M., REULEN, H.J., VOTH, D. (eds.), pp. 141-145. Berlin-Heidelberg-New York 1973
36. SEITZ, H.D. et al.: Klinische und tierexperimentelle Untersuchungen zum Hirnstoffwechsel und zur Hirndurchblutung beim Schädelhirntrauma. Neurochirurgia 6, 201-209 (1972)
37. TROUPP, H., VAPALAHTI, M.: Ventricular fluid pressure in children with severe brain injuries. In: Advances in Neurosurgery, Vol. 1. SCHÜRMANN, K., BROCK, M., REULEN, H.J., VOTH, D. (eds.), pp. 62-72. Berlin-Heidelberg-New York: Springer 1973
38. VAPALAHTI, M., TROUPP, H.: Prognosis for patients with severe brain injuries. Br. Med. J. 3, 404-407 (1971)
39. VECHT, Ch.J.: Disseminated intravascular coagulation and head injury. J. Neurol. Neurosurg. Psychiatry 38, 567-572 (1975)

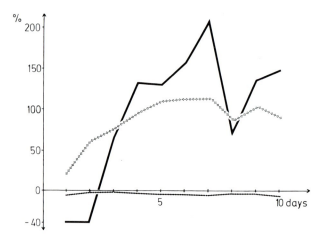

Fig. 1. Mean percentage deviation of total serum proteins, α-2-globulins, and haptoglobulin in a series of 33 patients, demonstrating increased α-2-globulins due to highly elevated haptoglobulin values

Fig. 3. CSF polyacrylamide gel electrophoresis
A Normal CSF
B 25-year-old woman, frontobasal depressed fracture, cerebral contusion, recovered within 4 weeks
C 48-year-old man, temporobasal skull fracture, epidural hematoma, multiple contusions, diffuse brain edema. Lethal outcome after 4 days

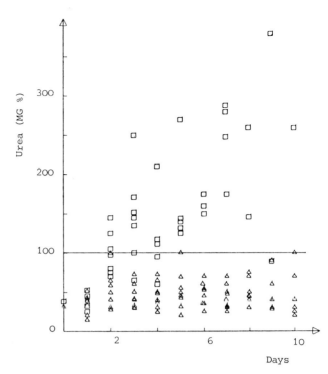

Fig. 2. Diagram of 29 patients with severe head injury, showing the trend of blood urea levels during the 1st week. A threshold between the two patient groups appears around 100 mg%
☐ Nonsurvivors
△ Survivors

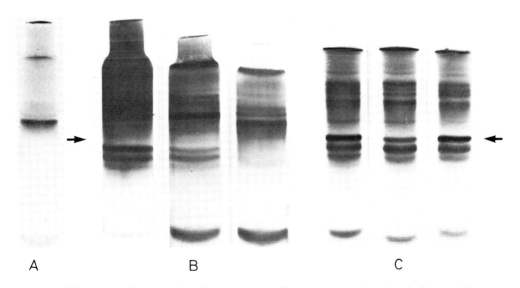

→ Normally nonexistent bands appear after severe brain injury. They disappear within the 1st week in survivors and persist in nonsurvivors

Changes in Lipid Metabolism in Experimentally Produced Head Injury: Qualitative and Quantitative Studies of Lipids

R. PREGER

Introduction

Numerous reports about the lipid and lipoprotein metabolism in the brain, cerebrospinal fluid (CSF), and serum of different cerebral diseases (1-5, 7, 9-14, 18) formed the background for our studies of lipid metabolism in cats after producing head injuries by acceleration. The report is limited to lipid changes.

Methods

Table 1 gives a general view of the number and the weight of the examined male cats, frequency of blows (repeated acceleration and decleration), survival time, and neurologic and histologic results. The cats were anesthetized with a sodium pentobarbital injection (25 mg/kg) and the head injury was produced by repeated acceleration of the cat's head with a model developed by Prof. BETZ (Tübingen)[1]. It is possible to produce standardized cerebral concussion (CC) and contusion (CT) in proportion to the number of blows. We observed and measured changes in the lipids and lipoproteins in the grey (BG) and white (BW) matter of the cerebrum, CSF, and serum (6, 8, 15-17, 19, 20). The lipids were separated by the thin layer technique on silica gel plains. They were identified by control lipids and by RF comparison with other reports on lipids.

Results

1. Cerebral Lipids

In Figure 1, the normal densitograms (DG) of BG and BW were contrasted, the indentified fractions recorded, and the sphingolipids (cerebrosides, sulfatides, sphingomyelines-SPH) accentuated by hatching. The increase of these lipids in BW in contrast to BG is clearly evident. In Figure 2, the DG of a case of CC (IA, IB) and a case of CT (IIA, IIB) were opposed. The DG of a CC is equal to that of the normal brain whereas the DG of a CT shows near equality between BG and BW. This agreement can be observed within 3 1/2 h after the acceleration head injury, although in this time no sure signs of an injury could be found histologically. In Table 2, the total lipid values of BG, BW, CSF, and serum are summarized. A mistake during the preparation of BG and BW with loss of water explains some abnormally high values. Because of only one normal cat, group A cannot be used for discussion. It must be expected that the lipid values of group B are to be compared with normal animals. By this conclusion, we observe in group C (CZ) an increase in the lipid values of BG and no changes in BW. In comparison with the above-mentioned DGs which showed an equality between BG and BW in the lipid pattern, two reasons for these changes can be assumed. First, there must be a myelin damage with spreading of SPH by diffusion, and second, a damage of the blood-brain barrier with transudation of serum lipoproteins and lipids.

---

[1] A report about this model was prepared.

Table 1. I: number of blows; II: survival time after head injury in hours; III: bodyweight before death in g; IV: neurologic results; V: pathologic results

No.	I	II	III	IV	V
Group A (cats without head injury)					
02	∅	∅	∅	None	Normal brain tissue
04	∅	∅	3100	Enteritis	Disseminated nerve cell damage, vacuoles
09	∅	∅	∅	None	Death without reason
Group B (cats with cerebral concussion)					
01	2	24	∅	None	Only some circumscribed nerve cell damages
03	5	25	∅	None	Normal brain tissue
05	5	28	2800	None	Slight edema and disseminated nerve cell damage
06	3	48	2400	None	Some disseminated nerve cell damages
Group C (cats with cerebral contusion)					
14	10	3.5	2800	Unconscious, trembling of the legs	Fresh edema, no severe cellular damage
08	8	23	2750	Unconscious, convulsions	Severe edema and cellular damage
07	5 (5)	50 (24)	2750	None	Extensive nerve cell damages, edema
11	9	49	2000	Apathetic, unsteady movements	Nerve cell damages, single bleedings in brain tissue
10	10	70	2150	Ocular pupillary reactions, aggressive	Severe edema and nerve cell damage
12	11	72	2910	None	Severe edema and nerve cell damage
13	15	c.2	2300	Unconscious, cerebral death spontanously	SAB and intracerebral bleeding, edema

2. CSF Lipids

In Figure 2, the DG of normal and pathologic CSF (IIIA, IIIB) and serum (IVA, IVB) of cat No. 7 (CT) are also copied from original curves. We found an increase in cerebrosides and cephalines in CSF after head injury, which means that there is probably a lipid dispersion from the brain into the CSF as well as a serum transudation. These changes could be explained by myelin damage as well as by the blood-brain barrier (BBB) damage and could offer a possibility for classification of severe head injuries. We found no explanation for the record of a special CSF lecithin and of a high unsaturated free fatty acid.

Table 2. I: total lipid values of grey matter in mg/100 mg wet weight; II: total lipid values of white matter in mg/100 mg wet weight; IIIA: CSF lipids before head injury in mg%; IIIB: CSF lipids after head injury in mg%; IVA: total serum lipids before head injury in mg%; IVB: total serum lipids after second control or after head injury in mg%

Group A						
No.	I	II	IIIA	IIIB	IVA	IVB
02	17.4	27.8	12.0	∅	644	688
04	33.7	18.1	∅	∅	715	1030
09	∅	∅	∅	∅	518	∅
Group B						
01	9.7	12.0	9.3	73.3	474	854
03	13.6	22.2	∅	∅	565	585
05	6.1	4.'	∅	∅	894	558
06	5.1	15.7	∅	∅	732	596
Average	8.6	13.7	9.3	73.3	666	648
Group C						
14	8.5	5.2	∅	∅	∅	469
08	18.5	6.4	∅	∅	509	704
07	20.3	12.5	∅	∅	389	274
11	10.1	20.9	∅	∅	∅	500
10	14.1	4.9	∅	∅	∅	283
12	28.9	32.4	∅	∅	∅	469
13	10.5	14.5	∅	∅	∅	0
Average	15.8	13.8	∅	∅	449	450

3. Serum Lipids

No cerebrosides and sulfatides could be found in normal serum in our studies (Fig. 2, IVA), but there could be found a clear cephalin band in DG. After CT, we observed a decrease or a loss of cephalin. It is now possible to identify cerebrosides which means that the lipids caused by the damage of myelin not only spread into the CSF but also into the serum. The loss of lipids in serum could be interpretated by a disturbance of lipid and lipoprotein synthesis in postcontusional shock as well as by influx (transudation) into the brain and perhaps into the CSF by BBB damage.

Discussion

Our studies show changes in cerebral lipid pattern beginning 3 1/2 h after severe head injury (CT). There is to be seen a spreading of SPH by diffusion and an increase of total lipid weights of BG. An increase of SPH could be found both in CSF and serum. In contrast, we also observed an influx of lipids into the brain and CSF. By means of change in lipid pattern, a classification of severe head injury can be made, and the effect of different treatment could probably be controlled. Exact explanation of lipid biodynamics is only possible in conjunction with studies in lipoprotein dynamics. Our studies will be continued and we will give further reports.

Summary

Lipid changes in experimental head injury of cats due to acceleration are reported. Our studies showed changes of total lipid values and single lipids in BG, BW, CSF, and serum. Remarkable changes were found in SPH as an effect of myelin damage. Cephalin changes accompanied by cholesterol and cholesterol ester could be explained by a BBB damage as well as by a disturbance of their synthesis during the post-contusional shock.

References

1. ALAJOUANINE, Th., FOURNIER, Et., GERVAIS, P.: Dysprotéinorachies, Presse méd. 68, 385-386 (1960)
2. BONZARTH, W.F., SHENKIN, H.A., GUTTERMANN, P.: Andrenal cortical response to neurosurgical problems, noting the effects of exogenous steroids. In: Steroids and Brain Edeme. REULEN, H.J., SCHÜRMANN, K. (eds.). Berlin-Heidelberg-New York: Springer 1972
3. DEBUCH, H., UHLENBRUCK, G.: Lipoide und Eiweißstoffe des Gehirns. In: Handbuch der Neurochirurgie I/2, pp. 213-269. Berlin-Heidelberg-New York: Springer 1968
4. DELANK, H.W., WREDE, M.Th.: Der klinische Wert quantitativ-immunochemischer Bestimmungen verschiedener Proteine in Liquor cerebrospinalis. Klin. Wschr. 47, 1270-1275 (1969)
5. DEMOPOULOS, H.B., MILOY, P., KAKARI, S., RANSOHOFF, J.: Molecular Aspects of Membrane Structure in Cerebral Edema. In: Steroids and Brain Edema. REULEN, H.J., SCHÜRMANN, K. (eds.). Berlin-Heidelberg-New York: Springer 1972
6. FRIED, R.: Methods of Neurochemistry, pp. 219-229. New York: Dekker 1971
7. GITLIN, D., LANDING, B.H., WHIPPLE, A.: The localization of homologous plasma proteins in the tissue of young human beings as demonstrated with fluorescent antibodies. J. Exp. Med. 97, 163-176 (1953)
8. HARZER, K., SANDHOFF, K., JATZKEWITZ, H.: Säulenchromatographische Darstellung von Phospatiden aus Gehirn-Gesamtlipoidextrakt. Hoppe Seyler's Z. Physiol. Chem. 348, 119-120 (1967)
9. HAUSDÖRFER, J., HELLER, W., JUNGER, H., PREGER, R.: Veränderungen des Lipidstoffwechsels nach akutem experimentellen Schädel-Hirn-Trauma. Med. Welt 27, 426-431 (1976)
10. HELLER, W., STOLZ, Ch.: Veränderungen des Fettstoffwechsels bei hypoxischer Hypoxie. In: Deutsche Gesellschaft für Anästhesie und Wiederbelebung. LAWIN, P., MORR-STRATHMANN, U. (eds.), pp. 212-216. Berlin-Heidelberg-New York: Springer 1974
11. HILL, N.C., GOLDSTEIN, N.P., McKENZIE, B.F., McGUCKIN, W.F.: SVIEN, H.J.: Cerebrospinal fluid proteins, glycoproteins and lipoproteins in obstructive lesions of the central nervous system. Brain 82, 581-593 (1959)
12. LATERRE, E.Chr.: Proteine im Liquor cerebrospinalis (I): Das normale Proteinspektrum. Laborblätter 25, 125-130 (1975)
13. LATERRE, E.Chr.: Proteine im Liquor cerebrospinalis (II): Laborblätter 25, 157-165 (1975)

14. MANUEL, J., ROUGEMONTE, J. de: Electrophorèse en gel d'amidon du liquide céphalo-rachidien dans le diagnostic des tumeurs intra craniennes. C.R. Soc. Biol (Paris), 1859-1862 (1962)
15. MARINETTI, G.V.: Lipid Chromatographic Analysis I. New York: Dekker 1967
16. MIESCHER, K.: Helv. Chim. Acta 29, 743 (1946)
17. MÜLLER, J., VAHAR-MATIAR, H.: Eine chromatographische Mikromethode zur Bestimmung der Lipide im Liquor cerebro spinalis. Z. Neurol. 23, 333-344 (1973)
18. PILZ, H.: Die Lipide des normalen und pathologischen Liquor cerebrospinalis. Berlin-Heidelberg-New York: Springer 1970
19. STAHL, E.: Dünnschichtchromatographie. Ein Laboratoriumshandbuch. Berlin-Göttingen-Heidelberg: Springer 1962
20. ZÖLLNER, N., EBERHAGEN, D.: Untersuchung und Bestimmung der Lipoide im Blut. Berlin-Heidelberg-New York: Springer 1965

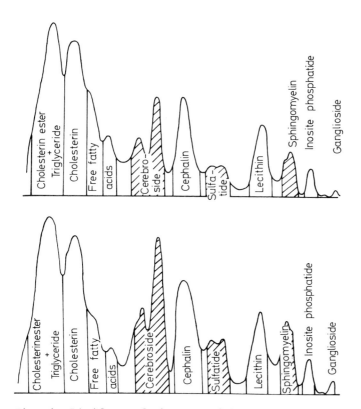

Fig. 1. Lipid DG of the normal brain of cat No. 2
Above: lipid pattern of grey matter
Below: white matter of cerebrum (λ = 550 nm-remission)

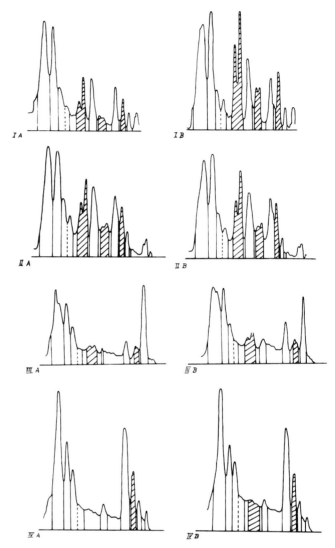

Fig. 2. Lipid DG from cat No. 3 from grey matter (*IA*) and white matter (*IB*) of cerebrum after CC; the same from cat No. 8 from BG (*IIA*) and BW (*IIB*) after CT; lipid pattern of CSF before (*IIIA*) and after head injury (*IIIB*) from cat No. 7; serum lipid pattern of serum (*IVA, IVB*) from the same cat

Cerebellum

Positive Ventriculography

Ventriculography With Resorbable Contrast Media: Field of Indication and Experience

St. Kunze and W. Huk

Since the beginning of 1971, we have been using central ventriculography for the visualization of the unpaired ventricles at the Neurosurgical University Clinic in Erlangen. After making a frontal burr hole over the nondominant hemisphere, a blunt cannula is introduced into the lateral ventricle under fluoroscopic control and then a thin catheter is advanced into the third ventricle. The contrast medium is now injected. Even in a nondilated ventricular system, the experienced investigator can advance the catheter quickly. As a rule, diffuculties are met only if the foramen of Monroe is blocked. Dimer-X is the contrast medium generally used; however, Amipaque has recently been employed on occasion. The epileptogenic effect of metrizamide is even lower than that of Dimer-X according to the animal experiments of GONSETTE (1). In 1972, we reported on the histologic examination of the ependymal lining of the ventricles as well as on the meninges of cats following the intraventricular injection of Dimer-X at the 23rd annual meeting of our society in Hamburg. Only in the first 48 h after contrast medium injection were infiltrates of leukocytes and lymphocytes to be found in the meninges.

The clinical side-effects of central ventriculography with water-soluble contrast media are nausea and vomiting at the end of the examination in about one-third of the cases. The most dangerous complication observed in the 415 examinations performed at our department was the occurrence of seizures in five patients, i.e., in just over 1%. Two of these patients were known to have had epileptic seizures previously. An injection of diazepam led to a cessation of the seizure in all cases.

The diagnostic accuracy of central ventriculography regarding the localization of a lesion is very high. The type of tumor, however, can only rarely by diagnosed, as for example in the case of an epidermoid in the fourth ventricle. The spotty appearance of the contrast medium is typical here.

In cases of midbrain tumor, positive ventriculography indicates the exact extent of the tumor and demonstrates the secondary stenosis of the aqueduct. The effect of radiation may also be shown in those cases where radiation is used (Figs. 1 and 2). In this case, the germinoma led to a therapeutically resistant metastases in the entire CSF space 4 1/2 years later.

The indication for central ventriculography with water-soluble contrast media has been made until now in cases of suspected space-occupying lesions of the third ventricle, the midbrain, and the posterior fossa. Since the introduction of computerized axial tomography, the question arises if central ventriculography is still necessary for planning an operative procedure.

Since July, 1975, we have investigated 35 patients with tumors of the posterior fossa (excluding neurinomas and brain stem lesions) at our department using computerized tomography as well as ventriculography. The diagnostic accuracy and information of computerized tomography was greater in 17 cases, that of ventriculography in 12 cases. In six patients, both methods of investigation were equally informative.

In cases of cystic lesions, i.e., angioblastomas, cystic astrocytomas, and meningiomas, computerized tomography was clearly superior. Possible, an improvement of the apparatus will improve the quality of the information about other lesions in the posterior fossa. The tomogram shown in Figure 3 was made with a finer matrix (256 x 256) on a patient with a cerebellar met metastasis in the upper medial portions of the left cerebellar hemisphere surrounded by a hematoma which extended as far as the vermis.

Today, ventriculography provides the greater amoung of information about tumors in and around the fourth ventricle, i.e. ependymomas, plexus papillomas and partly medulloblastomas. Especially in cases with a marked narrowing of the fourth ventricle, tomography often cannot exactly indicate the relationships to the floor of the fourth ventricle and the brain stem. In the ventriculogram, an ependymoma in the fourth ventricle can be clearly differentiated from a similar tumor originating from the lower vermis. In cases of disturbed CSF dynamics, ventriculography also provides more exact information, e.g., in the case of an incomplete CSF stop at the entrance of the fourth ventricle showing the position of the tonsils or a complete CSF stop at the exit of the fourth ventricle as in the case of the Dandy-Walker-Syndrome.

Although we can presently do without ventriculography in cases of menigiomas, angioblastomas, neurinomas, and occasionally spongioblastomas, we perform ventriculography with positive contrast media in all other cases right after computerized tomography. After the examination, the catheter can be withdrawn into the frontal part of the lateral ventricle and CSF drainage is performed via a valve until the time of operation.

References

1. GONSETTE, R.: Biological tolerance of the central nervous system to metrizamide. Acta radiologica (Stockh.) Suppl. 335, 25-44 (1973)

2. KUNZE, St.: Die zentrale Ventrikulographie mit wasserlöslichen, resorbierbaren Kontrastmitteln. Neurology Series 13. Berlin-Heidelberg-New York: Springer 1974

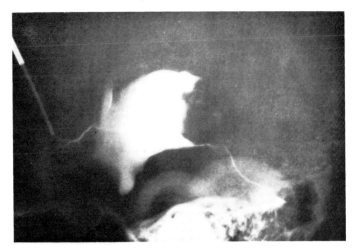

Fig. 1. Tumor of the pineal region. The extent of the tumor and the secondary stenosis of the aqueduct is demonstrated

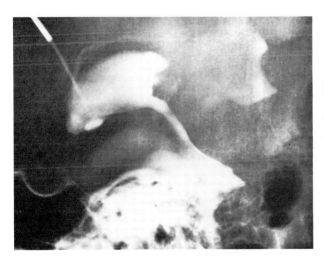 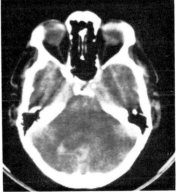

Fig. 2   Fig. 3

Fig. 2. Ventriculography 1 year later in the same patient. The effect of radiation is visible

Fig. 3. Computerized tomography (Siretom 2000) in a case with a cerebellar metastasis in the upper medial portions of the left cerebellar hemisphere surrounded by a hematoma which extended as far as the vermis

Ventriculography With Amipaque (Metrizamide)
H.-P. Richter and P. C. Potthoff

Introduction

Two different types of contrast media are available for positive ventriculography: *oily* contrast agents, such as Duroliopaque[R], bear the disadvantages of possible consequent arachnoiditis (3) and the necessity of complex movements of the patient and therefore long duration of the examination, whereas *water-soluble* contrast media as meglumine iothalamate (Conray) and dimeglumine iocarmate (Dimer-X) are often followed by adverse reactions like cerebral convulsions and spinal automatisms (1, 8, 11). This is a such report on our experience with the water-soluble contrast agent metrizamide (Amipaque) in ventriculography.

Material and Methods

Fifty-three patients were studied by ventriculography (24 children, 29 adults). After making a frontal burr hole, a thin ventricular catheter was introduced into the frontal horn of the lateral ventricle of the nondominant hemisphere. With the patient in a sitting position, Amipaque was injected under radiographic control. Usually, 6-10 cc were injected corresponding to an average concentration of 155-240 mg J/cc. Lateral and anteroposterior views as well as, if necessary, tomographic films were taken in this and often additionally in a reclined position (Figs. 1-4). Samples of ventricular CSF were examined for protein content and cell count before the ventriculography and compared to the findings some days later (17 patients).

Results

Out of 53 patients, 6 showed a normal ventriculogram. In 36 patients, a space-occupying lesion within the posterior fossa was demonstrated (Table 1). The injection of Amipaque[R] resulted in a good or very good visibility of the interesting structures in all cases of posterior fossa tumors and those around the third ventricle, unless there was a higher degree of hydrocephalus, which caused an excessive dilution of the contrast agent. The structures were clearly visible during 20-30 min, until the examination was finished. Except for reclination, additional movements of the patient were not necessary in our cases. Side-effects during or immediately after metrizamide ventriculography were slight and rare; some patients complained of dull headache during the injection of the contrast medium, which obviously was due to an overly rapid injection. No side-effects were observed which could be related to the contrast agent itself. We never saw hyperpyrexia, vomitus, cerebral convulsions, or spinal automatisms. Even though the protein content of the CSF was not altered after Amipaque ventriculography, a certain rise in the cell count (mostly granulocytes) was often observed but diminished some days after the examination (Fig. 5).

Table 1. Findings in 53 ventriculographies with Amipaque

Normal	6
Infratentorial mass (including two acoustic neurinomas)	36
Supratentorial mass	1
Internal communicating hydrocephalus	5
Arnold-Chiari malformation aqueduct stenosis	5

Discussion

According to our experience in 53 ventriculographies with Amipaque, we consider this water-soluble contrast medium to be superior to the other (oily and water-soluble) contrast agents. It allows a rapid investigation of the structures of interest without time-consuming and often stressing movements of the patient. It seems that cerebral convulsions can be provoked even by Amipaque, when injected into the cerebral subarachnoid space or if a neuroleptic drug is given simultaneously, which has been proven experimentally (7, 9, 14). Therefore, metrizamide should be regarded as slightly neurotoxic, but much less so than any other water-soluble contrast media known. From our observations with computerized axial tomography (CT), it can be stated that Amipaque enters the spinal and intracranial central nervous system from the subarachnoid space (5, 10) and can be visualized on CT much longer than by radiography. Our results are in accordance with those of other authors. Together with our material, 141 ventriculographies with Amipaque have been described (4, 6, 12, 13) without any serious complication. We consider it, therefore, to be the best contrast agent for ventriculography currently available.

Summary

Ventriculography with Amipaque has been performed in 53 patients, among these 36 patients with a posterior fossa space-occupying lesion. The interesting structure were well or very well visible in all these tumors. No serious side-effects have been observed. For the reasons documented here, Amipaque is considered superior to other contrast media for ventriculography.

References

1. AGNOLI, A., EGGERT, H.R., ZIERSKI, J., SEEGER, W., KIRCHOFF, D.: Diagnostische Möglichkeiten der positiven Ventrikulographie. Acta Neurochir. 31, 227-243 (1975)

2. ALLEN, W.E., VAN GILDER, J.C., COLLINS, W.F.: Evaluation of neurotoxicity of water soluble contrast agents by electrophysiological monitors. Radiology 118, 89-95 (1976)

3. CLARK, R.G., MILHORAT, T.H., STANLEY, W.C., DiCHIRO, G.: Experimental Pantopaque-ventriculography. J. Neurosurg. 34, 387-395 (1971)

4. CRONQUIST, S.: Ventriculography with Amipaque. Neuroradiol. 12, 25-32 (1976)

5. DRAYER, B.P., ROSENBAUM, A.E., HIGMAN, H.B.: Cerebrospinal fluid imagining using serial metrizamide CT cisternography. Neuroradiol. 13, 7-18 (1977)
6. GONSETTE, R.E. : Metrizamide as contrast medium for myelography and ventriculography. Acta Radiol. Diagn. Suppl. 335, 346-358 (1973)
7. GONSETTE, R.E., BRUCHER, J.M.: Potentiation of Amipaque. Epileptogenic activity by neuroleptics. Neuroradiol. 14, 27-30 (1977)
8. HEIMBURGER, R.F., CAMPBELL, R.L., KALSBECK, J.E., MEALEY, J., GOODALL, C.C.: Positive contrast cerebral ventriculography using water-soluble media. Clinical evaluation of 102 procedures using methylglutamine iothalamate 60%. J. Neurol. Neurosurg. Psychiatry 29, 281-290 (1966)
9. HINDMARSH, T., GREPE, A., WIDEN, L.: Metrizamide-Phenothiazine interaction. Acta Radiol. Diagn. 16, 129-134 (1975)
10. JOHNSON, R.: Personal communication
11. KUNZE, S., SCHIEFER, W.: Die Verwendung wasserlöslicher resorbierbarer Kontrastmittel zur zentralen Ventriculographie und Myelographie. Zentralbl. Neurochir. 35, 1-19 (1974)
12. SKALPE, O., AMUNDSEN, P.: Clinical results with metrizamide ventriculography. J. Neurosurg. 43, 432-439 (1975)
13. SUZUKI, S., ITO, K., IWABUCHI, T.: Ventriculography with non-ionic water soluble contrast medium Amipaque (metrizamide). J. Neurosurg. 47, 79-85 (1977)
14. WYLIE, J.G., AFSHAR, F., KOEZE, T.H.: Results of the use of a new water soluble contrast medium (metrizamide) in the posterior fossa of the baboon. Br. J. Radiol. 48, 1007-1012 (1975)

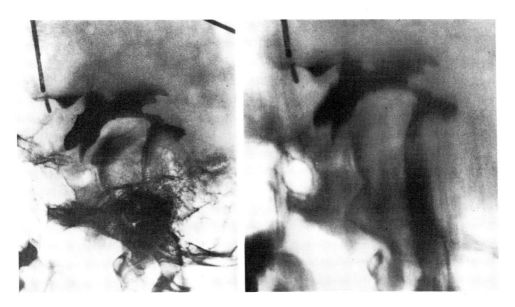

Fig. 1. T. J., 8 years: Amipaque ventriculography, lateral view (*left*) and median tomogram (*right*). Medulloblastoma of the fourth ventricle. No infiltration of the floor of the fourth ventricle on median tomogram

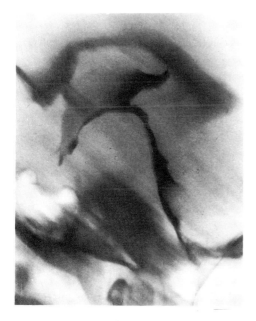

Fig. 2. St. J., 16 years: Amipaque ventriculography, median tomogram. Medulloblastoma of the fourth ventricle without infiltration of its floor

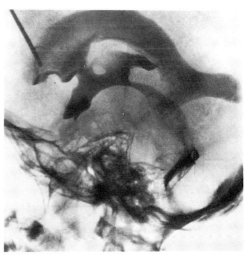

Fig. 3. M. Ch., 6 years: Amipaque ventriculography, lateral view. Astrocytoma grade I of pontine brain stem. Amipaque passes into cisterna magna and spinal subarachnoid space

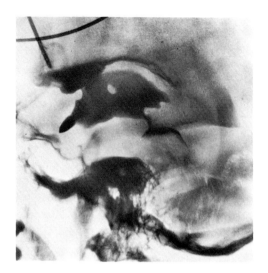

Fig. 4. K. C., 13 years: Amipaque ventriculography, lateral view. Polar spongioblastoma of vermis cerebelli infiltrating the adjacent brain stem. Complete blockage of the CSF pathways on the level of the fourth ventricle. Morbus Recklinghausen

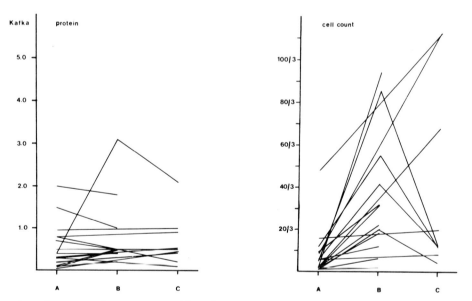

Fig. 5. Protein content (*left*) and cell count (*right*) in ventricular cerebrospinal fluid of 17 patients
A Before ventriculography with Amipaque
B 1-2 days after ventriculography
C 3-4 days after ventriculography

Value of Central Ventriculography With Dimer-X in the Differentiation Between Cerebellar Tumors and Caudal Brain Stem Tumors Before and After Radiation Therapy of So-Called Inoperable Midline Tumors

H. Altenburg and W. Walter

Despite modern progress in neuroradiology, central ventriculography with positive, water-soluble contrast media continues to be of great importance in the diagnosis of space-occupying or stenosing lesions of the midline structures, particularly of the midbrain, the oral and caudal brain stem, and the cerebellum, and in the planning and performing of the operative procedure (1, 3, 4, 8, 12).

Because of its almost exclusively neursurgical orientation in that it aims at clarifying the diagnosis and operability of a lesion, the indication for this examination should be posed only in a primarily neursurgical environment, where the conditions for a subsequent surveillance of the patient and, if necessary, for an immediate neurosurgical operation are given (13). Only if it is employed in the right manner does this method provide the maximum information in the hand of the experienced investigator (2, 9). It should be carried out only if all other possibilities have been exhausted.

Thanks to the clear visualization of the decisive structures, it can clarify the question of operability of a space-occupying lesion of the midbrain and cerebellum, in the latter case by demonstrating the relationship of the tumor to the floor of the fourth ventricle. Furthermore, it offers the possibility of rapid diagnosis of a space-occupying lesion in the posterior fossa in cases of greatest urgency, as in the case of impending or existing decerebration, i.e., in cases where the diagnostic measures are immediately followed by CSF drainage.

Typical ventriculographic pictures of cerebellar and caudal brain stem tumors are (6): 1) medial and lateral cerebellar tumors and tumors of the fourth ventricle (Fig. 1 shows a typical example of intraventricular tumor) and 2) caudal brain stem tumors (Fig. 2 demonstrates a typical ventriculogram for this type of tumor). Beyond this, central ventriculography makes it possible to show the effect of radiation therapy on midbrain tumors previously diagnosed by ventriculography (5, 7). SUZUKI and HORI (11) and PERTUISET and collaborators (10) are the only authors who have pointed out the value of control ventriculography with positive contrast media and to report their experience with pineal tumors.

We have also made it a rule to control the therapeutic success during and after radiation therapy with the help of ventriculography and to find an objective basis for the improvement, which may be attributed either to the shunt operation or to radiation therapy. If there is little or no reaction to the radiation, a neurosurgical indication must be posed. A typical picture of a patient before and after successful radiation treatment is shown in Figure 3.

In our opinion, central ventriculography provides the neurosurgeon with the decisive localizing signs for cerebellar and midbrain tumors, important in planning such a tumor operation. Exact information must be obtained about the relationship of the space-occupying lesions to the third ventricle, to the floor of the fourth ventricle, and to the aqueduct and, thus, to the vital midline regulatory centers.

References

1. AGNOLI, A., EGGERT, H.R., ZIERSKI, J., SEEGER, W., KIRCHHOFF, D.: Diagnostische Möglichkeiten der positiven Ventrikulographie. Acta Neurochir. 31, 227-243 (1975)
2. ANDREUSSI, L., CLARISSE, J., JOMIN, M., PASSERINI, A.: Ventriculography with watersoluble contrast in the diagnosis of posterior fossa tumors (107 cases). Neuroradiology 8, 25-38 (1974)
3. CRONQVIST, S.: Ventriculography with Amipaque. Neuroradiology 12, 25-32 (1976)
4. FINCK, M., VOGELSANG, H.: Experience with Dimer-X-ventriculography. Neuropädiatrie 6, 339-346 (1975)
5. JENNETT, B., JOHNSON, R., REID, R.: Postive contrast ventriculography of pineal region tumours. Acta Radiol. Diagn. 1, 857-871 (1963)
6. KUNZE, St.: Die zentrale Ventrikulographie mit wasserlöslichen, resorbierbaren Kontrastmitteln. Schriftenr. Neurologie, Bd. 13. Berlin-Heidelberg-New York: Springer 1974
7. KUNZE, St., SCHIEFER, W.: Ventrikulographie mit positiven Kontrastmitteln bei raumfordernden Prozessen der Mittellinie und im Bereich der hinteren Schädelgrube. Radiologe 9, 495-499 (1969)
8. KUNZE, St., KLINGER, M., SCHIEFER, W.: Central ventriculography with Dimer-X. Acta Neurochir. 28, 41-63 (1973)
9. LEONARDI, M., CECOTTO, C., FABRIS, G.: Corrales selective ventriculography in the study of posterior fossa pathology. J. Neurosurg. Sci. 21, 65-70 (1977)
10. PERTUISET, B., VISOT, A., METZGER, J.: Diagnosis of pinealoblastomas by positive response to cobalt-therapy. Acta Neurochir. 34, 151-152 (1976)
11. SUZUKI, J., HORI, S.: Evaluation of radiotherapy of tumors in the pineal region by ventriculographic studies with iodized oil. J. Neurosurg. 30, 595-603 (1969)
12. SUZUKI, S., KAWAGUCHI, S., MITA, R., IWABUCHI, T.: Ventriculography with methylglucamine iocarmate (Dimer-X). Experimental and clinical study. Acta Neurochir. 33, 219-231 (1976)
13. WINKELMANN, H.: Zentrale Dimer-X-Ventrikulographie. Indikationsstellung, Methodik und Aussagewert. Radiol. Diagn. 6, 825-835 (1975)

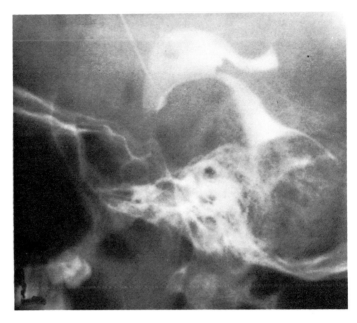

Fig. 1. Lateral view of Dimer-X ventriculogram showing a large tumor of the fourth ventricle and occlusive hydrocephalus

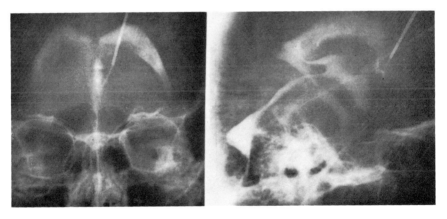

Fig. 2. Frontal and lateral view of a ventriculogram typical for a caudal brain stem tumor

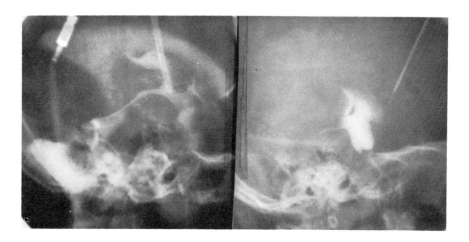

Fig. 3. Ventriculography before (*right*) and after (*left*) successful radiation therapy

Computer Tomography

Typical Findings With Computerized Tomography in Tumors of the Posterior Fossa

TH. GRUMME, A. AULICH, E. KAZNER, K. KRETSCHMAR, W. LANKSCH, and W. MEESE

The findings presented here are the result of computerized tomography (CT) in 398 tumors of the posterior fossa and represent a cooperative effort on the part of CT research teams in Berlin, Mainz, and Munich. The studies were performed solely in the horizontal plane, and each study was repeated after injection of a contrast medium (1 ml of 60%-66% contrast medium per kg body weight) when there was no contraindication to the procedure.

Interpretation of the computerized tomogram in tumors of the posterior fossa depends on direct demonstration of the tumor and its accompanying edema as well as on the relationship of neighboring structures, such as the fourth ventricle, the cisterns, the brain stem, and the cerebellum. One can also identify secondary effects on the supratentorial ventricular system (1, 2).

Table 1 summarizes absorption values, contrast enhancement, and frequency of localized edema in uncontrasted tomograms in 398 tumors of the posterior fossa. The following report will attempt to present characteristic tomographic findings for the individual tumor groups, although we are aware that considerable problems of differential diagnosis may be present in individual cases.

Medulloblastoma (Fig. 1a)

The medulloblastoma presents a fairly uniform picture with CT. Eighty-four percent of these tumors demonstrated homogeneous or slightly increased density in the plain scan. These areas consistently took up contrast media at an average rate of 3-8 EMI units. However, we observed two cases in which total necrosis resulted in diminished density in the plain scan as well as failure to take up contrast media. Primarily isodense tumors also concentrate contrast media well. Cysts calcification, and/or local necrosis occur in 20% of tumors. The medulloblastoma in children was almost always in contact with the fourth ventricle, while the tumor manifested itself more frequently in the cerebellar hemispheres in adults.

Spongioblastoma (Fig. 1b)

Spongioblastoma do not constitute a uniform group where absorption characteristics are concerned. One can differentiate three types:
1. Lesions with large cysts and diminished density. Only solid tumor tissue accepts contrast media, so the tumors appear as rings.

Table 1. CT findings in 398 tumors of the posterior fossa

Histologic diagnosis	No.	Absorption of tumor in plain scan			Tumor not visible in plain scan Ø	Contrast medium accumulation in tumor			Perifocal edema			
		In-creased	De-creased	Equal	Mixed		No.	Pos.	Neg.	grade No.	I	II	III
Spongioblastoma	37	2	16	8	11	2	32	26	6	8	8	–	–
Ependymoma	14	6	2	2	4	–	9	9	–	5	5	–	–
Medulloblastoma	44	28	2	5	9	1	42	40	2	16	14	2	–
Neuroma	107	15	10	62ª	7	61	105	92	13	28	24	4	–
Angioblastoma	22	1	18	1	2	1	22	6	16	3	3	–	–
Meningeoma	43	30	1	11	1	7	35	35	–	13	12	1	–
Sarcoma	9	3	1	1	4	1	9	9	–	5	5	–	–
Epidermoid	7	–	6	–	1	–	3	–	3	–	–	–	–
Metastases	53	16	18	10ᵇ	8	8	51	42	9	34	20	14	–
Other cerebellar tumors	28	9	5	3ᶜ	8	6	22	20	2	10	9	1	–
Tumors of unknown histology	34	10	18	4	2	2	33	23	10	11	8	2	1
Total	398	120	97	107	57	89	363	302	61	133	108	24	1
Percentage		30.2	24.4	26.9	14.3	22.4	91.2	83.2	16.8	33.4	81.2	18	0.8

ª Thirteen tumors were not detected.
ᵇ An incorrect slice in one case.
ᶜ Three tumors were not detected.

2. Tumors with isodense areas as well as areas of lower density. These lesions are composed mainly of solid tumor with a smaller cystic portion.
3. Isodense tumors and tumors with slightly reduced density which take up contrast media uniformly. These are solid tumors. The two cases which demonstrated increased density contained hemorrhages.

Angioblastoma (Fig. 2b)

The computerized tomogram most often reveals a circumscribed area of low density caused by cysts which make up the greater part of the tumor. The small solid portion is seldom demonstrated with contrast medium. The rare solid angioblastoma is characterized by strong, though inhomogeneous, uptake of contrast medium.

Ependymoma (Fig. 1c)

The absorption characteristics of ependymomas are not uniform. Our previous experience indicates that an ependymoma is most likely when many small calcifications are present in a tumor of slightly increased density found in a typical location. Certain differentiation from a medulloblastoma is often impossible. In contrast to the ependymoma, a choroid plexus papilloma of the fourth ventricle can be clearly delineated as a tumor with an irregular wooly surface surrounded on all sides by CSF.

Cerebellar Sarcoma

The cerebellar sarcoma is often cystic with a solid portion that readily takes up contrast media.

Metastases (Fig. 2d)

The absorption characteristics of metastases are extremely variable, and the contrasted tomogram produces widely varying results as well. One can find rings, solid and mixed tumors, as well as those that are only visible as a result of surrounding edema. We found the edema in two-thirds of our patients. It can be quite pronounced and is, therefore, the most typical characteristic of metastases. We rarely observed multiple metastases in the cerebellum, but we often found a combinnation of infra- and supratentorial lesions. Meningeal carcinomatosis cannot be demonstrated with first-generation scanners.

Acoustic neuroma (Figs. 2c and 3)

The absorption characteristics of the acoustic neuroma are to be found in Table 1. It is often impossible to demonstrate this tumor in the plain scan. In plain scans, 61 of 107 acoustic neuromas (57%) were not detected. Thirteen surgically verified acoustic neuromas (12%) went undetected even after injection of a contrast medium. With one exception, the diameters of these tumors were less than 1.5 cm. Evidence of indirect tumor signs, such as displacement of or inadequate demonstration of the fourth ventricle, hydrocephalus, or localized edema deserve special attention (1).

Meningeoma (Figs. 2a and 3)

A large majority of menigeomas (70%) demonstrated increased density in the plain scan. The isodense meningeoma is also typical: 26% had the same density as the surrounding cerebral tissue. Contrast enhancement was strong in every case. A localized edema is relatively rare in cases of infratentorial meningeoma in comparison with such tumors in the supratentorial area. The tentorium takes up contrast media readily and thus allows exact localization of the tumor. A malignant lymphoma cannot always be clearly distinguished from a meningeoma.

Epidermoid

The density of the epidermoid is the same as or less than that of the CSF. There is no uptake of contrast media. Peripheral calcification may be noted. Typical locations within the posterior fossa are the cerebellopontine angle and the fourth ventricle.

Concluding Remarks

Of 2000 brain tumors studied with CT at the university hospitals in Berlin, Mainz, and Munich, 291 (excluding acoustic neuromas) were located in the posterior fossa; 263 tumors (90.4%) were visible in the plain scan, and contrast enhancement raised the rate of detection to 96.6%. Results were poorer on inclusion of acoustic neuromas (107 cases), especially with plain scans. Only 77.6% of the tumors were demonstrated without contrast media (Table 2).

Many tumors show characteristic tomographic findings which provide diagnostically important indications of the tumor type. This is especially true of cerebellar tumors in children and of angioblastomas and meningeomas of the posterior fossa. Cystic and solid tumors can be differentiated preoperatively with a great deal of certainty. However, accurate preoperative histologic diagnoses are usually only possible in individual cases in which the patient's age and clinical evidence are also considered (Fig. 3). Localizing diagnosis permits accurate surgical therapy. Angiography of the vertebral artery is usually unnecessary in children with cerebellar tumors, but the procedure is recommended in adolescents and adults, especially in cases of tumors with strong uptake of contrast media. Ventriculography is usually unnecessary except in cases with ambiguous computer tomographic and angiographic results.

Table 2. Effectiveness of CT studies in tumors of the posterior fossa (with and without inclusion of acoustic neuromas)

	No.	Visible in plain scan No.	%	Visible after enhancement No.	%	Not visible in CT No.	%
Tumors of the posterior fossa without acoustic neuroma	291	263	90.4	281	96.6	10	3.4
Tumors of the posterior fossa with acoustic neuroma	398	309	77.6	375	94.2	23	5.8

References

1. GYLDENSTED, C., LESTER, I., THOMSEN, I.: Computer tomography in the diagnosis of cerebellopontine angle tumours. Neuroradiology 11, 191-197 (1976)
2. KAZNER, E., AULICH, A., GRUMME, Th.: Results of computerized axial tomography with infratentorial tumors. In: Cranial Computerized Tomography. LANKSCH, W., KAZNER, E. (eds.), p. 90. Berlin-Heidelberg-New York: Springer 1976

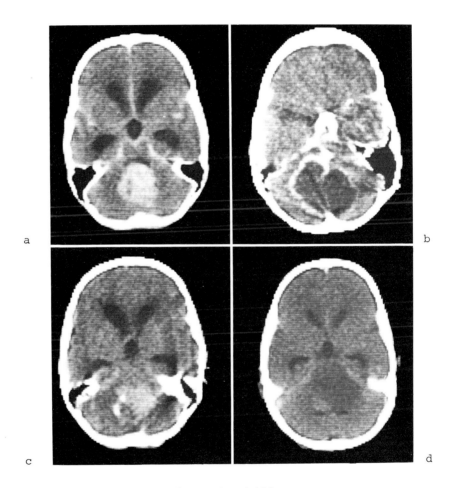

Fig. 1. Tumors of the posterior fossa in children
<u>a</u> Medulloblastoma   CT No. M 5322/76
<u>b</u> Spongioblastoma   CT No. B 339/76
<u>c</u> Ependymoma   CT No. M 4945/76
<u>d</u> Glioma of the brain stem CT No. M 5648/77

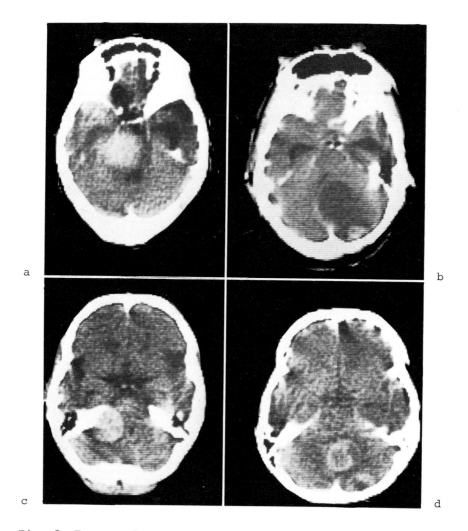

Fig. 2. Tumors of the posterior fossa in adults
a Tentorial meningeoma (*left*)   CT No. B   96/76
b Angioblastoma (*right*)   CT No. B 1253/77
c Acoustic neuroma (*left*)   CT No. B 463/77
d Cerebellar metastases   CT No. B 1838/76

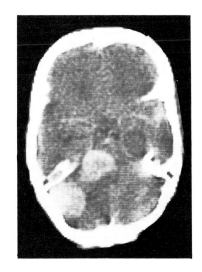

Fig. 3. Simultaneous presence of neuroma (medial tumor) and meningeoma (lateral tumor). CT No. B 2281/76

Limitations of Computerized Tomography in the Detection of Posterior Fossa Lesions

E. KAZNER, TH. GRUMME, W. LANKSCH, and J. WILSKE

By means of computerized tomography (CT), it is possible to directly demonstrate tumors and other lesions in the cerebellum and the caudal brain stem at a high percentage. Even the histologic diagnosis can be predicted correctly in many cases (1); however, the posterior cranial fossa undoubtedly forms the most difficult region within the cranial cavity for CT diagnosis. This is mainly due to the numerous bony structures of the skull base which may considerably affect the quality of CT scans. On the other hand, the percentage of isodense lesions (27%) is extraordinarily high in this region (acoustic neuromas included).

Frequent Artifacts

The most frequent artifact is a black horizontal line between the petrous bones - the so-called *Hounsfield* line - which can mask a lesion within the brain stem or the cerebellopontine angle (2). It is important to bear in mind the occurence of a radial artifact, originating from the inion (internal occipital protuberance). Erroneous positive findings may be simulated by this artifact. An "area artifact" (4) which occasionaly appears must also be mentioned here. It can cover a whole cerebellar hemisphere and thus simulate a large posterior fossa meningioma or a sarcoma.

Limitations of Tumor Detection

In some cases, an absolutely certain proof of a tumor is not possible even if the CT picture is analyzed subtly, contrast enhancement has been performed, intermediate slices have been scanned, and the investigation has been carried out under general anesthesia. Practically, this is true for all posterior fossa tumors with a diameter less than 1.5 cm. Without using contrast enhancement and scanning intermediate slices, a CT investigation must be considered as faulty today. Especially cerebellar metastases and acoustic neuromas may thus be missed in many cases.

However, in very rare cases, even cerebellar tumors of more than 15 mm in diameter elude CT detection if these are primarily isodense, do not show contrast medium uptake, and do not affect the neighboring structures.

Case Report

In a 7-year-old boy with distinct cerebellar symptoms pointing to a left-sided lesion, it was not possible to demonstrate the underlying tumor even by repeated CT investigations. The ventricular system was very small. Therefore, we performed an pneumencephalogram which only showed air within the cisterns. At a third CT study following intrathecal contrast medium injection, a slight torsion of the brain stem was suspicious. The ventricular system was somewhat enlarged compared with the initial CT scan (Fig. 1). Only by central ventriculography was it possible to diagnose with absolute certainty the cerebellar tumor which had shifted the fourth ventricle to the right and caused partial CSF blockage. At operation, a walnut-sized cerebellar astrocytoma grade II could be partially removed. The tumor had invaded the brain stem. Similar diagnostic difficulties occurred in three other patients in a series of 95 children with cerebellar tumors.

Vermian Pseudotumor

The diagnosis or exclusion of a vermian tumor may be extremely difficult, especially if the ventricular system is not dilated and the tumor exhibits only slight contrast enhancement, since the cerebellar vermis normally can show slightly increased absorption and distinct contrast medium uptake (Fig. 2). This potential pitfall of CT scanning has led to the term "vermian pseudotumor" (3). If, in addition, a hydrocephalus is present, we strongly recommend that a central ventriculography be performed. In the child whose CT scan is shown in Figure 3, the clinical data indeed pointed to a stenosis of the aqueduct; however, a vermian tumor could not be excluded from the CT scan. The ventriculogram shows the thread-like aqueduct to be the cause of the hydrocephalus (Fig. 3b).

Differential Diagnosis

The prediction of the differential diagnosis of cerebellar tumors based on the CT finding is limited by histologic peculiarities of some tumors. Thus, in necrotic medulloblastomas, contrast enhancement is lacking. The proportion of such tumors, however, is below 10%. With cerebellar astrocytomas, too, there may occur single cases without contrast medium uptake as was observed in a child with a solid, avascular, hyaline tumor which was identified as a variant of pilocytic astrocytoma. The CT scan showed only a large hypodense area which did not change its absorption after contrast medium application.

Differential diagnosis of lesions within the cerebellopontine angle also has its malices. It is not possible to dinstinguish between a neuroma or a meningioma since shape, site, absorption values, and the results of contrast-with-time studies are very similar. In one rare case, we observed a laterally developed giant basilar aneurysm which imitated an acoustic neuroma with regard to the clinical symptoms and the CT finding. Solid angioblastomas as well as melanoma metastases may simulate an acoustic neuroma in the CT scan.

Brain Stem Affection

Im some cases, the demarcation of cerebellar tumors against the brain stem, especially the lower part, is not possible with certainty. Since, in our experience, this question cannot be answered even by means of ventriculograms, it often happens that the neurosurgeon has to decide at operation if an tumor can be removed completely or not. In addition, the question of whether a lesion is situated intra-, para-, or prepontine cannot easily be answered on the basis of the CT finding. Thus, we suspected an intrapontine tumor in the case of a clivus chordoma. Because of the bad condition of the patient, further neuroradiologic investigations remained undone. At autopsy, an extremely thinned elevated pons covering the big basal tumor was found. Even knowing this result, it was not possible to interpret the CT scan correctly.

Cerebellar Hematomas and Infarctions

While the detection of freshly coagulated blood within the cerebellum or the brain stem does not cause any diagnostic problems, older intracerebellar hematomas may be missed because the x-ray absorption of such hematomas decrease continuously in the course of several weeks due to the catabolism of hemoglobin. Thus, the hematoma becomes isodense. In our series, we have missed three cerebellar hematomas which could be confirmed at operation or at postmortem examination. Recent cerebellar infarcts with compressing edema sometimes cannot be differentiated from a cerebellar tumor, especially if there is some contrast enhancement of the lesion. Hydrocephalus develops within hours. The infarcted area looks translucent after some hours. The decisive diagnostic pointer is offered by the case history.

Conclusions

Computerized tomography has greatly enriched the diagnostic equipment in our specialty and undoubtedly opened numerous new aspects. However, increasing experience with this still developing method has already shown some limitations of CT scanning. Numerous diagnostic errors will occur if not all clinical and paraclinical findings are considered. This underlines the fact that computerized tomography cannot replace the classic neuroradiologic methods in all cases.

References

1. KAZNER, E., AULICH, A., GRUMME, Th.: Results of computerized axial tomography with infratentorial tumors. In: Cranial Computerized Tomography. LANKSCH, W., KAZNER, E. (eds.), pp. 90-103. Berlin-Heidelberg-New York: Springer 1976
2. KAZNER, E., LANKSCH, W., STEINHOFF, H., WILSKE, J.: Die axiale Computer-Tomographie des Gehirnschädels - Anwendungsmöglichkeiten und klinische Ergebnisse. Fortschr. Neurol. Psychiatr. 43, 487-574 (1975)
3. KRAMER, R.A.: Vermian pseudotumor: a potential pitfall of CT brain scanning with contrast enhancement. Neuroradiology 13, 229-230 (1977)
4. LANGE, S., AULICH, A., LANKSCH, W.: Image artefacts in computerized tomography. In: Cranial Computerized Tomography. LANKSCH, W., KAZNER, E. (eds.), pp. 69-72. Berlin-Heidelberg-New York: Springer 1976

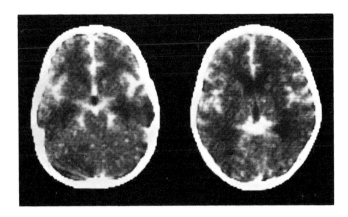

Fig. 1. CT scan of a 7-year-old boy with left-sided cerebellar tumor after intrathecal injection of Amipaque. Slight torsion of the brain stem. Slight enlargement of the anterior horns. No direct or indirect tumor demonstration (patient Ch. K., CT No. M 7148/77)

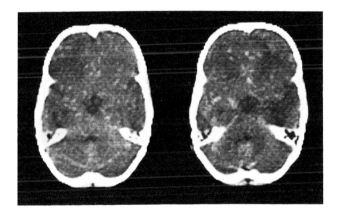

Fig. 2. Normal CT scan of a 7-year-old boy with "vermian pseudotumor." Distinct contrast medium uptake in the vermis (*right*). In the plain scan, the vermis is also slightly increased in absorption compared with the surrounding cerebellum (patient J. H., CT No. M 5521/77)

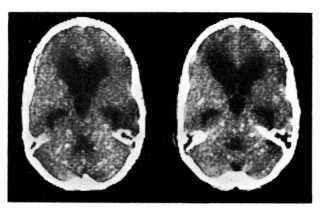
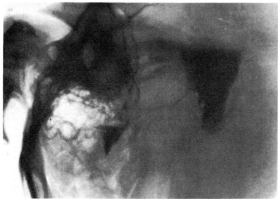

Fig. 3. *Above:* Vermian pseudotumor in the CT scan of a 13-year-old boy with stenosis of the aqueduct, before *(left)* and after *(right)* contrast enhancement (patient H. A., CT No. M 5470/77)
Below: Thread-like aqueduct visible in the ventriculogram with Dimer-X

Computerized Tomography of the Posterior Fossa and the Upper Cervical Spine

W. ISCHEBECK, H. U. THAL, and R. NABAKOWSKI

In spite of the diagnostic advantages of computerized tomography (CT), the posterior fossa and the upper cervical spine remain the most difficult regions to examine. Exact diagnosis is of utmost importance for the right choice of therapy (3). There has already been some improvement in the more recent CT scanners. Thus, it is now possible to extend the examination to the facial skull and the upper spine, water-coupling is no longer necessary, the scan and reconstruction time is much shorter, and the technical methods are much more variable. It is very important that the tentorium is clearly visible so that tumors can be shown in their actual connection to it. This applies, for example, to meningeomas and aneurysms so that the proper invasive neuroradiologic examination can be undertaken. The diagnostic results of the CT examinations are often limited by the difficulties presented by the Hounsfiled line and other artifacts in the regions under the tentorium. Therefore, it is, for example, very often difficult to decide whether or not there is a small acoustic neuroma in the cerebellar pontine angle. If the densities of the various tissues vary sufficiently, they can be shown on the CT without difficulty. Thus, it is no problem to differentiate CSF, cysts, or tumors of high density (e.g., cylindroma) growing from the mandibular angle to the posterior fossa through the foramen magnum. It is neither difficult to visualize the base of the skull nor to show its main cavities and foramina. Sometimes the contours of the cervical cord with its surrounding CSF can be shown, but very often it is disturbed by artifacts. It is rarely possible to documentate pathologic structures in plain scan and after contrast injection.

We suggest three additional means for improving the examination of these specific regions:
1. The positioning of the patient must be varied according to the region in which a lesion is suspected.
2. The lumbar or suboccipital puncture with metrizamide leads to better results, as reported by GREITZ and HINDMARSH (1).
3. An exact analysis of the absorption numbers and the histogram should be made.

In our experience, it has proved to be advantageous not to position the patient in the orbito meatal line. Retroflecting the head of the patient 15°-20° backward for scanning increases the distance between the protuberantia occipitalis interna and the petrosous bone, thereby minimizing the artifacts. To show the pons and the upper part of the cerebellar pontine angle, it is useful to cut the pyramid only partly. Thus, the basilar artery can be easily assessed.

An increasing number of authors suggest a position for the coronal section of the brain. As a rule, we do not think that this positioning provides improved information to any agreat extent. However, we must admit that we examined one patient with a very large oligodendroglioma of the left occipital region presenting the tentorium to such an extend that the fourth ventricle was displaced to the other side. We suspected an infratentorial growth of the tumor, which was not the case. In this instance, the coronal section would have been better, even though this position produces several artifacts.

The use of metrazamide is advantageous because the contours, especially of the cervical cord, are well-outlined (Fig. 1) and compressing lesions can be diagnosed easily. A lack of metrazamide resorption even enables us to diagnose tumors which are isodense and showing no enhancement after intravenous contrast-injection. The case of a patient with an astrocytoma of the cerebellar hemisphere, which is very rare, serves as an example. The 76-year-old man had all signs of a compressing lesion in the right cerebellar pontine angle and died soon after the CT scan was performed. Therefore, the anatomicopathologic specimen can be shown (Fig. 2). The exact cross-section makes it understandable that the histogram of the right side shows such a decreased density (Figs. 3 and 4). There was no enhancement after contrast, but the metrazamide was not to be seen on the CT in a large part of the right cerebellar hemisphere.

We do not find all tumors of the posterior fossa in CT. Therefore, when a ventriculography with water-soluble contrast medium has been performed, a CT scan should follow in order to ascertain the form and displacement of the fourth ventricle in an axial section.

A systematic evaluation of the CT absorption numbers in very important and facilitated by the exact determination of the regions under question (Figs. 3 and 4). The histogram shows the scale of the absorption numbers for the different tumors, and the extent of enhancement must be studied. It is also of considerable importance to allow differentiation between contusions and intracerebellar hemorrhages, which influences the indication of whether or not an operation should be performed.

To distinguish between tumor-cysts and ventricle or cysts of other origin, we found, for example, that the cyst of an astrocytoma of the cerebellum shows a much higher increase in density after contrast than the other structures do. This is especially interesting because the solid tumor parts of the spongioblastoma often cannot be shown in CT.

To find the correct preoperative diagnosis, more knowledge is necessary on the morphologic structures which can be seen in CT. On the one hand, that means cutting the brain in the exact parallel direction with a CT macrotome, and on the other hand, the postmortal scanning of normal and pathologic structures (Fig. 1) so that we may be able to learn which real absorption numbers of those regions are disturbed by artifacts. With a good brain phantom for CT scanners, even artifacts can be simulated. We can then obtain fundamental information to improve the computer program for the reconstruction of the pictures (2).

Summary

Possibilities to improve the results of computerized tomography in the infratentorial region and the upper cervical spine are discussed. The proper positioning of the patient, the intrathecal injection of metrizamide, and the exact analysis of the absorption numbers are the main points of discussion. Results of morphologic studies are shown.

References

1. GREITZ, T., HINDMARSH, T.: Computer assisted tomography of intracranial CSF circulation using a water-soluble contrast medium. Acta Radiol. 15, 497-507 (1974)
2. ISCHEBECK, W., THOERNER, G.: A new CT-Macrotome for the brain and a documentation system for the brain scanners of the new generation. Abstracts of the International Symposium and Course on Computed Tomography. Miami Beach, USA (1977) in J. Comp. Assoc. Tomogr. 1, 410 (1977)
3. KAZNER, E. AULICH, A., GRUMME, Th.: Results of computerized axial tomography with infratentorial tumors. In: Cranial Computerized Tomography. LANKSCH, W., KAZNER, E. (eds.), pp. 90-103. Berlin-Heidelberg-New York: Springer 1976

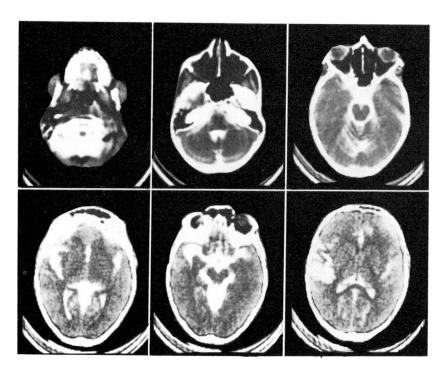

Fig. 1. CT after metrizamide. Especially the atrophy of the cerebellum and the left temporoparietal region is visualized

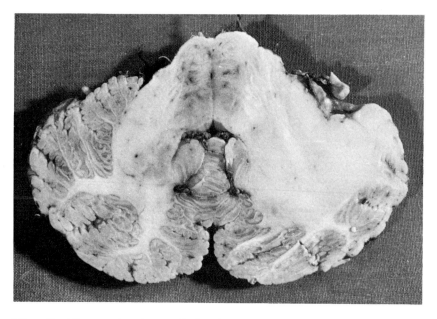

Fig. 2. The anatomicopathologic specimen of an amitotic astrocytoma of the right cerebellum

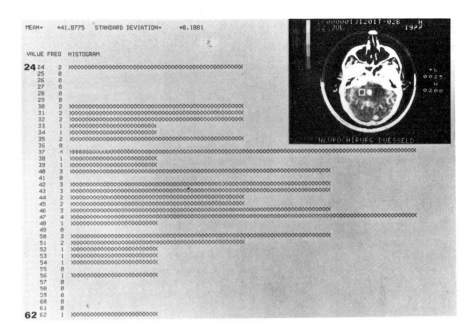

Fig.3

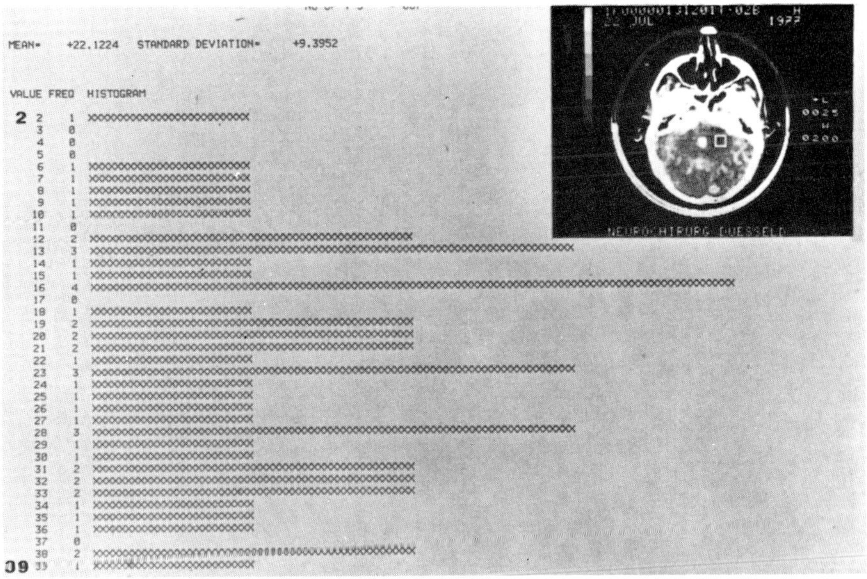

Fig.4

Figs. 3 and 4. Histogram of hypodense tumor (see Fig. 2) of the right cerebellum compared with the left side (after metrizamide)

Vascular Derformity of the Basilar Artery Which Gave the Clinical and Computerized Tomographic Impression of a Tumor

W. MAUERSBERGER

Only a few years after its introduction into neuroradiologic diagnostics, computer-assisted tomography has established a preeminent position in the field. However, it should not be forgotten that even this method has its limitations and that the results obtained can be misleading in some cases; thus, traditional neuroradiologic examination methods, especially angiography, retain their value.

We gained this experience in a particularly impressive way in the following case. A 45-year-old patient was referred to us by her attending physician because of impaired vision and difficulty in walking, which had persisted for several weeks. At the initial examination, hypertension with values of 140/110 mm Hg was noted among the internal results. On neurologic examination, we found bilateral reduction of visual acuity, choked optic disks bilaterally, and hypoesthesia of the left half of the face. The corneal reflex was not elicited on either side. Romberg's test showed moderate unsteadiness in standing; the gait was straddle-legged and staggering.

After an initial clinical diagnosis of a tumor of the posterior cranial fossa had been made, computerized tomography was performed. The tomogram showed bilateral hyperdense areas ca. 2 x 2 cm in size, which demonstrated positive enhancement after administration of contrast medium. In addition, the ventricular system was clearly enlarged (Fig. 1). The diagnosis of a bilateral tumor of the cerebellopontine angle thus appeared to be confirmed. Differential diagnosis suggested a meningioma because of noninvolvement of the acoustic nerve and positive enhancement in the computer tomogram.

Brachial angiography clearly showed widening of the intracranial segment of the internal carotid artery, with anterior and middle cerebral arteries of nearly normal width. The right vertebral artery and the basilar artery also appeared to be considerably widened and elongated. At the same time, the basilar artery described a widely projecting arc, which extented from the right far beyond the middle line almost into the left cerebellopontine angle and then returned from there to the midline. In addition, it was also striking that the contrast medium remained in the arterial vessels until late in the venous phase (Fig. 2). The areas of high density observed in the computer tomogram are to be interpreted as transverse sections of an extremely widened basilar artery and not, as originally assumed, as tumors.

Discussion

Extreme dilation and convolution of the vessels can simulate a compressing process, especially in the area of the posterior cranial fossa. This was reported by GREITZ and LÖFSTEDT (1) concerning five patients in whom enlargement of the ventricular system was caused by compression of the aqueduct. SCOTT and STAUFER (3) found that various cranial nerves were also impaired, in the case of a fusiform aneurysm of the basilar artery which simulated a compressing lesion in the pneumoencephalogram. WALLACE and JAFFE (4) observed a similar case. REUTER et al (2) reported two cases of vascular deformity of the posterior cranial fossa in which an initial diagnosis of tumor was made.

In the case presented here, the clinical findings as well as the computer tomogram were more indicative of a tumor. However, since the time we operated on another of our patients, in whom we had diagnosed an acoustic neurinoma on the basis of the clinical findings and the computer tomogram without further diagnostic measures, and found a huge aneurysm of the basilar artery extending into the crebellopontine angle (Fig. 3) at operation, we consider angiography to be an absolutely indispensable part of preoperative diagnostics, without which the operation of a tumor should not be performed.

Summary

In a 45-year-old patient with impaired vision and difficulty in walking which had lasted for several weeks, who appeared to have bilateral choked disks as well as damage to the trigeminal nerve, the computer tomogram revealed a bilateral hyperdense area with positive enhancement in the region of the cerebellopontine angle. Exclusion of a tumor and detection of a dolichomegabasilaris first was possible only with the aid of angiography. We concluded, therefore, that in every patient with the diagnosis of a tumor, arteriographic clarification of the findings in addition to computerized tomography should be undertaken.

References

1. GREITZ, T., LÖFSTEDT, S.: The relationship between the third ventricle and the basilar artery. Acta Radiol. 42, 85-100 (1954)
2. REUTER, S.R., NEWTON, Th., GREITZ, T.: Arteriovenous malformations of the posterior fossa. Radiology 87, 1880-1888 (1966)
3. SCOTT, M., STAUFER, H.M.: A case of aneurysmal malformation of the vertebral and basilar arteries causing cranial nerve involvement. Am. J. Roentgenol. 92, 836-837 (1964)
4. WALLACE, S., JAFFE, M.E.: Cerebral arterial ectasia with sacular aneurysms. Radiology 88, 90-93 (1967)

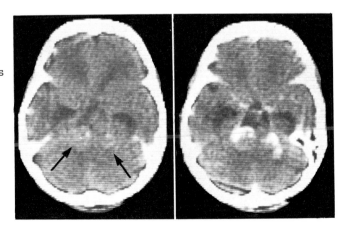

Fig. 1
Left: Native scan revealed bilateral areas of slightly increased density at the region of the cerebellopontine angle *(arrows)* and hydrocephalic dilatation of the ventricular system *Right:* Positive enhancement of the suspicious region after administration of contrast medium

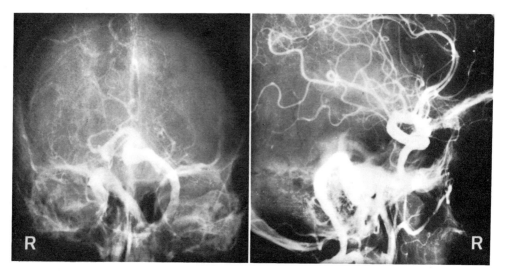

Fig. 2. Vertebral angiography demonstrated a dolichomegabasilaris and repudiated the theory of the existence of a tumor

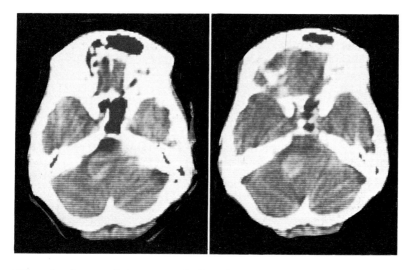

Fig. 3. Area of increased density at the left cerebellopontine angle (*left*), with strong positive enhancement after contrast medium application (*right*), corresponding to a giant basilar aneurysm which was misinterpreted as an acoustic neurinoma

Intracranial Pressure

Long-Term Measuring of Ventricular CSF Pressure With Tumors of the Posterior Fossa

K. E. RICHARD

Introduction

Among the patient material of the authors (2, 6, 7, 9), who have special clinical experience in methods and indication of measuring intracranial pressure, patients with space-occupying infratentorial processes form a relatively small group. This is quite surprising, as acute increase of CSF pressure after operation within the posterior fossa has been known for a long time and has been treated - according to CUSHING - by single or repeated drainage of CSF by puncturing the lateral ventricle.

Patient Material

In the course of 4 years, we examined ventricular fluid pressure (VFP) behavior in pre- and postoperative therapy with a total of 82 patients suffering from infratentorial space-occupying processes. Within the scope of this subject, we will deal with brain tumors of the posterior fossa only (Table 1).

We restrict ourselves to the following points:
1. Relationship between tumorous *dilatation of the ventricle* and *ventricular fluid pressure*
2. Importance of *ventricular fluid pressure* and *neurologic* or *metabolic disturbances under treatment*

Table 1. Tumors of fossa posterior (No. = 82)

Cerebellar tumors	Spongioblastoma	24	
	Ependymoma	5	
	Medulloblastoma	12	56
	Plexuspapilloma	4	
	Angioblastoma	5	
	Nonclassified tumors	6	
Extracerebellar tumors	Neurinoma	15	
	Meningioma	3	20
	Metastasis	2	
Intrapontine tumors		4	6
Aneurysm of basilar artery		2	

Total duration of VFP monitoring: 369 days
Mean duration: 4.6 days

3. Behavior of ventricular CSF pressure in *uncomplicated cases* and typical postoperative *complications*

Results and Discussion

1. VFP and Dilatation of the Ventricle

On observation of the ratio between mean VFP as measured before pressure-decreasing therapy and *dilatation of the ventricle* (Fig. 1) - represented by the thickness of the frontal brain mantle - we find that, on an average, higher pressure was measured with tumorous hydrocephali than with the ones that were not tumorous; apart from that, pressure of the hydrocephali was generally somewhat lower with cerebellar tumors than with hydrocephali of supratentorial or midline tumors. A hyperdilatation of the ventricle with a frontal thickness of the brain mantle of less than 2 cm was not frequent with tumors. Thus, tumorous hydrocephali correlated with higher pressures than the nontumorous ones. This difference can be due - as is suggested by experimental results obtained by OMMAYA et al.(10) - to differing increases of CSF volume with the different kinds of hydrocephalus. Tumors of the cerebral hemispheres and the midline lead to a more rapid increase of CSF volume by blocking CSF passage and thus - at least initially - to higher pressure than processes with gradually increasing volume.

2. VFP, Brain Function, and Course

On distributing the mean and maximum pressure values measured on individual days of preoperative, early postoperative, and late postoperative periods, according to the *clinical* course (survivals: primary, i.e., died within the 1st or 2nd postoperative week and secondary, i.e., died after the 2nd postoperative week), we will find the following relationships (Fig. 2a and b):

a) On preoperative days of measuring, mean VFP was generally between 16-30 mm Hg. The height of VFP and the state of consciousness do not show any relationship to the further process. Serious disturbance of brain function before operation was only to be assumed with one unconscious patient.
b) In the early postoperative process, i.e., up to the 4th postoperative day, mean VFP under therapy exceeded 30 mm Hg only on few days, and in none of the patients did it exceed 40 mm Hg. Acute and short increases of pressure exceeding 40 and even 60 mm Hg were much more frequent in both the surviving and the nonsurviving patients. It was only in very few cases that patients with favorable prognosis remained unconscious on days with increased pressure.
c) In the *later, postoperative process*, i.e., after the 5th day, mean VFP - especially in patients having an unfavorable prognosis - even exceeded 40 mm Hg on some days.

It is especially worth mentioning that prognosis was always unfavorable in such cases where high VFP was measured together with serious disturbances of unconsciousness. On the other hand, prognosis was only favorable in such cases where patients were fully conscious or just clouded when mean VFP was high.

These results show that recuperative capacity of the brain and prognosis are foremostly determined by the seriousness of brain dysfunction during the early postoperative course. It is also apparent that increased intracranial pressure, especially during late postoperative course and together with serious brain dysfunction, leads to a marked reduction of survival chances; it was only in cases of unimportant neurologic disturbances that increased pressure was survived. Here, the speed of intracranial pressure increase seems to play an important role.

3. Ventricular Lactate Concentration, VFP, and Course

To allow a judgement on the tendency of the course, *lactate concentration* of VF was evaluated as metabolic parameter (Fig. 3). During an early postoperative phase, we measured a severely increased lactate level in both patients with favorable and those with unfavorable prognosis. A progressing increase of the lactate level was found in lethal cases only, whereas extreme values showed a decreasing tendency in favorable cases. The relationship between VFP height and CSF lactate concentration proved to be dependent on the degree of brain dysfunction (Table 2).

Preoperative increase of lactate concentration with increased VFP is generally low (about 0.15 mmol/liter), whereas the postoperative increase is markedly higher (by about 2.37 mmol/liter on the whole). The highest CSF lactate measured on the 4th day after operation - in one of the favorable courses - was 5.5 mmol/liter. In this case, the condition of general brain function with normal VFP allowed recovery. But none of those patients survived, whose VFP increase exceeded 30 mm Hg after the 4th day and was combined with an increased lactate level.

4. Operability and VFP

It is also the kind and the preferred site of cerebellar tumors that give some hints for the clinical judgement of the disturbances of CSF pressure to be expected after operation. With *spongioblastoma* of the cerebellar hemispheres, uncomplicated processes (Fig. 4a) became distinct by the fact that mean VFP dropped to normal under early postoperative therapy and pressure peaks under the limit of 30 mm Hg. Acute pressure increase exceeding 60 mm Hg could be observed during early or late postoperative periods after extubation, interruption of external CSF drainage, or aseptic meningitis, especially with patients suffering from disturbed functions of caudal brain nerves (Fig. 4b).

In the case of a 37-year-old patient with an initially favorable course, we had to experience an aseptic meningitis with acute hydrocephalic crisis as well as respiratory paralysis, cardiac and circulatory arrest, and bilateral mydriasis after early mobilization. Immediate application of an external CSF drainage through the drill hole led to a successful reanimation of the patient. Also in a patient suffering from an *ependymoma* situated in the fourth ventricle, mean pressure of the early postoperative period sank to normal. Acute short-term increases of pressure were stated here with central and peripheral respiration disturbances. Only in one patient suffering from a medulloblastoma was it possible to avoid an acute increase of pressure by continous external CSF drainage after operation. A considerable increase of pressure was found in three other patients with favorable course after interrupting external drainage.

Postoperative course in patients with a *plexuspapilloma* was unfavorable because of intraoperative brain swelling, rebleeding of a residual

Table 2. Ventricular fluid pressure (= VFP) and CSF lactate concentration

Phase of treatment		VFP x̄ (mm Hg)				VFPmx (mm Hg)			
		0-15	16-30	31-40	41-60	0-20	21-40	41-60	>60
I preoperative CSF lactate (mmol/l)	N	16	37	28	12	18	34	35	6
	x̄	1.93	2.08	2.00	2.04	2.01	1.94	2.16	2.41
	SD	0.67	0.93	0.61	0.69	0.69	0.79	1.19	0.55
II post-operative CSF lactate (mmol/l)	N	59	112	47	14	49	114	51	18
	x̄	3.07	3.50	3.11	5.44	2.82	3.52	4.20	5.43
	SD	1.45	2.12	1.45	4.50	1.12	2.01	2.63	4.40

tumor, quickly progressing growth of a residual tumor, and after post-operative respiratory arrest.

In four patients - after total extirpation of an *angioblastoma* - the further course was without any complication. CSF pressure was normal under pressure-decreasing therapy. Two patients with acute respiratory arrest on the 2nd day after operation died during the primary or secondary course. With both patients, there had been no control of CSF pressure at the time of respiratory complication.

The course was unfavorable in patients suffering from a *tumor within the higher cerebellar sections*, either ventral or infratentorial. Even under intensive pressure-decreasing measures, we were not able to reach a normalization of intracranial pressure.

5. Postoperative VFP Control

These examples show that after extirpation of an infratentorial tumor and not only after partial resection, it is important to consider an immediate and sufficiently long CSF drainage to prevent CSF circulation disturbances as they often occur in such cases (11, 12). Application of a ventriculoatrial shunt (1, 3, 4) as suggested by different authors shows a high rate of complications and does not offer enough security against an acute increase in CSF pressure, if there is not continuous check on the pressure.

According to the statistics of SAYERS (13), application of a ventriculoatrial shunt bears the danger of mechanical complications in 39.8% and infection complications in 10.7% of the cases. There is a further 10% of late complications like hypotensive headache, chronic subdural hematoma, secondary block of aqueduct, pulmonary hypertension, shunt dependence, etc. Metastatic dissemination via the shunt is quite possible, especially with medulloblastoma (5, 7). In comparison, the rate of complications with pressure-controlled external CSF drainage carried out over a period of an average of 5 days together with the drainage system described in another paper is only 2.2% (11).

Summary

Among 82 patients suffering from a space-occupying process of the posterior fossa, 56 showed an extracerebellar tumor. Both the postoperative course and the prognosis were foremostly determined by the degree of the general brain dysfunction. Prognosis was always unfavorable with serious brain function disturbances lasting for more than 3 days and continued CSF pressure increase. CSF lactate concentration can supply valuable prognostic information after the 4th postoperative day.

It is foremostly patients with either inoperable or subtotally resected tumors who are threatened with an acute increase of VFP after operation. Especially for them, we suggest a pressure-controlled external drainage for a period of 3-7 days.

References

1. ABRAHAM, K., CHANDY, Y.: Ventricular-atrial shunt management of posterior fossa tumors. J. Neurosurg. 20, 252-253 (1963)
2. BECKER, D.P., HAROLD, F.Y., VRIES, J.K., SAKALAS, R.: Monitoring in patients with brain tumors. Clin. Neurosurg. 22, 364-388 (1975)
3. BÖHM, B., MOHADJER, M., HEMMER, R.: Preoperative continous measurements of ventricular pressure in hydrocephalus occlusus with tumors of the posterior fossa: The value of ventriculoauricular shunt. This volume, pp. 194-195
4. GRUSS, P., GAAB, M., KNOBLICH, O.E.: Disorders of CSF circulation after interventions in the area of the posterior cranial fossa with prior shunt operation. This volume, pp. 199-203

5. HOFFMAN, H.J., HENDRICK, E.B., RABIN, P.H.: Metastasis via ventriculo-peritoneal shunt in patients with medulloblastoma. J. Neurosurg. 44, 562-566 (1976)
6. JAMES, H.E., LANGFITT, Th.W., KUMAR, V.S., GHOSTINE, S.V.: Treatment of intracranial hypertension. Acta Neurochir. 36, 189-200 (1977)
7. JOHNSTON, I.H., JENNET, B.: The place of continuous intracranial pressure monitoring in neurosurgical practice. Acta Neurochir. 29, 53-63 (1973)
8. KESSLER, L.A., DUGAN, P., CONCANNON, J.P.: Systemic metastases of medulloblastoma promoted by shunting. Surg. Neurol. 3, 147-157 (1975)
9. LUNDBERG, N.: Continuous recording and control of ventricular fluid pressure in neurosurgical practice. Acta Psychiat. Scand. Suppl. 149, 36 (1960)
10. OMMAYA, A.K., METZ, H., POST, K.E.: Observations on the biomechanics of hydrocephalus. In: Cisternography and Hydrocephalus. HARBERT, J.C. (ed.), pp. 57-74. Baltimore 1972
11. RICHARD, K.E.: Liquorventrikeldruckmessung mit Mikrokatheter und druckkontrollierte externe Liquordrainage. Acta Neurochir. 38, 73-87 (1977)
12. RICHARD, K.E., FROWEIN, R.A.: Ventricular fluid pressure in posterior fossa tumors of childhood. Mod. Probl. Paediatr. 18 (1977)
13. SAYERS, M.: Shunt complications. Clin. Neurosurg. 28, 393-400. Baltimore (1976)

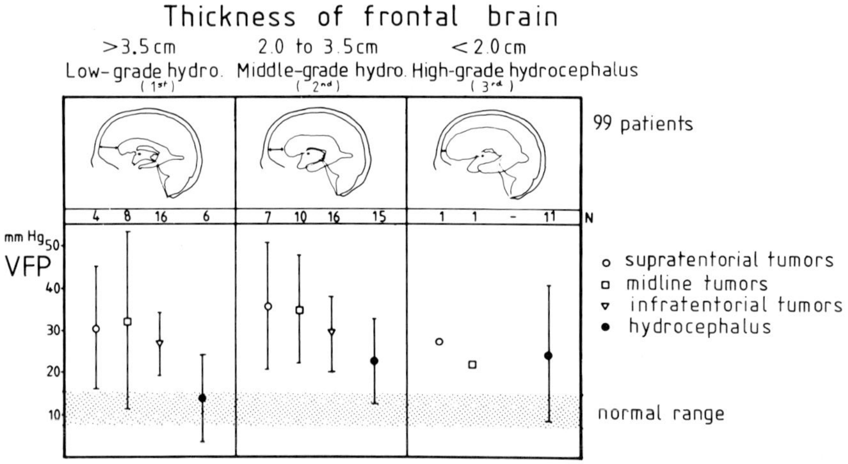

Fig. 1. Mean VFP is similarly high with infratentorial tumors, independent of the grade of hydrocephalus, but somewhat lower than with supratentorial tumors of the hemispheres or midline and markedly higher than with the nontumorous hydrocephali

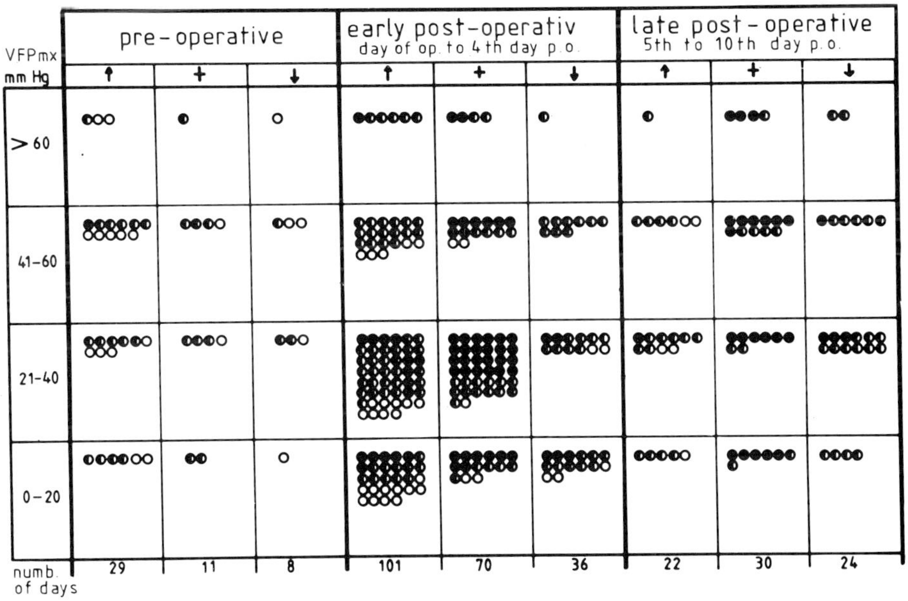

Fig. 2. Correlation of *mean VFP* (*a*) or *maximum VFP* (*b*), state of consciousness and prognosis in preoperative, early postoperative, and late postoperative phase of treatment

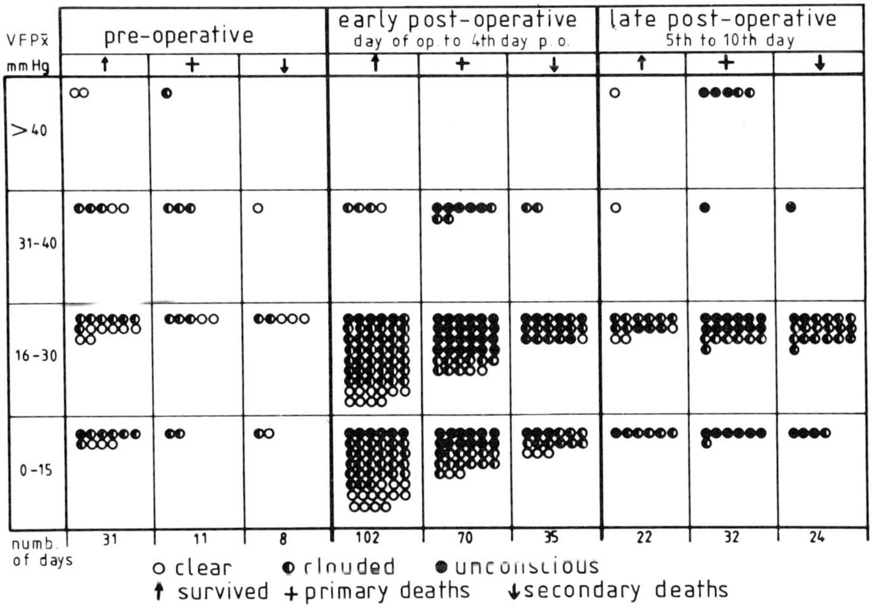

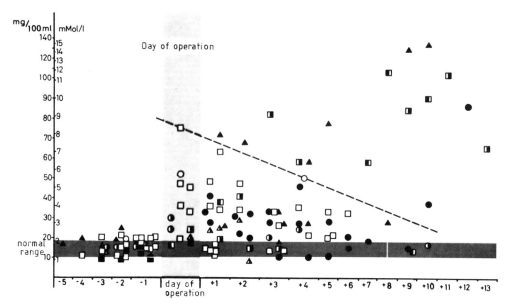

Fig. 3. Ventricular *concentration of CSF lactate* in pre- and postoperative course in patients suffering from tumors of the posterior fossa (39 patients, 121 measurings). *Open symbols*: values of patients surviving. *Semi- and completely filled symbols*: patients dying in either primary or secondary course. *Dotted line*: decreasing tendency of extreme values with favorable prognosis

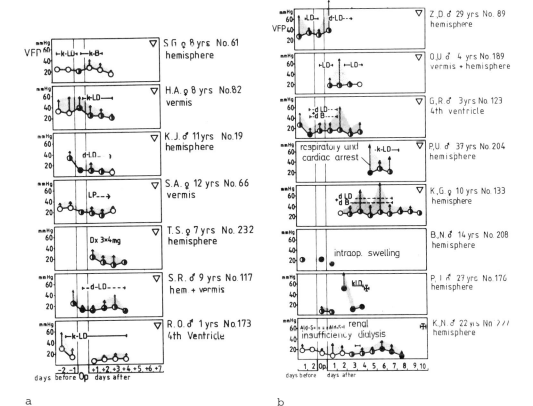

Fig. 4. Mean (*open and completely filled circles*) and maximum VFP (*arrows*) in the course of treatment in patients suffering from spongioblastoma
a Uncomplicated course
  ▽   Survived, ⊹ Deaths
  k-LD Continuous external CSF drainage
  k-B Continous ventilation
  d-LD Discontinous external CSF drainage
  Dx   Dexametasone
b Complicated course
  dB   Discontinuous ventilation
  Ald-S Aldactone-Saltucine

Circadian Occurrence of Pathologic Cerebrospinal Fluid Pressure Waves in Patients With Brain Tumor

M. Brock, W. M. Tamburus, C. R. Telles Ribeiro, and H. Dietz[1]

Introduction

Numerous biologic phenomena are subject to rhythmic circadian changes. Cerebrospinal fluid pressure (CSFP) variations have also been described which appear to be related to the day-night rhythm. COOPER and HULME (5) observed an increase in frequency, amplitude, and duration of pathologic CSFP waves in 15 neurosurgical patients. These authors state that plateau waves are only seldom observed in awake patients. MUNARI and co-workers (10) noticed an increase in CSFP during REM sleep in ten hydrocephalic adults while DI ROCCO and co-workers (12) observed the same in five hydrocephalic children. CSFP alterations during sleep have also been recorded occasionally by other authors (4, 6, 7, 9, 11, 13).

Since previous histographic studies have shown changes in the CSFP distribution pattern in the course of a 24-hour period in patients with brain tumor (3), we decided to study the circadian distribution of pathologic CSFP waves in such patients. We were unable to find similar detailed studies in the literature.

Material and Methods

The continuous ICP recordings of 103 patients with intracranial tumors, observed and treated in the Neurosurgical Clinic of the Hannover Medical School from January 1, 1971 to June 30, 1977, were submitted to a detailed analysis. ICP was recorded continuously for periods ranging from 2-26 days, either by means of an intraventricular catheter as described by LUNDBERG (9) or telemetrically (2). The tumor was supratentorial in 62 and infratentorial in 41 cases (Table 1). Fifty-three patients were male and 50 were female. All artifacts were carefully discarded. In the present study, the "day" period was considered to extend from 6:00 a.m. until 6:00 p.m. and "night" period from 6:00 p.m. until 6:00 a.m.

Three types of pathologic CSFP waves were studied as regards their frequency and duration:

Table 1. Continous recording of ICP in patients with brain tumor (No. = 103)

	♂	♀	Σ
Supratentorial	35	27	62
Infratentorial	18	23	41
Σ	53	50	

---

[1] The authors are indebted to Mrs. E. Hein, Miss B. Fülbier, and Miss E. Schmidt for their valuable help.

1. *Plateau waves* as defined by LUNDBERG (9). These are relatively rapid increases of CSFP to values above 40 mm Hg for a period of at least 2 min (Fig. 1).
2. *B waves* (9), which occure with a frequency of 1-2 per min, do not reach such highly values and are, by definition, associated with rhythmic respiratory variations (Fig. 2).
3. *Ramp waves* as defined elsewhere (1), which are frequently observed in patients with intermittently normotensive hydrocephalus. These waves are characterized by a progressive increase in CSFP to values up to about 40 mm Hg in the course of 1-2 min and by a subsequent abrupt return to control values (Fig. 3).

Results

Plateau waves were observed in 19 patients (Table 2). The sex of the patient as well as the location of the tumor (supratentorial or infratentorial) appeared to have no influence on the occurrence of plateau waves in our material.

B waves were recorded in 49 patients and are the most frequent form of supposedly pathologic CSFP waves observed in patients with brain tumor. They appear to be somewhat frequent in cases of supratentorial tumor, but this predominance is not significant.

Ramp waves were observed in only ten patients. Their frequency in males is four times higher than in females, a very striking finding despite the relatively small number of cases. Tumor location has no influence on the occurrence of ramp waves.

The circadian distribution of the 308 analyzed *plateau waves* shows no preferential occurrence of such waves during the night or during the day. The mean duration of the plateau waves during the day amounted to 7.1 min and was 1.0 min longer than at night. This difference is not significant (Table 3).

Although the *periods of B waves* are uniformly distributed during the 24 h, their mean duration during the night period is twice as long as it is during the day, a significant difference (Table 3). The opposite occurred with ramp waves; the mean duration of their periods showed no clear-cut day-night differences. Such periods were, however, more than twice frequent during the night (Table 3). We observed no preferential association of two of the above-mentioned types of waves.

Table 2

	♂	♀	Supra-tentorial	Infra-tentorial
Plateau waves (19 patients)	11	8	9	10
B waves (49 patients)	25	24	28	21
Ramp waves (10 patients)	8	2	5	5

Table 3

		No. of waves[a] or periods[b]	Total duration (min)	Mean duration (min)
Plateau waves	Night	165	1001	6.1
	Day	143	1013	7.1
B waves	Night	192	11440	59.6
	Day	187	6740	36.1
Ramp waves	Night	61	3680	60.3
	Day	26	1380	53.1

[a] In the case of plateau waves.
[b] In the case of B waves and ramp waves.

Discussion

The aim of this study was to search for a better comprehension of the pathophysiology of the different types of pathologic CSFP waves by studying the correlation between their occurrence and the seat of the tumor, the sex of the patient, and the day-night rhythm. The fact that, in contrast to some of the previous authors, we have found no influence of the analyzed parameters on the occurrence of plateau waves must be due, at least in part, to the fact that we have adhered strictly to the definition of plateau waves as originally given by LUNDBERG (9). The illustrations of some of the publications on this subject, on the contrary, show clear variance from this definition. Nevertheless, we had expected to observe circadian variations in frequency of plateau waves, since they are due to vasomotor phenomena, and hemodynamic parameters undergo definite circadien variations (8). The occurrence of plateau waves in about 20% of the patients with intracranial tumors is in agreement with the findings of others.

The fact that B waves occur in half the patients with an intracranial tumor and that the periods of such waves are almost twice as long during night time can be considered to be an expression of their relationship to respiratory phenomena. The ramp waves, hitherto considered to be B waves by some authors, are also related to respiratory changes. This is illustrated by the fact that the patient almost always presents a snoring breathing when they occur. This might also explain their clear-cut predominance in males. Nevertheless, ramp waves clearly differ from B waves by the fact that (1) they are significantly more frequent during the night hours and the duration of (2) their periods presents no day-night difference.

The pathophysiologic peculiarities of the various forms of waves become more evident when one considers the differences in frequency with which they occur in other groups of patients. Thus, for example, in a group of patients with intermittently normotensive hydrocephalus, we observed ramp waves in practically every patient and B waves in 80% of the cases.

In conclusion then, this study has confirmed the assumption that the different types of pathologic CSFP waves occur at different rates and has, furthermore, revealed that B waves and ramp waves have a circadian rhythmicity, strongly suggesting that they are the result of different pathophysiologic mechanisms.

Summary

Analysis of the CSFP recordings of 103 patients with intracranial tumors has revealed that plateau waves occur as often at night as during daytime. Their frequency is independet of the sex of the patient and of tumor location. Periods of B waves are also as frequent at night as during daytime, but their duration is significantly longer when they occur at night. B waves occur with the same frequency in male and female patients as well as in supratentorial as compared to infratentorial tumors. Ramp waves are much more frequent in males, and periods of such waves occur more than twice as often during the night. There is no day-night difference in the duration of ramp wave periods and no predominance among patients with supratentorial as compared to infratentorial tumors. These results are considered to mean that the various forms of waves studied have different pathophysiologic mechanisms.

References

1. BROCK, M.: Klinik und Therapie des intermittierend normotensiven Hydrocephalus. Radiologe 17, 1-6 (1977)

2. BROCK, M., DIEFENTHÄLER, K.: A modified equipment for the continuous telemetric monitoring of epidural or subdural pressure. In: Intracranial Pressure. BROCK, M., DIETZ, H. (eds.), pp. 21-26. Berlin-Heidelberg-New York: Springer 1972

3. BROCK, M., ZYWIETZ, C., MOCK, A., WIEGAND, H., ZILLIG, C., TAMBURUS, W.M.: Reliability and reproduceability of ICP frequency analysis. In: Intracranial Pressure III. BEKS, J.W.F., BOSCH, D.A., BROCK, M. (eds.), pp. 288-294. Berlin-Heidelberg-New York: Springer 1976

4. CHAWLA, J.C., HULME, A., COOPER, R.: Intracranial pressure in patients with dementia and communicating hydrocephalus. J. Neurosurg. 40, 376-380 (1974)

5. COOPER, R., HULME, A.: Intracranial pressure and related phenomena during sleep. J. Neurol. Neurosurg. Psychiat. 29, 564-570 (1966)

6. HAYDEN, P.W., SHURTLEFF, D.B., FOLTZ, E.L.: Ventriculuar fluid pressure recordings in hydrocephalic patients. Arch. Neurol. 23, 147-154 (1970)

7. HEMMER, R., MOHADJER, M., SCHIEFER, K.: Untersuchungen zur cerebralen Dysregulation bei Tumoren der hinteren Schädelgrube mit Hydrocephalus occlusus. Neurochirurgia 17, 96-106 (1974)

8. KHAIRI, I.M., FREIS, E.D.: Hemodynamic changes during sleep. J. Appl. Physiol. 22, 867-873 (1967)

9. LUNDBERG, N.: Continuous recording and control of ventricular fluid pressure in neurosurgical practice. Acta Psychiatr. Neurol. Scand. 149, 1-193 (1960)

10. MUNARI, C., CALBUCCI, F., VERSARI, P., BENERICETTI, E., COLUMELLA, F.: Pressione endocrania e variazioni del livello di vigilanza. Riv. Neurol. 45, 35-44 (1975)

11. NORNES, H., ROOTWELT, K., SJAASTAD, O.: Normal pressure hydrocephalus. Long-term intracranial pressure recording. Eur. Neurol. 9, 261-274 (1973)

12. DI ROCCO, C., McLONE, D.G., SHIMOJI, T., RAIMONDI, A.J.: Continous intraventricular cerebrospinal fluid pressure recording in hydrocephalic children during wakefulness and sleep. J. Neurosurg. 42, 683-689 (1975)

13. SYMON, L., DORSCH, N.W.C., STEPHENS, R.J.: Intracranial pressure monitoring in communicating hydrocephalus. Proc. R. Soc. Med. 65, 888-890 (1972)

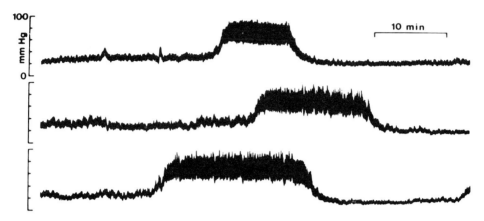

Fig. 1. Plateau waves in a patient with an angioblastoma of the cerebellar vermis

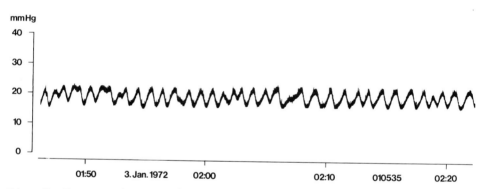

Fig. 2. B waves in a patient with a right-sided temporal multiform glioblastoma

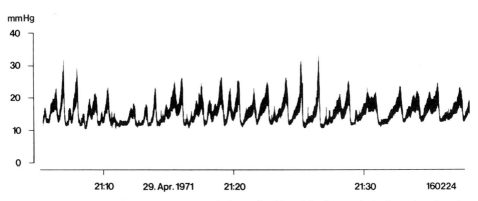

Fig. 3. Ramp waves in a patient with a left-sided parietal metastasis of a bronchial carcinoma

Preoperative Continuous Measurements of Ventricular Pressure in Hydrocephalus Occlusus With Tumors of the Posterior Fossa: The Value of Ventriculoauricular Shunt

B. BÖHM, M. MOHADJER, and R. HEMMER

Midline tumors of the posterior fossa are usually accompanied by a disturbance of CSF drainage in the area of the aqueduct and/or fourth ventricle and thus develop a hydrocephalus occlusus. One to three days after having relieved intracranial pressure, we carried out prolonged measurements of intraventricular pressure during nighttime in 13 patients with processes of the posterior fossa showing occlusion hydrocephalus verified by ventriculography .(4, 5, 6). The measurements took about 11 h. Thereby, a continuous rise in ventricular pressure averaging from 13-26 mm Hg was noticed, doubling the initial values (Fig. 1). This rise was accompanied in most of the cases by pressure waves type B and C as described by LUNDBERG. Plateau waves of pure form were present in only one of the cases (Figs. 2 and 3).

Electroencephalographic interval spectrum analysis did not reveal immediate reaction of the brain during pressure crisis or at the time of continous elevation of CSF pressure. Even during the extreme period of herniation of brain stem, no EEG findings differing from deep sleep changes could be found.

The course of the preoperative ventricular pressure justifies as first operative measure a ventriculoauricular drainage. In our hospital, this procedure has for years proved itself to be superior to previously used procedures like TORKILDSEN drainage or open CSF drainage. Other authors also prefer this procedure (1, 2, 3, 7). In our opinion, the following additional points speak for a closed CSF drainage:

1. Cautious normalization of increased intracranial pressure by selection of an adequate valve with 2-4 drops/min, up from 100 mm H_2O, corresponding approximately to a Holter normal or middle pressure valve with little drainage flow.
2. Lowering of risk of infection by elimination or reduction of a suboccipital CSF accumulation (CSF fistulas and meningitis).
3. Because for a considerable period of time the intracranial pressure is increased, the general state of health is usually weakened in children and adults. After shunting, significant improvement of the general physical condition ensues, partially also of the neurologic status, so that the operation of the lesion may take place under much more favorable conditions. Also, there exists the possibility of unlimited mobilizing exercises.
4. The CSF pressure does not show elevated levels during the postoperative phase either, so that crises with elevated intracranial pressure as noted by RICHARD (8) for one-third of the cases do not occur.
5. At any time, one may proceed with additional diagnostics of the CSF space with positive contrast media or air as well as with direct ventricular application of drugs (antibiotics, cytostatica, etc.) by means of a Rickham reservoir.

The main operation follows about 10-14 days after the recuperation of the patients. In rare instances, the interval was as long as several weeks.

For statistical purposes, 50 patients with tumor invasion of the midline and primary midline tumors (of the 5-year period 1972-1976) were examined. As complications, we saw a subdural hematoma and an infection in one of the cases, and a subcutaneous accumulation of CSF for a maximum of 3 days in three of the cases. In four patients, a shunt revision was necessary.

The comparison of this group of patients with 15 who were treated during the same period of time with open ventricular drainage showed that six had to be supplied by a ventriculoauricular drainage because of fluid accumulations which could not be otherwise removed. Thus, the proportion of CSF accumulation is 1:11 in patients with a preoperative shunt as compared with open ventricular drainage.

References

1. ABRAHAM, J., CHANDY, J.: Ventriculo-Atrial Shunt in the Management of Posterior-Fossa Tumours. J. Neurosurg. 20, 252-253 (1963)
2. ALBRIGHT, L., REIGEL, D.H.: Management of hydrocephalus secondary to posterior fossa tumors. J. Neurosurg. 46, 52-55 (1977)
3. GOUTELLE, A., FISCHER, G. et coll.: In: Les épendymomes intracraniens, intrarachidiens. Neurochirurgie 23, Suppl. 1, 138 ff (1977)
4. HEMMER, R., BÖHM, B.: Once a Shunt, Always a Shunt? Dev. Med. Child Neurol. 18 Suppl. 37, 69-73 (1976)
5. HEMMER, R., MOHADJER, M.: Hydrocephalus occlusus und Tumorentwicklung im Säuglings- und Kindesalter. Z. Kinderchir. 14, 1-11 (1974)
6. HEMMER, R., MOHADJER, M., SCHIEFER, K.: Untersuchungen zur cerebralen Dysregulation bei Tumoren der hinteren Schädelgrube mit Hydrocephalus occlusus. Neurochirurgia 17, 96-106 (1974)
7. LUYENDIJK, W.: The operative Approach to the Posterior Fossa. In: Advances and Technical Standards in Neurosurgery. KRAYENBÜHL, H. et al. (eds.), Vol. 3. Wien-New York: Springer 1976
8. RICHARD, K.E.: Liquorventrikeldruckmessung mit Mikrokatheter und druckkontrollierte externe Liquordrainage. Acta Neurochir. 38, 73-87 (1977)

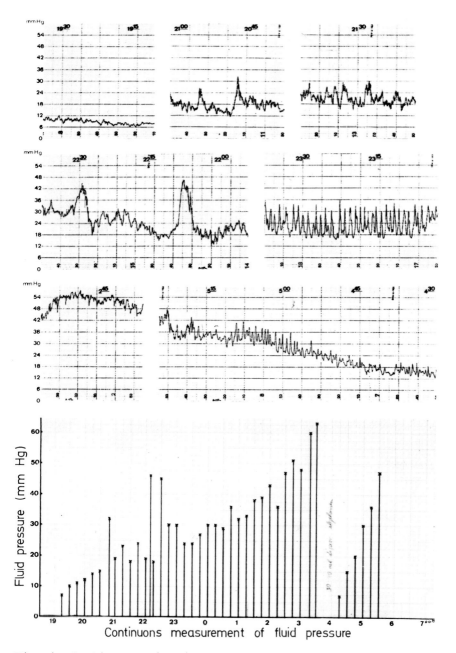

Fig. 1. Continuous rise in pressure, accompanied predominantly by B waves. Decrease in pressure from 67-15 mm Hg achieved by drainage with 35 ml fluid

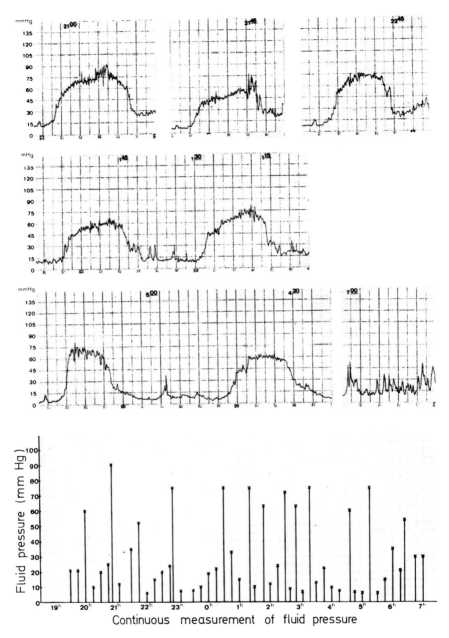

Fig. 2. Typical plateau waves up to 90 mm Hg and the course of the fluid pressure

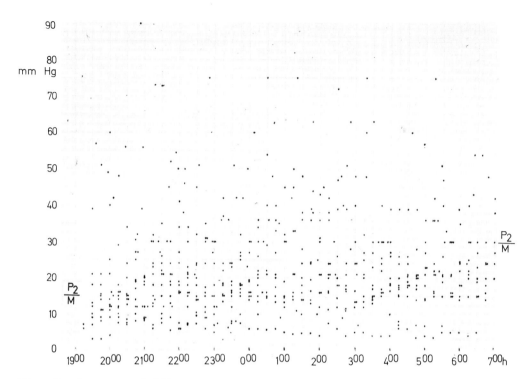

Fig. 3. Summary of 582 pressure measurements of 13 patients. The average initial value (P_1/M) of 13.38 ± 2.36 mm Hg was doubled (P_2/M) to 26.50 ± 3.46 mm Hg

Disorders of CSF Circulation After Interventions in the Area of the Posterior Cranial Fossa With Prior Shunt Operation

P. GRUSS, M. GAAB, and O. E. KNOBLICH

Introduction

Compressing processes in the posterior cranial fossa very often cause hydrocephalus (3). This frequently appears earlier than the "local signs," e.g., cerebellar ataxia, disorders of the eye, or cranial nerves. Since hydrocephalus is accompanied by raised intracerebral pressure, drainage of CSF from the brain ventricles can hardly be avoided:
1. In order to free the patient from brain pressure and thus improve his condition.
2. In order to relieve pressure for infratentorial exposure.

We almost always prefer shunt operation to open ventricular drainage, which is used only when the clinical picture has had a short course and a rapidly following subtentorial exposure is foreseen with certainty and can be assumed to eliminate the disturbance of CSF passage (1, 2). The shunt operation is especially advantageous before the exposure of slowly growing tumors with hydrocephalus, e.g., tumors of the cerebellopontine angle. It ensures that CSF pressure is reduced to physiologic values and diminishes the danger of pressure crises during the preoperative phase even with only slight hydrocephalus preoperatively.

Even though the method has its advantages CSF pressure normalizes reliably during the preoperative phase and at first also postoperatively, we noted complications in many cases a few days up to 1-2 weeks after removal of the infratentorial tumors, such as headache, vertigo, and hypotonic circulatory regulation (in some cases of an ominous kind), especially when attempts were made to stand up. We regarded the disorder as a consequence of low CSF pressure which had appeared in the meantime. This is illustrated by some CSF pressure measurements.

Results of Measurement

The first patient (W. H., 14.11.33) fell ill with a malignant spinal schwannoma. It was operated on twice but had spread to the posterior cranial fossa and brain stem despite irradiation after operation. A hydrocephalus with substantially raised CSF pressure arose. A shunt operation was performed on June 16, 1977. A Hakim high-pressure valve system was implanted. The CSF pressure was measured proximal to the valve system before insertion of the ventricular catheter. On perfusion of 60 ml NaCl/h into the system, the pressure was about 20 mm Hg in the horizontal position of the patient and then fell to almost -10 mm Hg when the patient rose up to 60°-70°. The CSF pressure rose slightly after the angle was reduced to 40° and then incompletely approached the initial value on renewed horizontal position (Fig. 1). The total duration of the intraoperative pressure measurement was about 15 min.

The second patient (female, K. M., 4.3.53) had an astrocytoma in the brain stem and hydrocephalus. At first, a shunt operation with Hakim extra high-pressure system was performed because of the appreciable hydrocephalus. The patient initially improved, then the tumor was stereotactically removed and ^{192}I was implanted. Six months later, the patient was readmitted with disturbances of balance, headache and disorders of vision. To investigate the question of low CSF pressure, continuous measurements were made via the antechamber of the shunt system: CSF pressure in the horizontal position was barely 10 mm Hg; when the feet were lower, CSF pressure fell to 3-5 mm Hg, whereas there was a corresponding rise in pressure when the head was low. The fall of CSF pressure to 10 mm Hg on standing is remarkable; it approximately normalizes on return to the horizontal position (Fig. 2).

The third patient (female, H. H., 26.9.19) had a tumor in the cerebellopontine area with hydrocephalus. At first, a shunt operation was performed, resulting in good regression of the slight brain pressure symptoms, and then the tumor was removed. After 1 week, headache and nausea occurred upon standing up and sitting down. Before clarifying the question of a local complication, CSF pressure was measured in the recumbent position after walking about for a short time. CSF pressure was still about -3 mm Hg. A positive CSF pressure built up slowly with regression of the headache (Fig. 3). There were no symptoms after removing the shunt system.

The CSF pressures were under 10 mm Hg in the patients with substantial low-pressure symptoms after shunt operation and removal of an infratentorial tumor. Pressure measurements were possible only after addition of fluid to the shunt system, although their accuracy is greatly limited by the added fluid and sucked in air.

Discussion

The syndrome of low CSF pressure after shunt operations is familiar (5, 6). In infants, the fontanelles are drawn in, often to an appreciable extent, and subdural effusions are observed. In older children or adults, headaches, nausea, disturbances of balance, and states of collapse occur. These phenomena must be explained by the construction of the shunt systems: with very low or negative pressure in the cardiac auricle, "suction" of the column of fluid in the cardiac catheter at the outlet valve arises. This can amount to a 25-cm column of water if the patient sits up in the full length of the cardiac catheter. Low-pressure conditions occur with greater frequency and intensity after operation in the region of the posterior cranial fossa with elimination of the hindrance to passage. We believe that this is related to two facts:

1. In operations to the posterior cranial fossa, a large part of the CSF flows away; there is a pronounced fall of CSF pressure in the sitting patient, so that the entire CSF system thus falls into a low-pressure state. With a well-functioning shunt system, a positive pressure cannot be readily built up (see also Fig. 3). Also, the high flow rate of many valve constructions must be borne in mind.
2. When a suboccipital craniotomy gap persists, atmospheric air pressure has at least a partial possibility of exerting a negative effect on the pressure of the CSF system.

Despite the low-pressure conditions observed postoperatively, we wish to adhere to our previously used procedure and initially treat hydrocephalus in compressing processes of the posterior cranial fossa with a shunt in most cases (except where the course is rapid). Our results indicate that the shunt system should be interrupted or removed in good time upon appearance of low-pressure conditions and when CSF passage has become free (4). We were unable to attain sufficiently good results with implantations of antisiphon systems ("low-pressure brakes"), which we performed twice. It is to be hoped that improvements are still possible here through new constructions (7).

References

1. ABRAHAM, J., CHANDY, J.: Ventriculo-atrial shunt in the management of posterior fossa tumors. J. Neurosurg. 20, 252-253 (1963)
2. HEKMATPANAH, J., MULLAN, S.: Ventriculo-caval shunt in the management of posterior fossa tumors. J. Neurosurg. 26, 609-613 (1967)
3. HEMMER, R., MOHADJER, M., SCHIEFER, K.: Untersuchungen zur cerebralen Dysregulation bei Tumoren der hinteren Schädelgrube mit Hydrocephalus occlusus. Neurochir. 17, 96-106 (1974)
4. LELAND, A., REIGEL, D.H.: Management of hydrocephalus secondary to posterior fossa tumors. J. Neursurg. 46, 52-55 (1977)
5. MAGNAES, B.: Body position and cerebrospinal fluid pressure. Part 1: Clinical studies on the effect of rapid postural changes. J. Neurosurg. 44, 687-697 (1976a)
6. MAGNAES, B.: Body position and cerebrospinal fluid pressure. Part 2: Clinical studies on orthostatic pressure and the hydrostatic in different point. J. Neurosurg. 44, 698-705 (1976b)
7. PORTNOY, H.D., SCHULTE, R.R., FOX, J.L. et al.: Antisiphon and reversible occlusion valves for shunting in hydrocephalus and preventing post shunt subdural hematomas. J. Neurosurg. 38, 729-738 (1973)

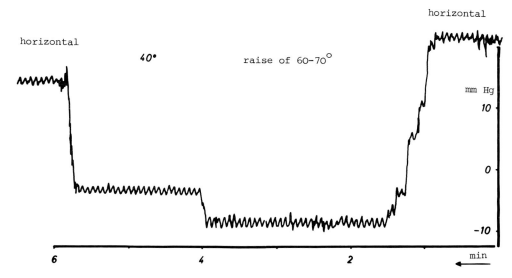

Fig. 1. Intraoperative CSF pressure measurement proximal to the valve system (ventricular catheter of the Hakim high-pressure system, ventriculoatrial shunt not yet applied). In the horizontal position, CSF pressure over 20 mm Hg on perfusion of 60 ml NaCl/min into the system. After raising the patient by 60°-70°, fall of the CSF pressure to about -10 mm Hg; slight rise after reduction of the angle and return of the pressure to about 15 mm Hg after resumption of the horizontal position

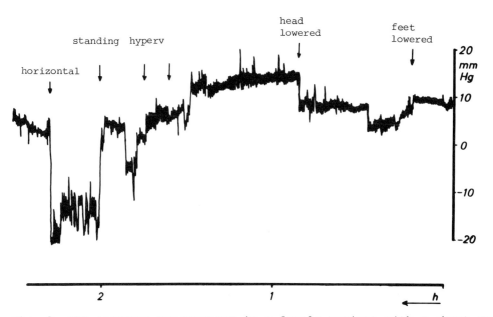

Fig. 2. CSF pressure measurement in a female patient with a shunt system in place via auricle (hydrocephalus in brain stem astrocytoma). CSF pressure in the horizontal position barely 10 mm Hg; slight fall in pressure when the feet are lowered and rise in pressure when the head is lowered. Slight fall in pressure on CO_2 rebreathing. Distinct fall in pressure to almost -20 mm Hg after standing up. The normal value is slowly reached again after return to the horizontal position

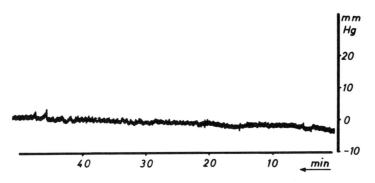

Fig. 3. CSF measurement in female patient after removal of an acoustic neurinoma with shunt still in place. Measurement in the horizontal position after the patient has been walking around: the pressure is negative at 3-4 mm Hg and only slowly approaches the zero line when the patient lies quietly

Ventricular Drainage in Patients With Posterior Fossa Tumors and the Problem of Intracranial Decompensation

J. ZIERSKI

Introduction

Plateau waves are an established clinical entity, but the mechanism by which they are created and their effect on brain function are still subject to investigation. In patients, appearance of such high pressure waves demands immediate therapy, usually in the form of control of IVP by drainage, which precludes systematic study of this phenomenon. The appearance of plateau waves has been explained by increase both in CBV and IVP and the decrease of CBF (7). In clinical practice, measuring of arterial pO_2, pCO_2, pH, and end-tidal CO_2 did not reveal any variations, although small variations or local tissue changes in these parameters, not detectable by the measurement technique, may be significant (3).

Experimental studies (8) on sympathetic vasoconstriction nerve activity showed that repeated insults of severe intracranial hypertension produce paralysis or temporary disappearance of sympathetic activity. This fact was considered as corresponding clinically to the occurrence of plateau waves. However, the study of behavior of vegetative parameters during occurrence of plateau waves observed in an unselected population of our patients failed to demonstrate any uniform pattern of reaction (4). This preliminary report deals with the description of effects of ventricular drainage in a selected group of patients with posterior fossa tumors upon the morphology of the pressure curve.

Material and Method

IVP was recorded in 22 patients harboring large posterior fossa tumors before and after the operation or before and after opening of the ventricular drainage. The pressure was recorded through a catheter placed in the frontal horn or through an Ommaya reservoir. Statham SP 37 transducer was placed over the frontral region and fixed to the head of the patient. The height of drainage was constant and was set at 15-17 cm above the level of the frontal horn. The details of our technique of registration have been published elsewhere (9).

In all of the patients, the posterior fossa mass produced displacement of the fourth ventricle and the brain stem as demonstrated by positive contrast ventriculography. The duration of pressure recording varied from 1-24 h before opening of the drainage and up to 5 days during functioning of the drainage or postoperatively.

Results

Out of 22 patients, 13 showed waves of increased IVP lasting from 10-20 min with a maximum mean pressure of 30-80 mm Hg. Seventy-seven pressure waves have been recorded in 229 hours of registration. They did not always correspond to the classic description given by LUNDBERG (5), as sometimes only high peaks of pressure with slow decline were demonstrated. The pressure waves usually occurred in series of 1-6 h with moderate elevation of basic pressure at the interval period. In two cases, plateau waves of 20-min duration followed each other (Fig. 1). As occurrence of such high pressure waves required therapeutic measurements, only short periods of recordings were possible. As expected, there was a considerable rise of pressure amplitude with the occurrence of pressure wave, the amplitude rising from 3-5 mm Hg to 25+ mm Hg within a few minutes. The opening of the drainage produced a rapid fall in pressure within a few minutes with further flat course of the pressure curve. Unexpectedly, this was not always the case. In some patients, in spite of functioning drainage, the pressure, after an initial drop, increased over the period of 1 h to 90 min reaching the values of the previous basic pressure. Although the very high pressure waves did not occur, wave form fluctuations of pressure of 20-min duration were recorded (Fig. 2).

The analysis of pressure classes before and after opening of the drainage sometimes showed that in spite of overall reduction of mean pressure there were still pressure increases (Fig. 3). Complete removal of posterior fossa tumor with apparent restoration of CSF pathways patency or inserting the Torkildsen drainage does not always mean that the IVP has been returned to normal. In spite of normal pressure values recorded in the first postoperative period, high pressure waves may appear on the 2nd and 3rd postoperative day.

It has also been noted that the reduction of pressure by drainage did not always abolished the occurrence of several, sometime rhythmic slow changes in IVP which had the form of abortive plateau waves (Fig. 4). Another form was the appearance of long-lasting pressure waves with a maximum mean pressure of 20 mm Hg, superimposing the flat monotonous pressure curve seen during the drainage.

Discussion and Conclusions

It seems that more attention should be drawn to the frequently reported fact that high pressure waves occur far more often in patients with posterior fossa tumors than in any other groups of patients with intracranial pathology leading to increased ICP, tumors, trauma, SAH, and obstructive and communicating hydrocephalus (1, 6). Drainage of intraventricular fluid causes a rapid fall of pressure after a small volume loss. However, further continuous recording during drainage or after the operation may sometimes reveal marked fluctuations of the IVP and not as expected a monotonous flat curve as seen in patients with non-tumorous hydrocephalus with a functioning shunt. These fluctuations resemble the abortive plateau waves. Further studies included the method of quantitative drainage as suggested by FUCHS (2) are necessary. Patients with posterior fossa tumors exhibit a striking frequency of rhythmic and arhythmic high pressure waves. The fact that in some patients rhythmic pressure increases occurred during the intraventricular drainage and in the postoperative period may suggest that these phenomena are connected with possible irritation of centers in the brain stem and are not exclusively related to the disturbed intracranial pressure (volume relationships).

Summary

Based on observations made on the behavior of intraventricular pressure in patients with large posterior fossa tumors, before and after opening of the ventricular drainage and before and after the operation, it is suggested that the mechanism of appearance of rhythmic plateau waves may be connected not only with the disturbed intracranial pressure and volume relationship but also with disturbance within the brain stem centers. This hypothesis needs further supporting evidence.

References

1. BROCK, M., ZILLIG, C., WIEGAND, H., ZYWIEC, C.: The influence of dexamethasone therapy on ICP in patients with tumors of the posterior fossa. In: Intracranial Pressure III. BEKS, J.W.F., BOSCH, D.A., BROCK, M. (eds.), p. 236. Berlin-Heidelberg-New York: Springer 1977
2. FUCHS, E.C.: Acute intracranial volume fluctuations. In: Advances in Neurosurgery, Vol. 4. WÜLLENWEBER, R., BROCK, M., HAMER, J., KLINGER, M., SPOERRI, O. (eds.), pp. 156-170. Berlin-Heidelberg-New York: Springer 1977
3. HOCHWALD, G.H., MARTIN, A.E., WALD, A.: Increases in ICP and development of plateau waves in decompensated hydrocephalic cats. A new model. In: Intracranial Pressure II. BEKS, J.W.F., BOSCH, D.A., BROCK, M. (eds.), pp. 37-41. Berlin-Heidelberg-New York: Springer 1976
4. LORENZ, R.: The cushing response. In: Intracranial Pressure III. BEKS, J.W.F., BOSCH, D.A., BROCK, M. (eds.), pp. 270-278. Berlin-Heidelberg-New York: Springer 1977
5. LUNDBERG, N.: Continuous recording and control of ventricular fluid pressure in neurosurgical practice. Acta Psychiatr. Scand. Suppl. 149 (1960)
6. NORNES, H., MAGNAES, B., AASLID, R.: Observations of intracranial pressure waves. In: Intracranial Pressure II. LUNDBERG, N., PONTEN, V., BROCK, M. (eds.), p. 421. Berlin-Heidelberg-New York: Springer 1975
7. RISBERG, J., LUNDBERG, N., INGVAR, D.H.: Regional cerebral blood flow volume during acute transient rises of the intracranial pressure (Plateau waves). J. Neurosurg. 31, 303-310 (1969)
8. TANAKA, H., HASHI, K., NISHIMURA, S., MATSUURA, S.: Changes of sympathetic vasomotor activity during increased intracranial pressure. In: Intracranial Pressure III. BEKS, J.W.F., BOSCH, D.A., BROCK, M. (eds.). Berlin-Heidelberg-New York: Springer 1976
9. ZIERSKI, J., BUSS, K.: Monitoring of intracranial pressure and other vegetative parameters in neurosurgical practice. Biomed. Tech. 21, 121-122 (1976)

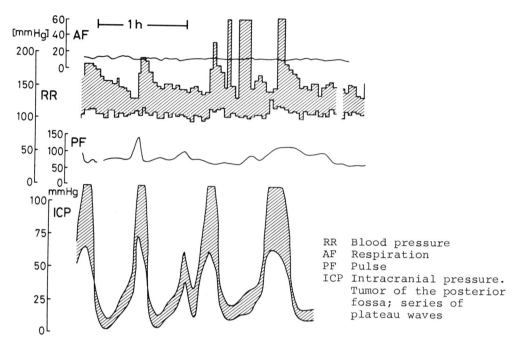

RR Blood pressure
AF Respiration
PF Pulse
ICP Intracranial pressure.
    Tumor of the posterior
    fossa; series of
    plateau waves

Fig. 1. Posterior fossa tumor. Recording before the drainage. A series of rhythmic plateau waves

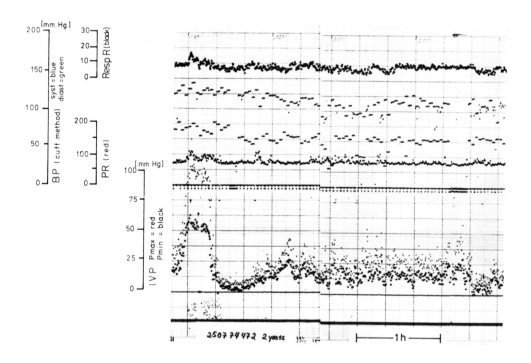

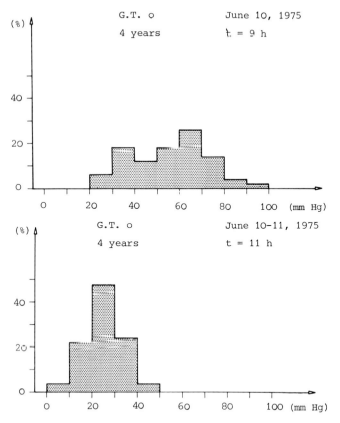

Fig. 3. Frequency distribution of pressure classes in a patient with posterior fossa tumor before and after opening of the drainage. *Above*: measurement with closed drainage; *below*: measurement with opened drainage

Fig. 2. Ependymoma of the fourth ventricle. High plateau wave with mean pressure of 75 mm Hg and pressure amplitude of 30 mm Hg. Decrease of pressure upon opening of the drainage with a slow rise followed by continuous wave form fluctuations of ca. 20-min duration

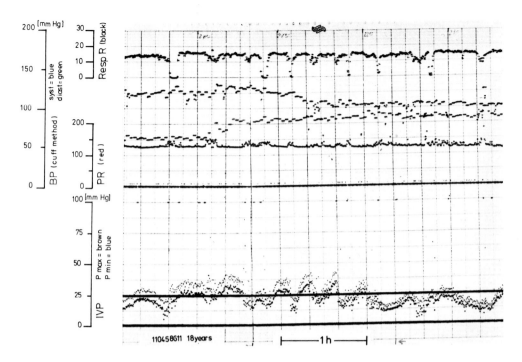

Fig. 4. Ependymoma of the posterior fossa. Functioning drainage. A series of four pressure waves (abortive plateau waves) followed by slow fluctuations

A Safe and Simple Method of Ventricular Drainage

N. O. Ameli and H. Rahmat

In 1943, J.L. POPPEN (3) published a paper on "Ventricular Drainage as a Valuable Procedure in Neurosurgery." Since then, its importance in preoperative and postoperative care of patients with lesions obstructing CSF flow has been universally recognized. There is no doubt that removal of such tumors is much safer when performed 7-10 days after ventricular drainage.

External drainage has many disadvantages. These include difficulties in nursing care, risk of infection, and loss of body fluid and important chemicals. The danger of infection is real. WYLER and KELLY (5) reported an 18% rate of infection in cases without prophylactic use of antibiotics, while SMITH and ALKASNE (4) reported 4.6% infection with the use of antibiotics. Three out of 65 cases developed frank meningitis, two of which died. Four other cases developed fever and CSF leukocytosis 7-14 days following venticulostomy removal. Internal drainage by ventriculoatrial or ventriculoperitoneal shunts (1) are major operations and rather expensive; there is also some danger of peritoneal metastsis (2). In the last 10 years, we have used a simple method of ventricular drainage by inserting a rubber catheter, one end into the ventricle and the other end into the subcutaneous tissue of the neck.

During the Second World War, when it was difficult to obtain apyrogenic fluids from Germany which supplied most of the medical needs of Iran and we were then still unable to produce our own, the subcutaneous route was commonly used to treat dehydration. By this route, large amounts of fluid can be absorbed over many days.

For ventricular drainage, subcutaneous tissues of the neck seem and ideal place, especially in children. At the same time, the resistance offered by these tissues does not allow rapid evacuation of the ventricles. The method is easy to perform and takes only a few minutes. A small burr hole is made in the posterior temporal region on the right side (Fig. 1). A rubber catheter size 8 or 10 is inserted into the ventricle and the other end is pushed into the tissues of the neck by a long-handled pair of forceps. In adults, a small incision in the upper part of the neck is needed. We have used this method in 24 cases without any complication. The catheter can be removed at the time of major operation or 1 week later under local anesthesia.

Recently, with the use of CAT, we have been able to demonstrate that even 3 days after the procedure the ventricles have become appreciably smaller (Figs. 2 and 3). In children, we are able to see the collection of fluid in the subcutaneous tissue and its gradual absorption (Fig. 4). In a case of tuberculous meningitis with severe hydrocephalus, this procedure was employed with success. Further experience may show that it is not only a cheaper but also a safer method than ventriculoatrial or ventriculoperitoneal shunts, which are now employed for treatment of these cases.

References

1. ABRAHAM, J., CHANDY, J.: Ventriculo-atrial shunt in the management of posterior fossa tumours. J. Neurosurg. 20, 252-253 (1963)
2. HOFFMAN, H.J., HENDRICK, E.B., HUMPHREYS, R.P.: Metastasis via ventriculo-peritoneal shunt in patients with medulloblastoma. J. Neurosurg. 44, 562-566 (1976)
3. POPPEN, J.L.: Ventricular Drainage as a valuable procedure in neurosurgery. Report of satisfactory method. Arch. Neurol. Psychiatry 50, 587-589 (1943)
4. SMITH, R.W., ALKASNE, J.F.: Infections complicating the use of external ventriculostomy. J. Neurosurg. 44, 567-570 (1976)
5. WYLER, A.R., KELLY, W.: Use of antibiotics with external ventriculostomies. J. Neurosurg. 37, 185-187 (1976)

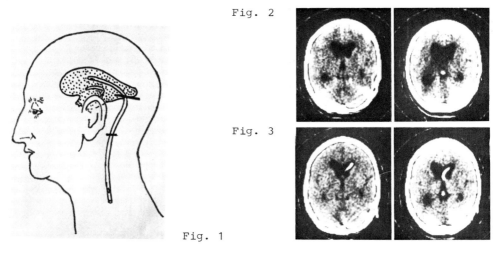

Fig. 1
Fig. 2
Fig. 3

Fig. 1. A rubber catheter is used to drain ventricular fluid into the subcateneous tissues of the neck

Fig. 2. CAT in a case of papilloma of the fourth ventricle

Fig. 3. The same as in Figure 2, three days after ventricular drainage showing smaller lateral ventricle

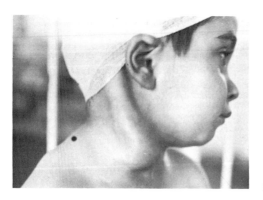

Fig. 4. Collection of fluid in the tissues of the neck following ventricular drainage. A case of medulloblastoma

Quantitative CSF Drainage in Cases of Posterior Fossa Tumor

E. C. Fuchs

We presented quantitative CSF drainage at the annual meeting of the German Society for Neurosurgery in Berlin in 1976 (2) (Fig. 1). Before we discuss the results achieved with this method in cases of posterior fossa tumor, a few remarks are necessary on the subject of indication for the procedure. Two technical innovations have significantly altered the indication for ventricular drainage in cases of tumor of the posterior fossa:

1. The development of a relatively safe surgical procedure for diversion of CSF by means of a ventriculoatrial or ventriculoperitoneal shunt. The method is certainly not without complications, including subacute infection. However, we believe that the complications most often encountered with this method result primarily from inadequate surgical technique.
2. World-wide use of computerized tomography, which allows detection of ventricular enlargement as soon as the slightest clinical suspicion arises. With careful application, it is often possible to demonstrate the tumor, either in the plain scan or with contrast enhancement. This is a great aid to clinicians, who can now dispense with echo encephalography, the accuracy of which has been overestimated where assessment of ventricular enlargement is concerned. Pneumencephalography and ventriculography, which are not only somewhat risky but also extremely painful, can henceforth be reserved for a few exceptional cases.

Many clinicians have used ventriculoatrial and ventriculoperitoneal shunts preoperatively in tumors of the posterior fossa in order to treat obstructive hydrocephalus, i.e., disturbances of CSF circulation, the existence of which has been suggested by clinical evidence and demonstrated in the computed axial tomogram. We do not perform primary shunt operation for two reasons:

1. Selection of a valve for the shunt operation implies presetting CSF pressure at a certain level. This makes individualized variation of CSF drainage impossible. However, we believe that precisely such individualized variation - depending on size, location, and type of the tumor - is necessary in order to bring imminent herniation at the tentorium or the foramen magnum under control. This is especially significant in cases of late diagnosis and advanced herniation, for individualized CSF drainage can return these patients to operable condition.
2. Only 70% of patients surgically treated for posterior fossa tumor need permanent CSF drainage. This means that a large percentage of patients would undergo a shunt operation which is unnecessary.

Our Procedure

One or two days before the main tumor operation, we perform ventricular puncture through a frontal burr hole and implant a quantitative CSF drain. Intracranial pressure determines the level at which we set the overflow drain: high pressure requires that the drain be initially set high. It often happens that very low or normal pressure is measured at operation despite extensive hydrocephalus and that pressure rises to high values in the hours after surgery. We are convinced that hyperventilation during anesthesia, accompanied by loss of small amount of CSF, produces these deceptive measurements.

Results

1. We have identified two types of volume curves in the 21 patients with posterior fossa tumors in whom we implanted a quantitative CSF drainage.
    a) One group demonstrated a clear decrease in the amount of CSF drained each day. The decline was relatively independent of the height of the drain, which ranged between 40 and 10 mm Hg. The tumor operation, which usually took place 2 days after implantation of the drain, did not influence the decrease in the amount of CSF drained. The CSF drainage can be removed 5 days after the surgical procedure in patients of this group with declined amounts of drained CSF (Fig. 2).
    b) In a second group, the amount of CSF drained each day remained fairly constant. Even a change in the height of the overflow drain from 10 to 40 mm Hg caused no significant change. (This means that the overflow drain was elevated from 13 cm to 52 cm above our reference line). Patients of this group, in which daily CSF drainage remains constant, require a permanent shunt upon which they are dependent. We follow standard procedures in implanting a Holter drain, usually with a medium pressure valve 5-8 days after surgery (Fig. 3).

2. An additional result of quantitative CSD drainage, observed in both patient groups, was the demonstration of periodic changes in intracranial volume, especially at night. LUNDBERG (7) has indirectly demonstrated this phenomenon in the form of plateau waves through measurement of intracranial pressure. He classified his results into three subtypes according to pressure and duration of the wave. LUNDberg (8), GROTE (4), MERREM (6), HEMMER (5), and many others used drainage to treat the often dangerous increase in intracranial pressure, the cause of which remained unexplained. Of course, such a dangerous increase in pressure never takes place with quantitative CSF drainage. One observes a sudden increase in the amount of drained CSF which cannot be explained by manipulation of the system or by the influence of other factors. Depending on the height of the overflow drain and the capacity for spontaneous resorption, volume fluctuations of 15-35 ml can be registered within a few minutes (Fig. 4). We are currently studying various CSF and serum fractions in a search for metabolites of vasoactive substances. We postulate that such large and rapid volume changes are only possible in the area of the cerebral vessels (8, 9). On first analysis of our data, we had the impression that normalization of CSF circulation can take place after CSF drainage in cases of rapidly growing tumors and hermorrhage, which can cause a total block of the basal cistern and acute obstructive hydrocephalus with all of its consequences (3). A review of our material, which now includes a much larger number of cases, indicates that damage to the cerebellum, subarachnoid hemorrhage, and location of the tumor negatively influence the possibility of spontaneous normalization of CSF circulation. This means that a preoperative prediction on the necessity of a permanent postoperative shunt operation is not possible.

Summary

Quantitative CSF drainage is a useful method of treating preoperative volume and pressure fluctuation in an individualized manner. Imminent tentorial herniation in the rostral direction can be treated or avoided by changing the height of the outlet drain. One can indentify patients with a disturbance of CSF circulation requiring a permanent shunt in the first few days after operation. Spontaneous volume fluctuation, which can result in critical situations when pressure alone is measured, can be registered without danger to the patient.

References

1. FUCHS, E.C.: Acute spontaneous volume fluctuation in the brain. A contribution to the interpretation of plateau waves. Neurochirurgia 19, 157-165 (1976)
2. FUCHS, E.C.: Acute intracranial volume fluctuation. In: Advances in Neurosurgery, Vol. 4. WÜLLENWEBER, R. et al. (eds.), pp. 156- 160. Berlin-Heidelberg-New York: Springer 1977
3. FUCHS, E.C.: Intrakranielle Volumenschwankungen. Acta Neurochir. (In press, 1977)
4. GROTE, W., WÜLLENWEBER, R.: Über - "Liquordruckkrisen" - spontane Druckschwankungen bei intrakraniellen Liquorpassagestörungen. Acta Neurochir. 9, 125-138 (1960)
5. HEMMER, R., MOHADJER, M., SCHIEFER, K.: Untersuchungen zur cerebralen Dysregulation bei Tumoren der hinteren Schädelgrube mit Hydrocephalus occlusus. Neurochir. 17, 96-106 (1974)
6. MERREM, B.: Die Liquordruckkrise. Zentralbl. Neurochir. 32, 245-257 (1971)
7. LUNDBERG, N.: Continous recording and control of ventricular fluid pressure in neurosurgical practice. Acta Psychiat. Scand. (Suppl. 149) 36, 1-193 (1960)
8. LUNDBERG, N., KJÄLLQUIST, A., KULLBERG, G., PONTEN, U., SUNDBÄRG, G.: Non-operative management of intracranial hypertension. In: Advances and Technical Standards in Neurosurgery, Vol. 1. KRAYENBÜHL, H. (ed.), pp. 3-59. Wien-New York: Springer 1974
9. RISBERG, J., LUNDBERG, N., INGVAR, D.H.: Regional cerebral blood volume during acute transient rises of the intracranial pressure (plateau waves). J. Neurosurg. 31, 303-310 (1969)

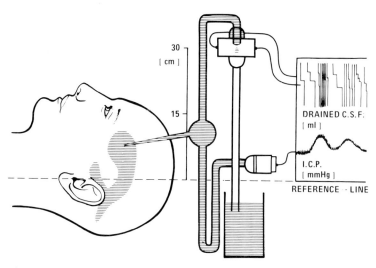

Fig. 1. Schematic diagram of quantitative CSF drainage. The ICP below the limit set by the level of the overflow drain is registered as well

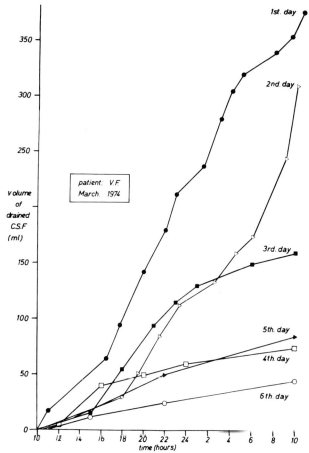

Fig. 2. This curve shows the typical decline in volume of drained CSF, in group I patients (not shunt-dependent)

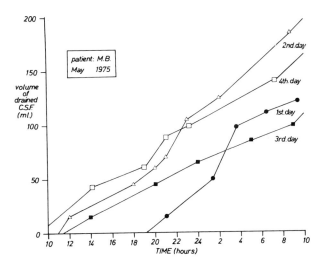

Fig. 3. The parallel slopes of the curves indicate that the volume of CSF drained each day remains constant (shunt dependency)

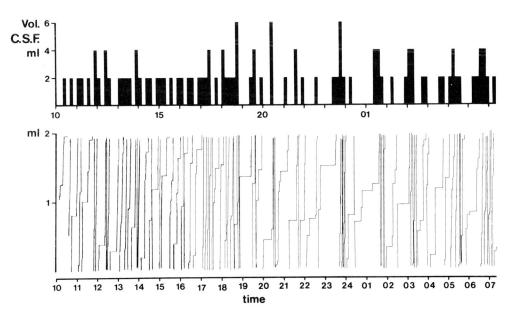

Fig. 4. Note the nocturnal periodicity of drained CSF. The lower part of the Figure reproduces the original tracing

Catheterization of the Aqueduct in Certain Lesions of the Posterior Fossa

M. SCHÄFER, C. LAPRAS, and H. RUF

Insertion of a thin rubber tube for treatment of aqueduct stenosis or obstructive cerebellar tumors was described as early as 1920 by DANDY (3). The material he used, as well as the tantalum spiral that was used by LEKSELL (6) in 1949, were not appropriate to be left in place for a longer time because of their rigidity and tissue incompatibility. In recent years, smooth siliconized ventricle catheters have become available. Making use of these, we have reestablished this operation method, encouraged by the results of CROSBY et al. (2) and THURNBULL et al. (9).

Material and Method

In 113 patients of the Neurosurgical University Hospitals of Frankfurt and Lyon, we performed catheterization of the aqueduct during the last 4 years. Indications were: tumors in 50, Arnold-Chiari-malformations in 47, and aqueduct stenosis in 16 cases (Table 1).

We utilize a smooth, siliconized, and barium-coated ventricle catheter[1] of 11-12 cm length, as aplied for ventriculoatrial shunts. All patients of more than 1 year of age are operated on in a sitting position (4, 5). After lifting the roof of the fourth ventricle, the aqueduct is placed into position and a catheter without mandarin is inserted into the third ventricle. The distal end is left in the subarachnoid space at the level of C2 or C3 without fixation. Thus, a direct connection between the third ventricle and the spinal subarachnoidal space has been created. Tissue compatibility of the catheter is excellent even after many months in situ, as shown by autopic examination of the ependyma. One of the patients with tumor developed a postoperative Staphylococcus aureus meningitis. He was successfully treated with chloramphenicol, and operative revision was not required. In two cases of Arnold-Chiari malformation with a largely dilated aqueduct, the catheter inadvertently slipped into the caudal space without eliciting local symptoms. In such cases, we now recommend a ventricle catheter with lamellae.

Results

In all tumor cases, a recurrency was to be expected, either because of the nature of the tumor (7) or, in cases of infiltration of the brain stem, because of incomplete extirpation (Table 2; Figs. 1 and 2). In

Table 1. Indications for intubation of the aqueduct (No. = 113)

1. Posterior fossa tumors	50
2. Arnold-Chiari malformations	47
3. Aqueduct stenosis	16

---

[1] Ventricle catheter manufactured by CODMAN and SHURTLEFF, Randolph, Mass./USA.

Table 2. Histology of posterior fossa tumors, treated by intubation of the aqueduct (No. = 50)

Spongioblastomas	15
Medulloblastomas	14
Ependymomas	6
Brain stem tumors	7
Ca metastases	4
Sarcomas	2
Oligodendroglioma	1
Neuroblastoma	1

these cases, catherization of the aqueduct seems to be the method of choice since the complication rate is much lower than in cases of Torkildsen drainage (8) or ventriculoatrial shunt. No death was related to the procedure of intubation of the aqueduct. In three cases, we had to insert a ventriculoatrial shunt at a later date because of recurrent symptoms of increased intracranial pressure.

In 47 of 91 patients operated on for Arnold-Chiari malformation, we finished with intubation of the aqueduct. The standard procedure consists of removal of the occipital squame up to the transverse sinus, enlargement of the occipital foramen, dissection of arachnoidal adhesions at the end of the fourth ventricle, and a lyophilized dural graft. Four patients died 3-12 months after the operation. Their death was not directly related to the intubation of the aqueduct. We have grouped the results according to preoperative clinical symptoms and compared the two surgical procedures within these groups (Tables 3-6).

Table 3. Results according to clinical symptoms and surgical procedures

Torticollis, cerebellar syndrome, bulbocerebellar syndrome (No. = 17)

Posterior fossa decompression (No. = 11)		Posterior fossa decompression and intubation (No. = 6)	
Good	10	Good	6
Poor	1	Poor	0

Table 4 Intracranial hypertension and posterior fossa tumor symptoms (No. = 11)

Posterior fossa decompression (No. = 6)		Posterior fossa decompression and intubation (No. = 5)	
Good	3	Good	4
Poor	3	Poor	1

Table 5. Spinal cord Syndrome and vestibular cerebello pyramidal syndrome (No. = 20)

Posterior fossa decompression (No. = 4)		Posterior fossa decompression and intubation (No. = 16)	
Good	0	Good	8
Poor	4	Poor	8

Table 6. Syringomyelia (No. = 31)

Posterior fossa decompression (No. = 15)		Posterior fossa decompression and intubation (No. = 16)	
Good	4	Good	10
Poor	11	Poor	6

In the first group, there is no important difference between the two surgical procedures. In all other cases, average results are less satisfactory, particularly when spinal cord symptoms are present. In these cases, however, there is a better improvement after intubation of the aqueduct combined with posterior fossa decompression. The procedure prevents secondary blockage of cerebrospinal fluid (CSF) flow in the area operated on caused by new arachnoidal adhesions. In cases associated with syringomyelia or syringobulbia, the CSF bypass of the fourth ventricle seems to be of particular advantage. An abrupt increase of pressure is not transmitted to the syrinx since the CSF from the third ventricle is directly drained to the cervical subarachnoid space.

Six cases of Arnold-Chiari malformation were complicated by *aqueduct stenosis*. The stenosis was always short as shown by combined ventriculography and pneumencephalography. In intubating the aqueduct, the two problems were solved by the same procedure. In three of the cases, a metallic guide was needed to cross the stenosis. This could be done without any complication.

The last group of our series comprises aqueduct stenosis not caused by tumor (1) (Table 7). Only exceptionally was there an indication for intubation of the aqueduct; in six cases, a posterior fossa tumor was suspected, and in three children 4-5 years old, a valve defect produced acute intracranial hypertension without ventricular dilatation. Only seven patients were operated on primarily for a short membranous obstruction. One patient died immediately after the operation. In two cases, we later had to insert a ventriculoatrial shunt. All other patients are alive, and no other intervention was necessary.

Discussion

Among the different operations for drainage of the CSF, the intubation of the aqueduct has its firm place. In our experience of 113 patients in 4 years, we feel that this method is superior to other shunt operations in infiltratively growing tumors, Arnold-Chiari malformations, and aqueduct stenosis. As described by other authors (1, 9), the tissue compatibility is excellent even over long periods. The insertion of a smooth catheter at the end of an exploration of the posterior fossa does not imply any difficulties for the surgeon and can be quickly and safely performed. This method does not require any additional manipulations such as puncture of the lateral ventricle and repositioning of the patient. Further shunt operations become unnecessary because in the long-term follow-up the complication rate is much lower than in valve operations.

Table 7. Nontumoral stenosis of the aqueduct in children and adults (No. = 16)

1-15 years	6
Over 15 years	10

Summary

The results of 113 operations of the posterior fossa in which intubation of the aqueduct was performed are reported. Indication for this procedure was given in 50 posterior fossa tumors, 47 Arnold-Chiari malformations, and 16 aqueduct stenoses. The overall mortality was 4.4%. A later shunt operation with valve was necessary in 6.2% of our cases. Incompatibility reactions of the smooth, siliconized material were not observed.

References

1. BENNETT, R.T., ALLEN, P.B.R., MILLER, J.D.R.: Non tumoral stenosis of the aqueduct in adults. Surg. Neurol. 4, 524-527 (1975)
2. CROSBY, R.M.N., HENDERSON, Ch., PAUL, R.L.: Catheterization of the cerebral aqueduct for obstructive hydrocephalus in infants. J. Neurosurg. 38, 596-601 (1973)
3. DANDY, W.E.: The diagnosis and treatment of hydrocephalus resulting from strictures of the aqueduct of sylvius. Surg. Gynecol. Obstet. 31, 340-358 (1920)
4. LAPRAS, C., LEPOIRE, J.: Traitement de l'hydrocêphalie non tumorale du nourrisson par la dérivation ventriculo-atriale. Neurochirurgie 13, 209-342 (1967)
5. LAPRAS, C., POIRIER, N., DERUTY, R., BRET, Ph., JOYEUX, O.: Le cathérérisme de l'aqueduc de Sylvius. Sa place actuelle dans le traitement chirurgical des sténoses de l'aqueduc de Sylvius, des tumeurs de la fosse cérébrale postérieure et de la syringomyélie. Neurochirurgie 21, 101-109 (1975)
6. LEKSELL, L.: A surgical procedure for atresia of the aqueduct of sylvius. Acta Psychiatr. Neurol. Scand. 24, 559-568 (1949)
7. THOMALSKE, G., SCHÄFER, M., BECKER, H.: Diagnostic différentiel des tumeurs intraventriculaires par la tomodensitométrie. Neurochirurgie 23,1, 81-91 (1977)
8. TORKILDSEN, A.: A new palliative operation in case of inoperable occlusion of the sylvian aqueduct. Acta Chir. Scand. 82, 117-124 (1939)
9. TURNBULL, I.M., DRAKE, C.G.: Membranus occlusion of the aqueduct of sylvius. J. Neurosurg. 24, 24-33 (1966)

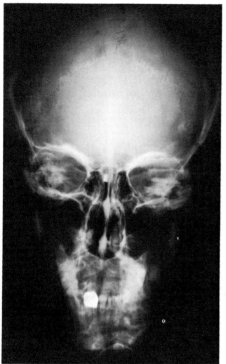 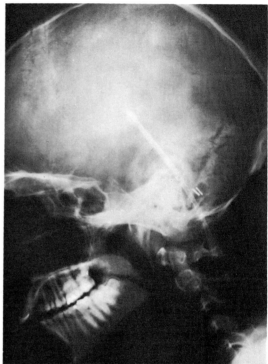

Fig. 1. X-ray image supplied by Prof. Dr. Hacker, director of the Department of Neuroradiology at the University Clinic in Frankfurt/Main) in anterior-posterior projection, showing postoperative catheter control in a 14-year-old boy with medulloblastoma of the vermis

Fig. 2. Same image in lateral view, showing catheter in correct position

Clinical Aspects and Anatomy

Electromyographic Analysis of Brain Nerve Reflexes in Posterior Fossa Processes

D. LINKE

Introduction

Processes in the posterior fossa do not only influence the function of the cerebellum and the long pathways but also frequently alter the afferents, efferents, and relay centers of the brain nerve reflexes. A clinical testing of these reflexes is much more difficult than in cases of the spinal nerves. An electromyographic registration and evaluation, therefore, seems appropriate.

Methods

We investigated the brain nerve reflexes in five patients with posterior fossa processes; four pontine tumors and one unknown process with symptoms of the posterior fossa. The blink reflex, the silent period of the masseter, and a tongue reflex were tested. The registration was made with a four-channel oscilloscope. In some cases up to ten reflex tests were averaged.

The blink reflex was elicited by stimulation of the supraorbital nerve. The activity of both orb. oculi was recorded with surface electrodes. For recording of the silent period of the masseter, muscle needle electrodes were used. The tongue, the second root of the trigeminal nerve, and the masseter itself were stimulated to evoke the silent period. Investigation of the tongue was made by stimulating the hypoglossal and the lingual nerves in the mandibular angle and recording the response from the tongue surface by a suction electrode system.

Results

The blink reflex was altered in its second component in all five cases. As an example, the case D. H. may be quoted. In this 10-year-old patient with a pontine tumor, the second component of the blink reflex was retarded on the left side up to 44 ms. In contralateral stimulation, this effect was given more pronounced. In clinical examination, no alteration of the blink reflex could be seen, although hypaesthesia in the area of the left trigeminal nerve could be demonstrated.

In computerized tomography, which was performed in the same week as the electromyographic investigation, there was no pathologic finding, but weeks later the full symptomatology of a pontine tumor developed. The silent period of the masseter muscle was altered significantly in only one case (Fig. 2). In one case, no deviations could be found, in spite of hypaesthesia in one side of the face. The tongue reflex was retarded in only one case (from 8-10 ms). Clinically, there were no peculiarities about the tongue in this case.

Discussion

The blink reflex seemed to be the most sensitive of the tested reflexes, because it was altered in all five cases and it was also altered when there were no clinical peculiarities about it. Furthermore, the normal values and physiologic basis are well-known for these reflexes (2, 3). The evaluation of the silent period of the masseteric muscle seems to be less important, because the normal values vary greatly (1).

Especially important is the fact that this inhibitory reflex was not changed in the case of trigeminal hypaesthesia. The tongue reflex was changed in one case, although no clinical peculiarity was to be observed. Normal values have been established for comparison (4, 5, 6, 7).

In summary, electromyographic investigation of brain nerve reflexes in cases of processes in the posterior fossa can demonstrate pathologic changes although there may be no clinical alterations. This is of special importance, because the possibilities of computerized tomography are limited in cases of posterior fossa processes. The electromyographic investigation may be an additional aid to early diagnosis. For exact differential diagnosis, further experience is necessary.

References

1. HUFSCHMIDT, H.-J., LINKE, D.: A damping facotir in human voluntary contraction. J. Neurol. Neurosurg. Psychiatry 39, 6, 536 (1976)

2. KILIMOV, N., LINKE, D.: Blink-reflex in facialhypoglossic anastomosis. (In preparation)

3. KUGELBERG, E.: Facial reflexes. Brain 75, 385-396 (1952)

4. LINKE, D.: The silent period in human intrinsic tongue muscles. Eur. J. Physiol. Suppl. Vol. 362 (1976a) R 35

5. LINKE, D.: Die Sprechmotorik. Habilitationsschrift Med. Fak. Bonn (1976b)

6. LINKE, D.: Motor control of the human tongue. Proceedings of the international union of physiological societies, XIII (1977a)

7. LINKE, D.: Electromyography of the tongue. Electroencephalogr. Clin. Neurophysiol. 43, 621 (1977b)

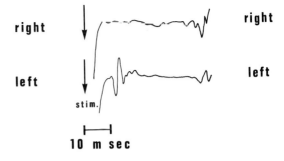

Fig. 1. Blink reflex

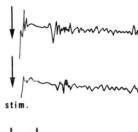

Fig. 2. Masseteric silent period

Prepontine and Parapontine Tumors

H. STEFAN, J. WAPPENSCHMIDT, and W. FRÖSCHER

Prepontine and parapontine tumors are the most frequently occuring ones among the extracerebral tumors around the brain stem. Histologically, they are (classified according to topographic points of view):

1. Extradural tumors originating from the bone-like osteoma and osteosarcoma, tumors within the bone-like chordoma and metastases, osteochondroma originating from synchondroses, and glomus tumors originating from the ganglia of the vegetative nerves.
2. Mengingeoma, neurinoma, epidermoids, and dermoids within the subarachnoidal space as well as angiomas and aneurysms simulating compressing lesions.
3. Tumors extending from the extracranial adjacent area into the cranial cavity like tumors of the epipharynx and sinus tumors as well as processes of the tympanum and internal ear.

Contrary to the most frequently occuring cerebellar tumors, the medulloblastoma and spongioblastoma, they rarely become clinically manifest until middle or later age. A differentiation between prepontine and parapontine tumors and the intracerebral brain stem tumors is clinically not possible. However, due to the different therapeutic measures - extracerebral tumors can be treated surgically but not intracerebral ones - a differentiation is important. So far, the conventional contrast media techniques were the safest methods for such a differentiation. The ventral extracerebral tumors cause a posterior or posteriolateral displacement of the brain stem. Typical (i.e., the most frequent) arteriographic signs of this are the dorsal and lateral displacement of the basilar artery and due to the flattening of the brain stem, compressed, shorter appearing arterial segments of the upper and lower cerebellar arteries surrounding the brain stem. Other indicative signs are pathologic stainings via vessels, which supply the bones and meninges. Due to their topographic-anatomic position, they demonstrated a dorsal or dorsal and lateral displacement of the aqueduct and fourth ventricle in the encephalogram, in which case the more cranial ones displace the aqueduct and the more caudal ones displace the fourth ventricle to a greater extent. A posterior displacement of the internal liquor spaces is, however, also caused by brain stem tumors. Different and therefore decisive for the diagnosis is the appearance of the outer liquor spaces: the intracerebral tumor distends the brain stem and thus constricts the ventral cisterns, while the extracerebral process dilates the cisterns above and below the tumor due to the displacement of the brain stem. This leads to the very important consequence that an extracerebral tumor can only be diagnosed with certainty in the encephalogram, when the tumor-free residual lumen of the cisterns is sufficiently filled with air. One can identify the cranial and caudal surface of the tumor in the tomoencephalogram and thus recognize the sagittal expansion of the tumor. Misinterpretations occur when little or no air reaches the outer liquor spaces due to the size of the tumor. As is demonstrated by the following examples, the arteriogram can be a decisive aid in this case. In Figures 1a and 1b, the lateral pneumograms indicate the ventral position of a tumor by a posterior displacement of the aqueduct and fourth ventricle. In case 1a, the constriction of the pontine cistern and the broadening of the pons shadow definitely indicate an inoperable brain stem tumor. The poor filling of the basal cisterns with air in case 1b could simulate a similar location of the tumor. The arteriogram of the two cases prevents misinterpretation. In the case of Figure 2a, the diagnosis of a pontine tumor is confirmed by a displacement of the basilar artery toward the clivus; in the case of Figure 2b, however, the arteriogram confirms the extracerebral location of the tumor due to the posterior displacement of the basilar artery. In this case, the tumor proved to be a chordoma.

On the other hand, the arteriogram may result in misinterpretations when only the displacement of the basilar artery is taken into consideration. There are localized glious pontine tumors, on the one hand, which protude from the anterior surface of the pons with nodular protuberances, grow around the basilar artery, and displace it in a posterior direction. The arteriogram, however, demonstrates a definite elongation and dilation of the vessels around the brain stem in the sagittal and lateral view. This means that a broadening of the brain stem is caused by an intracerebral tumor. Misleading dislocations of the basilar artery can occur in glious and paraglious tumors with an atypical ingrowth from the fourth ventricle through Luschka's foraminae into the cerebellopontine angle. On the other hand, parapontine epidermoids have been described with an atypical growth between the basilar artery and pons, causing a ventral displacement of the basilar artery in the arteriogram. This means that both contrast media methods must be used in doubtful cases. A definite arteriographic criterion for an extracerebral localization is met, however, when the dilated supplying arteries of the tumor originate from vessels which are physiologically supplying the dura or the tentorium. It must be emphasized in this case that branches of all three cephalic arteries, the vertebral artery, the external, and internal carotid artery, contribute to the blood supply of the dura mater. The best results are, therefore, seen from selective and superselective angiograms.

Finally, vascular malformations can only be demonstrated arteriographically. In this case, the large aneurysms around the bifurcation of the oral basilar artery lead to a depression of the posterior part of the floor of the third ventricle. When the circummesencephalic cisterns are not filled or not sufficiently filled, a differentiation between extracerebral and penducular tumors is not possible (Figs. 3a and 3b). Generally, it is not easier to determine size and extension of the extracerebral tumors in the arteriogram than in the pneumencephalogram. Tumors of the tentorial fissure can be recognized from the lifting of the prepeduncular segments of the posterior cerebral artery, the ipsilateral supra- and infratentorial extension of the tumor from the displacement of vessels of the vertebral and carotid circulation. The extradural tumor growth can also be recognized arteriographically without doubt from the displacement of the pre- and intracavernous carotid segments. These changes, which are often not taken into consideration, were observed in our patients in cases of chordoma, chondroma, trigeminus neurinoma, and tumors of the epipharynx and meningioma.

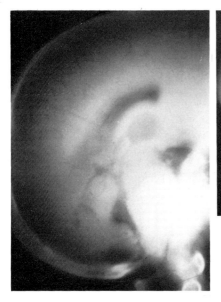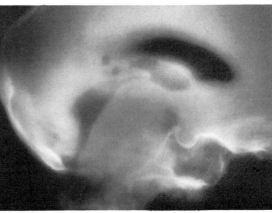

Fig. 1. *a* Pneumencephalogram showing a glioma of the pons   Fig. 1. *b* Poor filling of the basal cisterns; no correct diagnosis possible

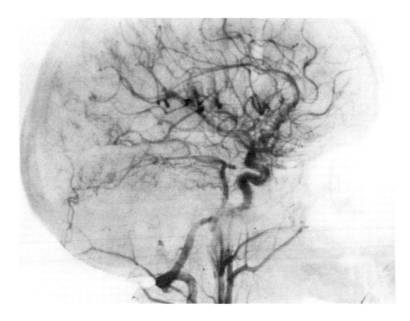

Fig. 2. *a* Basilar artery pressed toward the clivus due to glioma of the pons

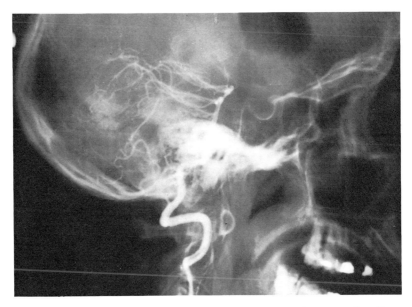

Fig. 2. *b* Posterior displacement of the basilar artery due to chordoma

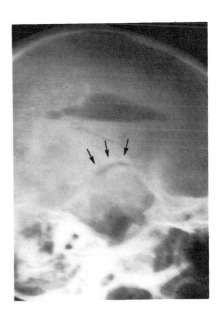

Fig. 3. *a* Elevation of the floor of the third ventricle, simulating a tumor of the peduncle

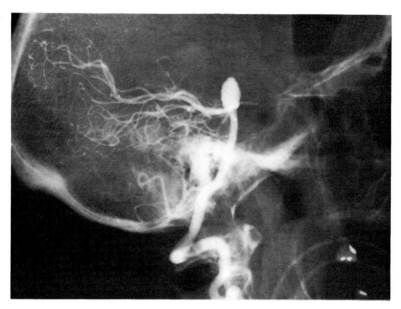

Fig.3. *b* Angiogram of the same case showing a large aneurysma of the basilar artery

The Role of Angiotomography in the Evaluation of the Posterior Fossa
K. SARTOR, E. FLIEDNER, N. FRECKMANN, and K. MATSUMOTO

LAFONT et al. (2) were the first to perform tomography on cerebral vessels. Since that time (1956) cerebral angiotomography (AT) has been used routinely only in a relatively small number of neuroradiologic departments. The reason is mainly to be found in the fact that it was only rarely that suitable tomographic equipment was available in the angio-room. Therefore, other techniques of image enhancement and various methods of obtaining information on complex vascular structures were preferred. AT, however, can be a very effective means of solving certain angiographic problems, particularly in the posterior fossa. It is not a difficult procedure and does not require very sophisticated apparatus, at least in its most simple forms.

Material and Methods

During the last 5 years, we have performed cerebral angiotomographic studies in more than 200 patients. In about 60 patients, predominantly tumor cases, the posterior fossa was evaluated. In the majority of studies linear single-phase AT using a Neurodiagnost (Philips) armed with a multisection cassette containing five layers was done, the arc of tube movement usually being 10º-12º. In a small number of cases, serial lateral midline magnification auto-AT was applied instead.

Results

In posterior fossa compressing lesions, AT improved mass localization and determination of the extent of neovasculature, if present. It also showed cystic tumor components that could only be suspected on conventional angiograms (Fig. 1). The method was found particularly helpful in the evaluation of nine aneurysms in various locations of the vertebrobasilar system (8). In these, a better definition of the relationship between the angiodysplasia and parent or neighboring arteries was achieved than with conventional angiographic studies alone. Special projections, magnification, and subtraction were unnecessary in almost all cases.

In one patient, who had a complex sceletal deformity at the craniovertebral junction, AT clearly showed major features of the anomaly and at the same time the exaxt relationship between the dysplastic bones and the abnormally coursing vertebral arteries.

In a larger number of cases, later reported as normal, AT proved its ability to show vascular details that could not be appreciated on the conventional studies, even after subtraction, e.g., the vein of the lateral recess of the fourth ventricle on the lateral view and intrapontine veins on the Towne view. Occasionally, the fourth ventricle could be seen very clearly on lateral midline angiotomograms.

Discussion

Lateral midline auto-AT and single-phase AT with the Neurodiagnost (3) can be performed very quickly, usually requiring only one or two additional injections of contrast medium. Using the Neurodiagnost, AT may be done in almost any projection. For better correlation with the topography of the classic angiographic views, however, we prefer in most cases performance of lateral and/or sagittal AT; AT in oblique planes is rarely used by us. The timing of injection and tube movement (tomographic exposure) has to be learned by experience, hand injections are probably better than automatic injections.

AT has its best results where vessels overlying the vessels in the plane of interest are to be eliminated without a change of projection. In fact, AT is the only angiographic technique with which this can be achieved. In addition, bony structures overlying the region of interest are blurred to a sufficient degree, even when using relatively small arcs of tube movement, e.g., $10°-12°$. Our own experience is that such small sweeps of the x-ray tube produce the best compromis between contrast and tomographic effect (6, 7).

A third major advantage of AT is the improved definition of small details similar to magnification angiography, as has been shown by FREYSCHMIDT and RITTMEYER (1). Also, one gains from a synopsis of a set of five angiotomograms produced simultaneously a three-dimensional impression of the vascular anatomy in and around the plane of interest (6, 7).

One may well say that up to a certain degree, AT includes the individual advantages of tomography, stereography, magnification, subtraction, and of selective/superselective injections and special projections (5, 6, 7).

Since the advent of the CT scanner, the necessity of using AT in the localization of posterior fossa masses has been reduced. There are, however, still cases where AT proves helpful when trying to correlate CT with angiographic findings. In the evaluation of predominantly or purely vascular problems, AT remains a method still unsurpassed in many respects (6, 7, 8). Relatively sophisticated apparatus for serial AT is already available. A simple device for this purpose that could be used in every angio-room along with conventional cerebral angiography, is still needed, however.

Summary

Angiotomography is a radiographic technique that combines, to a certain degree, the individual advantages of tomography, stereography, magnification, subtraction, selective injections, and special projections. In the posterior fossa, it is particularly useful when predominantly or purely vascular processes have to be evaluated. It may, however, still prove to be of value for correlation of angiographic and CT findings in mass lesions.

References

1. FREYSCHMIDT, J., RITTMEYER, K.: Experimentelle Untersuchungen zur Auflösung von Detailgrößen und -kontrasten im Angiotomogramm. Fortschr. Röntgenstr. 123, 262-267 (1975)
2. LAFONT, R., BETOULIERES, P., TEMPLE, J.P., PELISSIER, M.: Angiographie carotidienne et tomographie simultanée. Rev. Neurol. 94, 263-267 (1956)

3. NADJMI, M., PÖSCHMANN, A.: Angio-Tomographie am Diagnost-N. Radiologe 12, 437-440 (1972)

4. NADJMI, M., PÖSCHMANN, A.: Über ein Gerät zur Serien-Angio-Tomographie. Fortschr. Röntgenstr. 123, 299-301 (1975)

5. NADJMI, M., BUSHE, K.A., RATZKA, M., MOISSL, G.: Angiotomographische Aspekte der zerebralen Aneurysmen und Angiome. Fortschr. Röntgenstr. 125, 428-437 (1976)

6. SARTOR, K.: Angiotomographische Detaildiagnostik bei Aneurysmen an der Hirnbasis. Fortschr. Röntgenstr. 122, 506-510 (1975)

7. SARTOR, K.: Zerebrale Angiotomographie mit dem Neuro-Diagnost. Röntgenstr. 35, 11-17 (1976)

8. SARTOR, K.: Zur Angiographie bei intrakraniellen Aneurysmen im vertebrobasilären System. Fortschr. Röntgenstr. (In press)

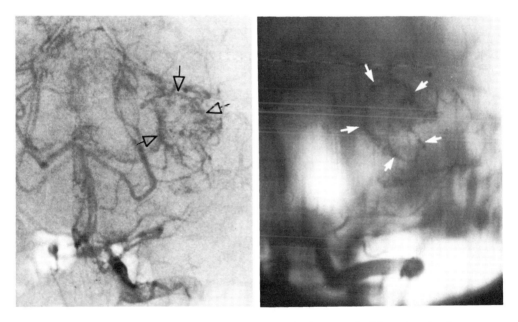

Fig. 1. Cystic hemangioblastoma in the left cerebellar hemisphere. On the conventional subtraction angiogram (*left*), the cystic component of the mass (*arrows*) can only be suspected. On the AP angiotomogram (*right*), the cyst (*arrows*) is clearly shown

Medulloblastomas

Studies on the Biology of Medulloblastoma
W. MÜLLER, F. SLOWIK, and R. SCHRÖDER

Since the typization of the medulloblastoma by BAILEY and CUSHING in 1925 (2) it has been confirmed that this neoplasm is a neuroectodermal tumor of the cerebellar midline prevailing in children. But when referring to broader statistics, it becomes evident that both the manifestation in older patients and the localization in the hemispheres of the cerebellum are not exceptions but facts which were emphasized as early as 1930 by CUSHING (6). In 1964, RUBINSTEIN and NORTHFIELD (14) convincingly explained that the tumor introduced by FOERSTER and GAGEL (9) and found mostly in middle-aged persons as "umschriebenes Arachnoidalsarkom des Kleinhirns" is in reality a variation of the medulloblastoma (without neglecting the occurrence of true mesodermal sarcomas in the posterior fossa). Histologically, this type of medulloblastoma is characterized by a very intense production of mesodermal fibers, so that a probable reason for this phenomenon, as is the case in other neoplasms, is to be seen in a stimulation through the tumor cells. RUBINSTEIN and NORTHFIELD (14), in contrast to the classic type, termed this variant of medulloblastoma "desmoplastic." Additional "transitional" types can be observed.

Besides these different morphologic aspects, important clinical ones, especially those concerning the prognosis, must be added. Thus, it has been well-known for a long time that the medulloblastomas in children and of the midline have a worse prognosis than the so-called medulloblastomas of adults with frequent localization in the hemispheres (e.g., 4, 5, 7, 12). These statements are in contrast to the conclusions of other investigators (e.g., 1, 3, 6). But, since tumors in the hemispheres apparently often represent the desmoplastic variant of the medulloblastoma, other authors considered the question of whether the different biologic behavior was not particularly caused by this fact (e.g., 4, 8, 10, 11).

Without regard to the clinical problems based on a greater number of cases - half of them from the Neurosurgical Clinic of the University of Cologne and half from the Hungerian National Institute of Neurosurgery in Budapest - the parameters, i.e., classic and desmoplastic midline and hemispheric medulloblastoma in relation to age and sex distribution, are compared, and where possible, their significance is explored.

From a total of 327 cases, the sex distribution of 202 males and 125 females is in agreement with other reports. Setting the age limit of childhood at 15 years, 74 of the 327 cases (22.7%) were older (Fig. 1). In 55 of the 327 cases (16.8%), the tumor location was in the hemispheres, 30 in the males and 25 in the females. Statistically, the sex distribution represents no difference in the case of midline tumors.

Therefore, it should be desirable to check this relationship in a greater number of cases.

Regarding the age of patients with hemispheric tumors in comparison to those with midline tumors, we can confirm a different distribution (Fig. 2). Considering all medulloblastomas beyond the 15th year, a lateral localization exists in 41.9%; during childhood, this value amounts to only 9.5%. Statistically, these values are of high significance.

It was possible to classify 272 of the medulloblastomas histologically. Fifty-seven, nearly one-fifth, were desmoplastic with a sex distribution of 38 males and 19 females. The age distribution was the same as in the group of classic medulloblastomas. Figure 3 demonstrates - within the age distribution of 272 tumors - the relationship between the midline localization (narrow hatching) on the one side and the classic (unhatched) and the desmoplastic (broad hatching) tumor variant on the other side. The increase of the hemispheric localization in adolescent and adult patients is prominent. Beyond that, we state that hemispheric localization and desmoplastic variants are by no means concurrent. On the basis of the frequencies determined statistically, we can expect the coincidence of desmoplastic variant and hemispheric localization in 3.5%. The real coincidence of these two parameters of 5.1% signifies an almost complete congruence with the expected value; therefore, it is only an accidental coincidence.

In summary, we can demonstrate in this comparatively extensive group of patients that the desmoplastic type actually represents a variant of the classic medulloblastoma, both histologically and statistically. A peculiar biologic significance can, therefore, probably be denied. Compared to this and according to the different age distribution, the localization for the clinical behavior seems to be of more fundamental importance. Further investigations have be carried out to analyze the relationship between localization and clinical course.

References

1. ALEKSEEVA: Medulloblastome der hinteren Schädelgrube beim Erwachsenen. Vopr. Neirokhir. 6, 30-33 (1959) (russ.)
2. BAILEY, P., CUSHING, H.: Medulloblastoma cerebelli, common type of midcerebellar glioma of childhood. Arch. Neurol. Psychiatr. 14, 192-224 (1925)
3. BERGER, E.C., ELVIDGE, A.R.: Medulloblastoma and cerebellar sarcomas: clinical survey. J. Neurosurg. 10, 139-144 (1963)
4. CHATTY, E.M., EARLE, K.M.: Medulloblastoma. A report of 201 cases with emphasis on the relationship of histologic variants to survival. Cancer 28, 977-983 (1971)
5. CHRISTENSEN, E., ALS, E.: Medulloblastomas. Acta Psychiatr. Scand. Suppl. 108, 87 (1956)
6. CUSHING, H.: Experiences with cerebellar medulloblastoma: critical review. Acta Pathol. Microbiol. Scand. 7, 1-86 (1930)
7. CUTLER, E.C., SOSMAN, M.C., VAUGHAN, W.W.: Place of radiation treatment of cerebellar medulloblastoma: report of 20 cases. Am J. Roentgenol. 35, 429-453 (1936)
8. DEXTER, D., HOWELL, D.A.: Medulloblastomas and arachnoidal sarcomas. Brain 88, 367-374 (1965)

9. FOERSTER, O., GAGEL, O.: Das umschriebene Arachnoidealsarkom des Kleinhirns. Z. Gesamte Neurol. Psychiatr. 164, 565-580 (1939)
10. KUNICKI, A., STEFANKO, St., KUKULSKA, Z.: Morphologic peculiarities of anaplastic cerebellar tumors and their prognostic significance. Acta Med. Pol. 12, 319-337 (1971)
11. LINS, E.: Das Medulloblastom des Erwachsenen. Acta Neurochir. 31, 67-72 (1974)
12. MILES, J., BHANDARI, Y.S.: Cerebellar medulloblastoma in adults: review of 18 cases. J. Neurol. Psychiatry 33, 208-211 (1970)
13. POTTHOFF, W.: Beitrag zur Architektur zweier Medulloblastome anhand von Serienschnitten. Inaug. Diss. Univ. Köln (1971)
14. RUBINSTEIN, L.J., NORTHFIELD, D.W.C.: The medulloblastoma and the so-called "arachnoidal cerebellar sarcoma". Brain 87, 379-412 (1964)

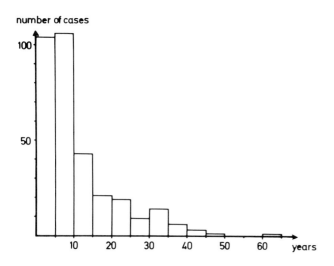

Fig. 1. Age distribution of 327 medulloblastomas

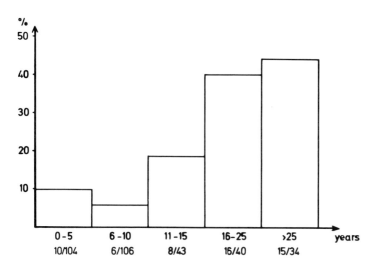

Fig. 2. Percentage of patients with hemispheric medulloblastoma. Below the abscissa, the absolute numbers are indicated (No. = 327)

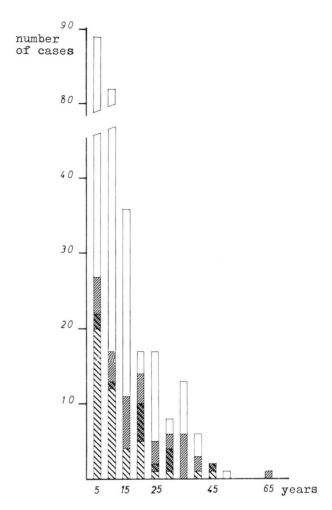

Fig. 3. Age distribution of 272 histologically classified medulloblastomas (classic = unhatched; desmoplastic = broat hatching). Superimposed is the hemispheric localization (narrow hatching). The parameters desmoplastic variant and hemispheric localization are not in predominant coincidence

Immunoelectrophoretic Evaluations in Posterior Fossa Tumors

D. K. Böker, W. Entzian, and F. Gullotta

An immunoelectrophoretic investigation on brain tumors is presently being carried out on a large scale in our institutions. The findings on all of the 25 posterior fossa tumors (Table 1) are reported here. Our interest was particularly focused on the immunologic behavior of "medulloblastomas," as it is well-known that the nature and origin of this tumor is still controversial (1, 2).

Material and Methods

Tumor tissue was cut to small pieces and homogenized at 0°C. After adding an aliquot of physiologic saline, the material was stored 24 h at +4°C, being agitated occasionally. After centrifugation at 20,000 xg for 30 min, the overnatant was considered to contain all the "soluble antigen." The protein quantity was adjusted to 10 mg/ml. Immunoelectrophoresis was carried out using a serum gained from rabbits previously immunized by injection of a glioblastoma extract, suspended in complete Freund's adjuvant.

The sera of the animals were pooled, and immediately before use, they were absorbed with pooled lyophilized human plasma in order to clear them from nontumor precipitations. The electrophoretic separation of "soluble antigens" took place in agar solution (1.5%) in Michaeli's buffer. After electrophoresis, grooves were cut into the gel. They are filled with the pooled rabbit serum and left overnight. The experiment was ended after the appearance of a precipitate in the positive control, after 16 h at the latest. "Positive control" means that a precipitation is to be expected from the extract of the glioblastoma used to immunize the rabbits and the pooled serum of these immunized rabbits.

Results

1. Positive reactions, i.e., precipitation line at adequate position in the immunoelectrophoresis of the extracts of the tumors and of the positive controls, were found in all tumors of ectodermal origin as spongioblastomas, ependymomas, plexuspapillomas, and neurinomas (Fig. 1).
2. Angioblastomas (Lindau tumors) showed different reactions, as the precipitation line was positioned too far away from the precipitation

Table 1. Findings on 25 posterior fossa tumors

Spongioblastomas	5
Ependymomas	5
Papilloma of plexus	2
Neurinomas	2
Angioblastomas (Lindau)	3
Medulloblastomas	8

line of the positive control to be considered the effect of identical antigen (Fig. 2).
3. Out of eight medulloblastomas, four showed a positive and four a negative reaction (Table 2).

Discussion

In a previous series of immunoelectrophoresis, the serum of glioblastoma-inoculated rabbits had proved its specifity against approximately 120 tumors of neuroectodermal origin. A positive immunoreaction was found in all examined extracts of glioblastoma, astrocytoma, oligodendroglioma, ependymoma, and spongioblastoma, and a negative reaction was found in all the examined extracts of tumors of mesodermal origin such as meningeoma and intracerebral metastases.

In this series there is also no wrong reaction in immunoelectrophoresis, especially of those tumors whose histogenetic order is established without doubt, i.e., a positive precipitation line was found in all cases of spongioblastoma, ependymoma, plexuspapilloma and neurinoma, as to be expected.

Somewhat surprising, at first glance, were the precipitation lines of angioblastoma because their positions were located apart from those of the posterior controls. The reason for these results, which were confirmed by control studies, might be the reaction of an antigen against reactive glial tissue or cerebral tissue. In our opinion it is a reaction against the tissue of the vascular wall. This observation, however, should be confirmed by further examinations.

The results in medulloblastomas were inhomogeneous and gave cause for considerations. If the medulloblastoma was a tumor or neuroectodermal origin, the precipitation line of the tumor extract should be identical to that of the positive controls. However, the extracts of the four tumors K. E., H. K., M. M., and T. K. did not correspond to the schedule. It seems probable that these four tumors are not of neuroectodermal origin and that they contain neuroectodermal tissue of only minor amount. This suggestion supports the results of GULLOTTA (1).

The histologic specimens of all "medulloblastomas" were reexamined - without knowledge of their immunobiologic behavior - especially concerning the existence of neuroectodermal or mesenchymal structures. The morphologic results are compares with the immunoelectrophoretic results in Table 2. Tumors of glial origin or mixed tumors with predominant glial tissue showed positive precipitation lines; sarcomatous tumors or mixed tumors with predominant sarcomatous tissue never

Table 2. Medulloblastomas

	Imm. electr.	Histol.
K. E.	∅	Sarc.
H. K.	∅	Sarc. > gliom.
M. M.	∅	Sarc. > gliom.
T. K.	∅	Sarc.
M. U.	+	Gliom.
B. P.	+	Gliom.
F. A.	+	Gliom. > sarc.
O. A.	+	Gliom.

showed a precipitation. From this experience, it may be presumed that the evidence of antigens depends on the amount of neuroectodermal tissue and of the concentration of antigen.

Concerning the nature of the antigens only surmises can be discussed. Probably, natural antigens against glial tissue become efficient and not tumor-specific antigens. Concerning the nature of the medulloblastoma, it is suggested that these results correspond to the theory of the "overgrowth sarcoma." It should be concludable that the definition of "medulloblastoma" covers a group of tumors of different histogenesis.

References

1. GULLOTTA, F.: Das sogenannte Medulloblastom. Berlin-Heidelberg-New York: Springer 1967
2. GULLOTTA, F., KERSTING, G.: The Ultrastructure of Medulloblastoma in Tissue Culture. Virchows Archiv Abt. A, Pathol. Anat. 356, 111-118 (1972)

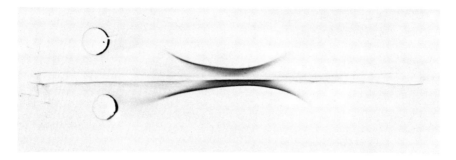

Fig. 1. The precipitation line of a glioma corresponds to that of the control

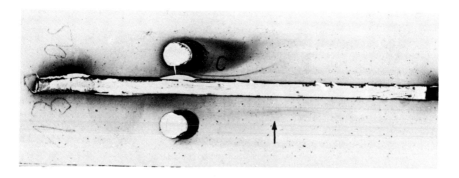

Fig. 2. Tumor of Lindau. The precipitation line of angioblastoma (*arrow*) does not correspond to that of the control (*c*)

The Clinic of Medulloblastoma

O. WILCKE and U. FUHRMANN

On evaluating the literature on the clinic of medulloblastoma published in the recent 25 years, we find that there are remarkable approaches for improving the prognosis of this highly malignant tumors. Observations of about 2500 cases reported in literature allows some precise statements. We find, for instance, that 4% of all CNS tumors are medulloblastomas; 20% of infantile brain tumors are medulloblastomas; 80% of which are found in children under 16 years of age. There is a predominance of boys over girls, the ratio being 7:3 (2, 5, 6, 11, 28).

Two-thirds of the medulloblastomas originate in the vermis and one-third in the cerebellar hemispheres. Only about 3% originate in the brain stem (8, 9, 20). The highest rate (Fig. 1) is to be found between 3-10 years, whereas no age disposition is visible in the 20% of medulloblastomas observed in patients over 16 years of age (10). Clinical experience shows that prognosis is less favorable in younger patients than in older ones, and long survival times were quite frequent in adult age (1, 6, 7, 8).

We will not go into detail as to the *symptomatology*, which is well-known. Both the short anamnesis of the quickly progressing syndrome and the quickly developing signs of intracranial pressure are characteristic, and in 90% of the cases we have to deal with papilledema. Similarly often, vomiting, ataxia, and headache are the first symptoms. In about 40% of the cases, the first symptoms are cranial nerve deficits.

In most cases, preoperative *differential diagnosis* on the medulloblastoma is not possible. In nearly 100% of the cases, EEG shows general changes, sometimes with special lateral stress. The *echo* generally indicates increased intracranial pressure by showing a dilated third ventricle. According to our own experience, 80% of the medulloblastomas can be diagnosed under the *isotope test* but do not allow a sure differential diagnosis. Neither is it possible to come to a sure differential diagnosis by vertebral angiography, which only shows the narrowing process. We will have to wait and see to what extent computerized tomography will improve the differential diagnostic forecast in combination with clinical diagnosis. Most detailed and operation-determining information is generally achieved by the ventriculogram, especially with positive contrast medium, in which detailed ventricles, angulation of the aqueduct, contours in the fourth ventricle, and blocked CSF drainage allow both localization and diagnosis of a tumor.

Surgical treatment of medulloblastoma has not produced any new developments in recent years, apart from a general technical improvement. Altogether, medulloblastomas have a high rate of operation mortality - 32% as already indicated by CUSHING (11) - partly because of their unfavorable initial condition at an advanced stage and partly because of the extension of the tumor affecting important vessels. In the literature, we find that it ranges from 0%-52%, always depending on the time definition of the term operation mortality (2, 5, 6, 18, 19). Like other important clinics, we count all those patients who die within the first 4 weeks after operation among operation mortality and have identical results. Autopsy of 201 patients who died within the first 4 weeks also revealed a rate of 35% (9). The clinical experience that operation mortality is higher with subtotal tumor removal than with total removal has been confirmed by many authors (2, 8, 13, 20, 22).

As medulloblastomas have a tendency toward recidivity and metastases formation, *radiotherapy* is of decisive importance in postoperative treatment after radical removal of the tumors. Medulloblastomas belong to the most radiosensitive kinds of tumor of the CNS (6, 8, 14, 16, 26), and presently available results of radiotherapy definitely prove that postoperative survival time depends to a great extent on sufficient postoperative irradiation. With about 30% of the medulloblastoma patients without intensive radiotherapy, the formation of metastases in the spinal sphere was to be observed (24), and it was more frequent than with all other tumors of the CNS that extracerebral or extraspinal metastases - mainly osteolytic skeleton metastases in the pelvic region - were observed (3, 4, 5, 21, 25, 27). HENDRIK and co-works (13) observed metastases in the peritoneal cavity in 6 out of 40 medulloblastomas with ventriculoperitoneal shunt.

Postoperative radiotherapy has to include both the tumor bed and the spinal region, the latter being the favored site for the formation of metastases. Considering that the maximum tolerance dosage of the brain stem is 5000 rad in 6-7 weeks with telecobalt or supervolt, a 4000-4500 rad irradiation is possible. Most favorable long-term results can be achieved with this dosage. Survival chances are markedly less favorable with lower dosages of less than 3500 rad or higher dosages of more than 5000 rad. Dosage for the spinal region is 2000-2500 rad after radiotherapy of the skull. Some others recommend postirradiation of the posterior fossa at 1800-2000 rad in general or if neurologic symptoms reappear (6, 8, 21, 26). This postoperative radiotherapy, though practiced in most cases, does have its complications such as radiation necrosis with disturbances of mental development, attacks, and pareses. According to BLOOM and co-workers (6), brain damage was found in 18% of the children who received intensive postirradiation. LAMPE and co-workers (16) observed such damage in four out of seven long-term survivors. However, it is beyond doubt that postoperative irradiation brings about an improvement of survival chances. Among 147 patients with medulloblastoma (Fig. 2), long survival was only achieved by those who received an intensive postirradiation of more than 3000 rad. Of those who were just operated on but did not receive postirradiation, only one patient survived for 3 1/2 years. Long survival times could only be achieved if postirradiation was sufficient and if the patient was beyond childhood (1, 7, 8, 15, 19, 22). During infancy - up to 3 years of age - we were only very seldom successful in achieving a long survival. Our statistics are in accordance with the findings of other authors (2, 6, 8, 26). Additional chemotherapy did not seem to have any especially marked influence on our patients.

At present, there are no figures to show to what extent additional chemotherapy may improve therapeutic measures in general. Individual observations of recurrent medulloblastomas and metastases seem to indicate a certain efficiency of chemotherapy, and experiments on animals confirm the therapeutic effects on embryonic tumors (12, 17, 23, 27). A triple polychemotherapy parallel to and after radiotherapy for a total of 1 year (12) was recommended by the International Society of Pediatric Oncology. Limits are set to cytostatic treatment by both the individual tolerance and the general toxicity, especially the toxic influence of the medulla.

Finally, on establishing a survey of the present stage of therapeutic success with medulloblastomas (Fig. 3), conclusions drawn from 2000 cases in the literature show that - apart from the high rate of operation mortality - about 30%-40% of the patients were able to survive the 3rd year after operation and about 26% survived the 5th year; 12% of our patients survived for more than 10 years. The cases evaluated by pathology (9) show - in accordance with a partly negative choice of patients with insufficient treatment - that survival chances exceeding 5 years were only 12%.

In summary, we may say that the high rate of operation mortality with medulloblastomas can probably be improved by early diagnosis. There are clear guidelines for the radiotherapy necessary in postoperative treatment which will influence the survival time considerably and may lead to permanent cure. Further investigations will show to what extent cytostatic treatment may improve current therapeutic treatment.

References

1. ARNOLD, G.: Cerebellar medulloblastoma in adults with cerebrospinal low level glucose and unusual ophthalmologic aspect. Rev. Otoneuroophthalmol. 43, 46-50 (Jan.-Febr. 1971)
2. ARON, B.S.: Medulloblastoma in children. Twenty two years experience with radiation therapy. Mer. J. Dis. Child. 121, 314-317 (April 1971)
3. BANNA, M.: Radiological study of skeletal metastases from cerebellar medulloblastoma. Br. J. Radiol. 43, 173-179 (May 1970)
4. BATES, T.: Extracranial metastases from a cerebellar medulloblastoma. Proc. R. Soc. Med. 66, 652-654 (1973)
5. BERGER, E.C., ELVIDGE, A.R.: Medulloblastoma and cerebellar sarcomas. A clinical survey. J. Neurosurg. 20, 139-144 (1963)
6. BLOOM, H.J.G., WALLACE, E., HENK, J.M.: The treatment and prognosis of medulloblastoma in children. A study of 82 verified cases. Am. J. Roentgenol. Radium Ther. Nucl. Med. 105, 43-62 (1969)
7. BORGHI, G., CHIORINO, R.: Medulloblastomas in adults. Neurochirurgia (Stuttg.) 7, 8-17 (1964)
8. CHANG, C.H.: An operative staging system and a megavoltage radiotherapeutic technic for cerebellar medulloblastoma. Radiology 93, 1351-9 (Dec. 1969)
9. CHATTY, G.M., EARLE, K.M.: Medulloblastoma. A report of 201 cases with emphasis on the relationship of histologic variants to survival. Cancer 28, 977-83 (Oct. 1971)
10. CRUE, B.L.: Medulloblastoma. Springfield, Ill.: Charles C. Thomas 1958
11. CUSHING, H.: Experiences with cerebellar medulloblastoma. A critical review. Acta Pathol. Microbiol. Scand. 7, 1-86 (1930)
12. NEIDHARDT, M.: Maligne Tumoren im Kindesalter. DMW 95, 153-158 (1970) (1970)
13. HENDRIK, E.B., HOFFMANN, H.J., HUMPHREYS, R.P.: Treatment of intratentorial gliomas in childhood. Recent Results in Cancer Research: Gliomas. HEKMATPANAH, J. (ed.). Berlin-Heidelberg-New York: Springer 1975

14. JENKIN, R.D.T.: Medulloblastoma in childhood: radiation therapy. Canad. Med. Assoc. J. 100, 51-53 (11. Jan. 1969)
15. KING, G.A.: Late recurrence in medulloblastoma. Am. J. Roentgenol. Radium Ther. Nucl. Med. 123, 7-12 (1975)
16. LAMPE, I., McINTYRE, R.S.: Experiences in the radiation therapy of medulloblastoma of the cerebellum. Am. J. Roentgenol. 71, 659 (1954)
17. LASSMANN, L.P., PEARCE, G.W., GANG, J.: Effect of vincristine sulphate on intracranial gliomata of childhood. Br. J. Surg. 53, 774-777 (1966)
18. LAUSBERG, G.: Symptomatology, therapy and prognosis of cerebellar medulloblastoma. Z. Kinderheilkde. 102, 193-203 (1968)
19. McFARLAND, D.R., HORWITH, H., SAENGER, E.L.: Medulloblastoma - a review of prognosis and survival. Br. J. Radiol. 42, 198-214 (Mar. 1969)
20. MILES, J.: Cerebellar medulloblastoma in adults: Review of 18 cases. J. Neurol. Neurosurg. Psychiatry 33, 208-211 (April 1970)
21. PATERSON, E., FARR, R.F.: Cerebellar medulloblastoma: treatment of irradiation of whole central nervous system. Acta radiol. 39, 323-336 (1953)
22. PROBERT, J.C., LEDERMAN, M., BAGSHAW, M.B.: Medulloblastoma - treatment and prognosis. A study of seventeen cases in ten years. Dept. Radiol. Div. Rad. Ther. Stanford Univ. School, Med. Sao Paulo. Calif. Med. 118, 14-17 (1973)
23. ROSENBAUM, M.L., REYNOLDS, A.F., SMITH, K.A., RUMACK, B.H., WALKER, M.D.: Clorethyl-cyclohexyl-nitrosourea (CCNU) in the treatment of malignant brain tumors. J. Neurosurg. 39, 306-314 (1973)
24. RUBINSTEIN, L.J., NORTHFIELD, D.W.C.: The medulloblastoma and so-called arachnoidal cerebellar sarcoma. A critical re-examination of a nosological problem. Brain, 87, 379-412 (1964)
25. SMITH, C.E., DONLIN, M.L., JONES, T.K., SEYMOUR, H.L.: Experiences in treating medulloblastoma at the University of Minnesota Hospitals. Radiology 109, 179-182 (1973)
26. TAVERAS, J.M.: Radiotherapy of brain-tumors. Clin. Neurosurg. 7, 200-213 (1961)
27. WILSEN, C.B.: Medulloblastoma current views regarding the tumor and its treatment. Oncology 24, 273-290 (1970)
28. ZÜLCH, H.J.: Atlas of Gross Neurosurgical Pathology. Berlin-Heidelberg-New York: Springer 1975

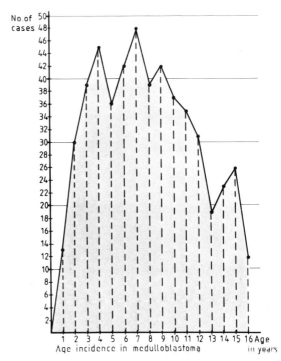

Fig. 1. Age distribution of medulloblastomas (CRUE series and own cases)

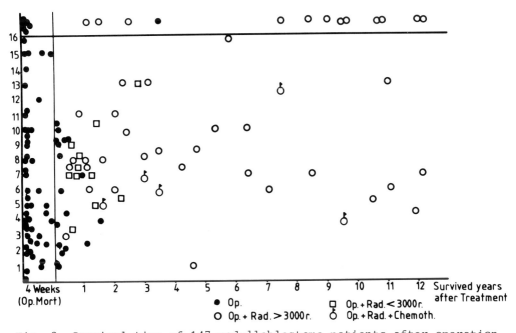

Fig. 2. Survival time of 147 medulloblastoma patients after operation

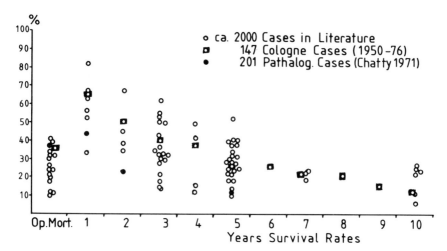

Fig. 3. Rate of survival of 2000 medulloblastoma patients in the literature; 147 own cases and 210 cases from the Pathological Institute (9)

Management and Prognosis of Medulloblastomas: Review Series of 80 Cases

N. KLUG

Eigthy patients with histologically verified medulloblastomas were treated in the Department of Neurosurgery of the University of Giessen in the years 1951-1977. There were 29 females (37.5%) and 51 males (62.5%). Age and sex distribution are presented in Figure 1. The average age was 11 3/4 years for females and 12 1/2 years for males; 52.5% of the patients were less than 10 years old, and 79% of the patients were under 20 years of age. There were only eight patients aged over 30; the oldest was 64 years old.

Follow-up data were available for 73 patients. The mean survival time among 60 nonsurviving patients was 11 months. Five patients (6.3%) survived more than 5 years; of them, two patients are still alive with a postoperative survival time of 10 and 18 years. The mean age of five patients with tumors localized in the cerebellar hemisphere (24 7/12 years) was markedly higher than the mean age of patients with tumors of the vermis (10 8/12 years). Eight patients aged over 30 had a longer survival time (25 months) than younger patients. There was no difference in survival among patients with tumors in the cerebellar hemisphere and in the vermis.

The review of the cases is presented in Table 1. The division into three groups is based on the development of the Neurosurgical Department in Giessen: 1951-1960 was the developmental phase, 1961-1967 was the period during which limited postoperative intensive care was possible, and 1968-1977 was the period during which postoperative care in the intensive care unit with all the modern possibilities of monitoring and therapy were available. Table 1 shows that the postoperative mortality diminished progressively with the improvement in postoperative care. However, as far as overall mortality is concerned, no significant change was noted.

The follow-up study compared 27 patients in whom preoperative ventricular drainage was employed to 48 patients in whom no preoperative drainage was performed. No positive influence of preoperative drainage on operative mortality was found. In both groups of patients, papill edema before operation was 1-2 dptr.

Table 2 shows the details of surgical procedures. On 20 occasions, total removal of the tumor was performed macroscopically: on 45 occasions, subtotal tumor resection - in 17 cases combined with the Torkildsen drainage - was performed. Seven patients had a biopsy combined with Torkildsen drainage and two patients had a biopsy only. Five patients died in the hospital before the operation could be performed. It seems that the subtotal resection of the tumor combined with Torkildsen drainage is superior to any type of surgery as far as the immediate postoperative mortality and survival time is concerned. Thirty-nine patients received radiotherapy. As can be seen in Table 3, radiotherapy positively influences the survival time. On the other hand, extension of survival time is combined with local recurrence in 25% of the patients and with one metastases or more in 41.6% of the patients.

Table 1. Early and late prognosis of patients with medulloblastoma (No. = 80). Mortality in patients with medulloblastoma over the years 1951-1977

	No.	Follow-up	Dead	<1 Month	2-12 Months	>12 Months	>5 Years	Alive
1951-1960[a]	20	20	19	9	4	6	1	1
1961-1967[b]	25	24	23	6	10	7	1	1
1968-1977[c]	35	29	18	4	7	7	3	11
Total	80	73	60	19	21	20	5 (6.3%)	

[a] Developmental phase.
[b] Limited possibilities.
[c] Modern intensive care.

Table 2. Type of operation and survival. Influence of Torkildsen-drainage upon survival

	No.	Follow-up	Dead	<1 Months	2-12 Months	>12 Months	Average survival (months)
Total removal	20	17	12	5	5	2	8
Subtotal ⟨-⟩No drainage	28	25	22	4	11	7	11
Removal ⟨-⟩Torkildsen-dr.	17	16	12	2	4	6	15
Biopsy a. Torkildsen-dr.	7	7	6	1	2	3	14
Biopsy	2	2	2	2	–	–	1
No surgery	6	6	6	6	–	–	1
	80	73	60	20	22	18	

Table 3. Influence of radiotherapy upon survival

	No.	Follow-up	Dead	Average survival (months)	Recurrence	Period (months)	Metastases	Period (months)
Operation + radiotherapy	39	36	26	19	9	15	15	20
Operation only	35	32	29	4	2	–	2	–
No surgery	6	6	6	1	–	–	–	–

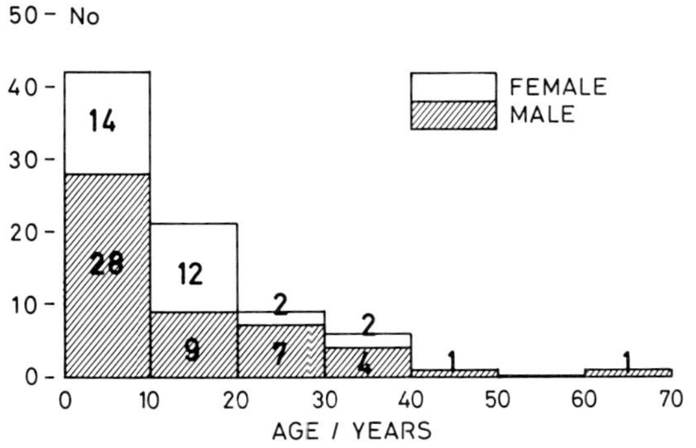

Fig. 1. Age and sex distribution of 80 patients with medulloblastoma (Department of Neurosurgery, Giessen, 1951–1977)

Table 4. Influences of type of resection. Torkildsen-drainage, and radiotherapy upon survival

Type of surgery	Additional	No.	Follow-up	Dead	Dead <1 Months	Dead 2-12 Months	Dead >12 Months	Dead (Months)	Alive	Alive (Months)
Subtotal removal	Radiotherapy Torkildsen-dr.	10	7	5	–	1	4	22	2	79 48
	Radiotherapy	13	13	10	–	3	7	19	3	120 30 29
	Torkildsen-dr.	9	9	7	2	3	2	8,8	2	37 6
	–	13	12	12	4	8	–	2,5	–	
Total removal	Radiotherapy	12	9	6	1	4	1	11,6	1	216 60 17
	–	8	8	6	4	1	1	4,4	2	12 4

Seventeen patients showed metastases of medulloblastoma's. In seven patients, the secondaries were multiple, and in ten patients, they were isolated. In 11 patients, secondary deposits occurred within the spinal canal and on four occasions in the supra- or infratentorial compartment. One patient had a metastasis in the basis of the skull and one patient had multiple metastases in the bones. Eight spinal metastases were treated with radiotherapy in seven cases, six in remission, i.e., with disappearance of neurologic signs. In one patient, the improvement was minimal and in one patient radiotherapy showed no effect.

Table 4 summarizes the survival time in relation to different operative methods and postoperative treatment. Operative treatment combined with Torkildsen drainage and followed by radiotherapy seems to provide the best chance for the longest survival. The longest survival was registered in the group of patients in whom subtotal removal of the tumor combined with Torkildsen drainage was followed by radiotherapy of the whole CNS axis. The mean survival time in this group of patients was 22 months. However, the two cases with longer survival had no Torkildsen drainage.

The clinical course and findings in one of our patients with medulloblastoma were so unusual that we find it worthwhile to report the case here.

Case Report

A 15-year-old girl was admitted to the Department of Pediatrics with a 4-months' history of headache, nausea, vomiting, double vision, and gate disturbances. In spite of all these signs and symptoms, she attended school until the last day before admission. In the morning of the day of admission, she was drowsy and her speach was slurred. Shortly before arriving at the hospital, she became comatous and both her pupils did not react to light stimuli. Profound coma and respiratory arrest occurred 1/2 h after admission. She was put on a ventilator, and ventricle drainage was established as an emergency measure. The ventricular fluid was blood stained, and after draining on 15 ml, the intraventricular pressure was still 50 mm Hg. Computerized tomography was performed (Fig. 2) and showed a tumor within the fourth ventricle. Blood clots in the fourth ventricle, lateral ventricles, and basal cisterns could be seen. Her condition improved slightly for a few hours but worsened again. At this stage, exploration of posterior fossa was performed. The tumor filled the fourth ventricle completely and showed large areas of infarction. The sylvian aqueduct was filled with blood clots which were removed. Free passage of the CSF was established. The child showed no improvement after the operation and died with signs of bulbar syndrome on the 5th postoperative day. Histologic examination confirmed the clinical diagnosis of medulloblastoma.

Discussion

The data provided by our series correspond with those found in the literature concerning the early and late prognosis of patients with medulloblastoma. SPITZ et al. (11) and GRANT (6) as well as others reported that the survival of patients with medulloblastoma is longer in older age groups. CHRISTENSEN (2) mentioned that the mean of age of patients harboring a tumor localized in the cerebellar hemisphere is higher than in the group of patients with vermian tumors. Our data support these views; however, we found no difference in survival between the group of patients with hemispheric and vermian tumors.

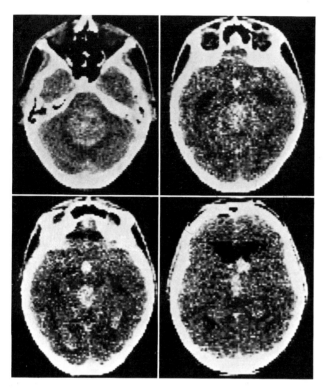

Fig. 2. Medulloblastoma of the fourth ventricle; intratumoral and ventricular bleeding

Of our patients, 6.3% survived more than 5 years. Almost identical figures were reported as early as 1939 (9). Two of our patients are alive 10 and 18 years after the operation, respectively. CUSHING (3) reported in 1931 on one patient who survived 14 years and GRANT in 1956 (6) on three patients surviving 9, 12, and 17 years, respectively. INGRAHAM and BAILEY (1944) (cited after BUCHMANN and ZÜLCH (1)) described one patient who was alive 22 years after the operation and another who died 19 years following surgery. PENFIELD and FEINDEL (1947) reported a 17-year survival. Further cases of long survivals were reported by SMITH et al. (10) in 1969, STOLZENBERG (12) in 1970, and DEBMAN and STAPLE (4) in 1973. In some of these cases, false diagnosis of medulloblastoma had probably been made (1, 9). On the other hand, exceptional biologic factors and changes of growth potential following radiotherapy must be taken into consideration (1, 9). Further confusion is caused by the different histologic classifications used. We did not consider the so-called cerebellar arachnoidal sarcomas described by FOERSTER and GAGEL (5).

In 17 of our patients, secondary metastases occurred and in one case multiple bone deposits. The description of medulloblastoma metastases by WOHLWILL in 1930 (14) was accepted with considerable caution, but the concept of metastases of neuroectodermal tumors was revised in the middle of the 1950s, after TOMPKINS et al. (13) had reported deposits of pinealoma and ZÜLCH described metastases of medulloblastoma. Apart from metastases in the nerve roots and infiltration of the nerve root pockets according to ZÜLCH (15) in some cases, hematogenic metastases are possible. GRIEPENTROG and PAULY (7) reported intra- and extracranial medulloblastoma metastases in twins. There are single reports about metastases occurring through ventriculoatrial and lumboperitoneal shunts (8). In our material, no such cases were found.

There is a strikingly high number of spinal metastases in patients who received radiotherapy prophylaxis. We are of the opinion that both local radiotherapy and the site of operation are certainly indicated; the analysis of our material seems to indicate that prophylactic radiotherapy of CSF pathways so far employed is of doubtful value in preventing metastases. It seems more justified to start with radiotherapy after the manifestation of signs of secondary deposits.

Summary

The analysis of 80 patients harboring medulloblastomas and treated in the Department of Neurosurgery in Giessen in the years 1951-1977 is presented. Postoperative mortality has decreased in recent years thanks to better intensive care. Late prognosis and survival time are the same as 25 years ago. The best results are achieved by large resection of the tumor combined with Torkildsen drainage and local radiotherapy. Of the patients who received radiotherapy to the whole CSF axis, 41.6% showed secondary deposits of the tumor. Prophylactic irradiation of the CNS axis should not be considered as a routine method of treatment. It seems more justified to stark with radiotherapy after the manifestation of secondary deposits.

References

1. BUCHMANN, E., ZÜLCH, K.J.: Zur Frage der postoperativen Überlebensdauer und zur Fernmetastasierung beim Medulloblastom des Kleinhirns. Acta Neurochir. 7, 263-273 (1959)

2. CHRISTENSEN, E.: Medulloblastomas. Excerpta Med. (Amst.) Sect. VIII, 8, 815 (1955)

3. CUSHING, H.: Experiences with cerebellar astrocytomas. Surg. Gynecol. Obstet. 52, 129-204 (1931)

4. DEBMAN, J.W., STAPLE, T.W.: Osseous metastases from cerebellar medulloblastoma. Radiology 107, 363-365 (1973)

5. FOERSTER, O., GAGEL, C.: Das umschriebene Arachnoidalsarkom des Kleinhirns. Z. Neurol. 164, 565-580 (1939)

6. GRANT, F.: A study of the results of surgical treatment of 2326 consecutive patients with brain tumor. J. Neurosurg. 13, 479-488 (1956)

7. GRIEPENTROG, F., PAULY, H.: Intra- und extracranielle frühmanifeste Medulloblastome bei erbgleichen Zwillingen. Zentralbl. Neurochir. 17, 429-440 (1957)

8. KESSLER, L.A., DUGAN, Ph., CONCANNON, J.P.: Systemic Metastases of Medulloblastoma Promoted by Shunting. Surg. Neurol. 3, 147-152 (1975)

9. PIA, H.W.: Hirntumoren im Kindesalter. In: Die Prognose chronischer Erkrankungen. LINNEWEH, F. (ed.), p. 298. Berlin-Göttingen-Heidelberg: Springer 1960

10. SMITH, D.R., HARDMAN, J.M., EARLE, K.M.: Metastasizing neuroectodermal tumors of the central nervous system. J. Neurosurg. 31, 50-58 (1969)

11. SPITZ, E.B., SHENKIN, H.A., GRANT, F.C.: Cerebellar medulloblastoma in adults. Arch. Neurol. Psychiatry. (Chicago) 57, 417-422 (1947)

12. STOLZENBERG, J., FISCHER, J.J., KLINGERMAN, M.M.: Extradural metastasis in medulloblastoma 10 years after treatment. Ann. J. Roch. Rad. Ther. Nucl. Med. 108, 71-74 (1970)

13. TOMPKINS, V.N., HAYMAKER, W., CAMPBELL, E.H.: Metastatic pineal tumors. J. Neurosurg., Springfield 7, 159-169 (1950)

14. WOHLWILL, F.: Zur pathologischen Anatomie der malignen medianen Kleinhirntumoren der Kinder. Z. Neurol. 128, 587-614 (1930)

15. ZÜLCH, K.J.: Die Hirngeschwülste in biologischer und morphologischer Darstellung. Leipzig: Barth 1951

Results of Medulloblastoma Treatment Under the Influence of Modern Therapy

H. ARNOLD, G. GRUBEL, H. FRANKE, I. GROSCH, and G. MARSMANN

Ninety-two cases of medulloblastoma of the last 25 years were evaluated, 88 of which we were able to follow up. As expected, the operation lethality including the first 6 weeks after the operation and the lethality within the first 6 months was highest in the groups of the 0-4-year-old and the 4-8-year-old children (Fig. 1). Surprisingly, the group of the 8-16-year-old patients exhibited the best long-term results. After 10 years, 5 out of 21 patients were still alive. The only adult who so far survived for more than 10 years died after 10 1/2 years from recidivation.

Looking at the different periods of treatment (Fig. 2), it is obvious that the survival rate of 50% within the first 6 months during the 1950s increases to 70-80% in the 1960s. An impressive improvement occurs in the 1970s; operation lethality is 0, and 19 out of 21 patients are still alive after one year. The age distribution was the same in the four different treatment periods. We conclude that the improvement of the results is not due to an overbalance of older patients in the time between 1971 and 1976.

There must be more than one cause for the improvement in the results of the last period. The three factors possibly influencing these results are: (1) technique of operation in combination with anesthesia and intensive care, (2) chemotherapy, and (3) radiotherapy. The influence of the refined neurosurgical and anesthesiologic possibilities is deductable from the remarkable decrease in the operation lethality and during the first 6 months after the operation. Within the first 6 months 22 patients died whose tumors had been removed incompletely. In the group of patients whose tumors were macroscopically totally eradicated, only four died. Whereas up to 1970, only 40% of the tumors could be completely removed, since we introduced microsurgical methods the rate increased to 60%. This is hoped to also have a positive effect on long-term results, as patients who undergo a operation are shown to survive for a longer time. Of those surviving the first 6 months, there were still 65% alive after the 2nd year in comparison to 52% who had not undergone a radical operation. After 5 years, 39% of the totally operated group were still alive in contrast to 14% in the other group (Table 1).

During the period 1971-1976, 15 patients, exclusively children, were given combined chemotherapy using methotrexate, Endoxan, and vincristine. Methotrexate (0.5 mg/kg body weight) was given intrathecally once a week only during radiation therapy. Vincristine was given in repeated 4-week periods every week alternating with Endoxan. The dosage was

Table 1

Tumor removal	No. of patients surviving	
	2nd year	5th year
Complete	22/34 (65%)	12/31 (39%)
Incomplete	12/23 (52%)	3/22 (14%)

0.05 mg/kg once a week of vincristine and 10 mg/kg once a week of
Endoxan, respectively. These 15 patients were compared to an equally
large group of children treated without chemotherapy and undergoing
the same mode of radiotherapy. Children who died during the first 6
months after the operation are excluded. The group of patients treated
with chemotherapy seemed to fare better during the first 3 years,
whereas after 3 years no difference was left. However, it must be considered that 13 children of the control group belong to the treatment
period 1966-1970. As shown in Figure 2, the survival rate in this group
was lower than it has been since 1971 due to less refined neurosurgical
and anesthesiologic treatment techniques. Therefore, we conclude that
our findings do not prove a significant effect of chemotherapy.

A trial was made to analyze the influence of radiation therapy thought
to be indispensable in the treatment of medulloblastoma. Of the patients who did not get x-rays, only two survived the first 6 months
after the operation. Not considering the patients who died during the
first 6 months, 60 patients remain whose data can supply us with
information on the effects of radiotherapy (Table 2). Thirty-six patients received 5000 rad on the focus, 4000 rad on the cerebral CSF
system, and 3000 rad on the spine. The other 24 patients received
4000-5000 rad on the site of the focus and ca. 3000 rad on the spine;
a few of them only got focal x-ray treatment. Of the patients who had
received incomplete radiotherapy for 5 years, 10 out of 24 were still
alive in contrast to 5 out of 27 patients with complete radiotherapy
who had been operated on 5 years ago. In addition, there are nine patients of the latter group who could potentially reach the 5-year
mark. These findings are contrary to our expectations. In our patients,
modern radiation therapy does not seem to be more effective up to 1976
than the incomplete one that was used before. On the other hand, there
is no doubt that radiation therapy of the cerebral CSF system is
indicated, as is also proved by autoptic findings of supratentorial
seeding in our patients. The present results may be explained by a
mistake caused by the small number of patients.

Summary

The outcome of medulloblastoma treatment has improved considerably
during the last 6 years regarding operation and first-year lethality.
This can be largely explained by refined operation techniques in combination with modern anesthesia and intensive care. A positive effect
of chemotherapy could not be ascertained. Our material does not prove
any superiority of modern radiotherapy with radiation of the focus, the
cerebral CSF system, and the spinal canal over the older technique of
focal and spinal radiation treatment. This finding is in contrast

Table 2

Radiotherapy	No. of patients surviving		
	6 months	2nd year	5th year
Focal + spinal	24	15 (62%)	10 (42%)
Focal + spinal + cranial	36	19/31 (61%)	5/27 (19%)

to communications dealing with this topic. To obtain more evidence about the effect of radiotherapy and chemotherapy, a larger group has to be examined. Therefore, a cooperative study of several hospitals would be desirable.

References

1. BLOOM, H.J.G.: Cancer 35, 111-120 (1975)
2. CHANG, C.H., HOUSEPIAN, E.M., HERBERT, C.: Radiology 93, 1351-1359 (1969)
3. HOPE-STONE, H.F.: J. Neurosurg. 32, 83-88 (1970)
4. MILES, J., BHANDARI, Y.S.: J. Neurol. Neurosurg. Psychiatry, 33, 208-211 (1970)
5. SMITH, C.E. et al.: Radiology 109, 179-182 (1973)

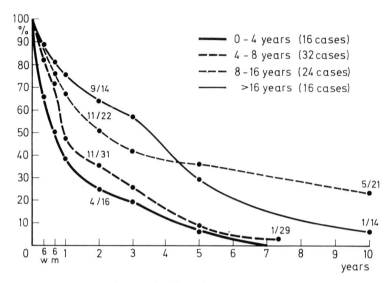

Fig. 1. Age and survival rate

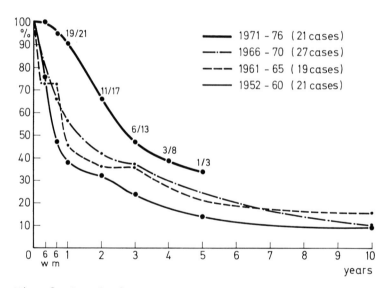

Fig. 2. Survival rates

Successful Treatment of Childhood Medulloblastoma – and What Thereafter?

P. GUTJAHR and D. VOTH

Therapeutic progress, which has increased cure rates in many of the childhood malignancies, has also improved the former poor prognosis of cerebellar medulloblastoma. As the number of long-term survivors and permanent cures grows, the problem of possible late effect of tumor and/or treatment becomes more and more important. We have studied late effects in long-term survivors of medulloblastomas at the Mainz University Hospitals.

Among 139 children under 16 years of age with primary tumors of the CNS - all being cared for by neurosurgeons and pediatricians - 37 had medulloblastomas of the cerebellum (27%). Boys were affected twice as often as girls; the youngest patient was 2 and the oldest 15 8/12 years old.

Before 1967, therapy consisted of a most radical surgical procedure and local radiotherapy to the posterior fossa (usually 6000 rad) and mostly a single-agent chemotherapy with cyclophosphamide. All 12 children of this group died within the 1st year after diagnosis. Craniospinal irradiation has been performed since 1967 after a more restrictive operation; 4000 rad of 60 Co were applied to the whole CNS and another 2000 rad were added to the posterior fossa (duration of radiotherapy 6-8 weeks). Chemotherapeutically, intrathecal methotrexate was used (once every week during the phase of radiotherapy, 10 mg/m^2 body surface), and a systemic cytotoxic chemotherapy was performed (vincristine, 1.5 mg/m^2 plus cyclophosphamide, 600 mg/m^2 every 2 weeks) for a total of 18 months. Since mid-1976, cyclophosphamide was replaced by the more promising nitrosoureas (CCNU, 150 mg/m^2 every 4 weeks).

The treatment results of this second group of 23 children - two recent boys are not shown in the survival curve - proves therapeutic progress: 8 of the 23 children survived more than 1 year (35%), seven of them without recurrence. The difference is statistically significant. Future cure rates with the therapeutic regimen in use seem possible in the range of 45%-56%, the more so since operative procedures and postoperative intensive care have also improved, by means of a restrictive operation, craniospinal radiotherapy, and chemotherapy with vincristine, CCNU, and intrathecal methotrexate.

Treatment of childhood malignancies means treatment of the whole child. Therefore, we feel that it is absolutely necessary - in order to care for the child's somatic and psychosocial future - to analyze late consequences of tumor and/or therapy routinely and thoroughly so that the results of these findings may form a basis for rehabilitation of the child itself and be integrated into thoughts about future treatment concepts.

Twelve of our medulloblastoma children were studied 1 year after diagnosis or later for late effects. Neurologic abnormalities were present in all cases: in four children they were discrete, in five severe, and one child had a complete cervical cord compression due to early tumor seeding via CSF. Walking disabilities and altered cranial nerve function may mostly be a late consequence of pretherapeutically increased intracranial pressure. In cerebellar astrocytoma children, however, we did not find such a great number and severity of late changes, although intracranial pressure increase probably lasted longer in the latter. EEG findings gave good results; none of the children had convulsive seizures or electroencephalographic foci. Diffuse changes, which were present in 50% of the cases before treatment, had regressed completely in all cases. Genetic and immunologic late consequences for the risk of a second malignant tumor have not proved to be of significant importance until now. We would estimate, however, that this future risk will be in the range of 5%.

There was one boy with severe chronic progressive - probably transfusion-related - hepatitis. This is not an exception in survivors of childhood tumors: we investigated 160 patients after childhood tumors and found 18% to have chronic hepatitis. As a consequence of spinal irradiation, 4 of the 12 survivors of medulloblastoma had a complete growth arrest of the vertebral column. Vertebral changes are not always this severe after spinal radiotherapy. Frequently, there are discrete growth disturbances such as transverse lines and the so-called vertebra-in-vertebra indicating a brief growth arrest. Other growth disturbances included a deficit in human growth hormone (HGH); three children had a complete growth arrest due to HGH deficiency. In comparison, 6 out of 12 children with craniopharyngeoma had HGH deficiency after operation and radiotherapy with 6,000 rad 60 Co. Response to substitution of HGH is good. LH and FSH were normal in all cases.

Partial irradiation of the thyroid gland cannot be avoided in spinal irradiation. As a consequence function tests of TSH secretion gave elevated concentrations of TSH after stimulation with TRH in the serum of irradiated medulloblastoma children compared with a control group. The mean values, however, were lower than after mantle irradiation of malignant lymphomas. Two children had a partial hearing loss; visual problems were of minimal importance, which is a finding quite in contrast to the cerebellar astrocytomas.

The major problem among the late sequelae is in our opinion the late psychosocial and intellectual effects. Of the 12 1-year survivors, two did not yet attend school and one had already left school. Of the remaining nine, two failed high school, and six attend special schools for backward children. Until now, only one can follow his former school activities. We feel that greater problems will arise in employing these patients later, and even more so in providing them with an adequate professional education. For this reason, we recently established an outpatient service for rehabilitation problems. The late psychosocial and intellectual situation in children after brain tumors contrasts significantly with those of children suffering from tumors in other locations and leukemias. Even among the other brain tumors, we did not notice late effects to such degree. It seems worth mentioning that, with minor exceptions, the world literature does not report on the problem. The Psychologic analysis further showed that the children also had marked neuroticism, different kinds of phobias, and a reduced intellectual capacity. As for psychomotoric activities, their level is at the 98th percentile compared with normals of the same age.

More and more children with malignant neoplasias - about 2000 every year in West Germany - have the chance to be permanently cured, if treated adequately and at a center. Of our 139 children with primary brain tumor, 50% are presently alive. Improvement of survival curves, however, should not be the only goal of modern pediatric oncologic therapy. It must also be aimed at recognizing and treating the numerous and possibly severe late effects. Tumor therapy has its price.

Surgery of Extensive Glomus Jugulare Tumors

J. Menzel, H. J. Denecke, and H. Penzholz

Glomus jugulare tumors are locally invasive tumors in the region of the middle ear and relative newcomers to the medical scene. Even though VALENTIN (10) had described a ganglion-like formation at the beginning of the tympanic nerve in 1840, over 100 years passed before GUILD (5) in 1941 described structures in close relation to the bulb of the jugular vein which he named the glomus jugulare. ROSENWASSER (9) presented the first tumor of the glomus jugulare in 1945. Glomic tissue may be found not only in the jugular bulb, but also along the course of the tympanic nerve in the middle ear and along the course of the auricular branch of the vagus nerve to the stylomastoid foramen (Fig. 1). Although glomus jugulare tumors are generally considered benign, they exhibit invasive growth and have a marked tendency to recur. Metastasizing cases are on record, and FRIEDMANN (3) found ten cases with metastases to the regional lymph nodes, liver, bones, and lungs. Beyond that, the course of these tumors is slowly but always progressive. In the final stage, the tumor compresses the cerebellopontine angle and the pons causing acute hydrocephalus.

These facts require surgical treatment of glomus jugulare tumors because irradiation therapy is ineffective (6, 7, 8). The small tumors in the middle ear are an otologic problem. They can be removed by the transmeatic approach. If the tumor extends to the hypotympanic cavity, a retroauricular way is recommended. The cases with marked intracranial extension require the cooperation of otologist and neurosurgeon (2, 4).

Clinical Aspects

The differentation of neurologic signs and symptoms shows that these can be divided into two groups:
1. Those due to the tumor bulk in the middle ear, i.e. conductive hearing loss, tinnitus, bleeding, aural pain, aural drainage, and aural polyps.
2. Those due to tumor extension, i.e. aural pain, neurosensory deafness, vertigo, and neurologic signs. The latter can be the result of either peripheral nerve involvement or the extension to the central nervous system.

According to the literature, about 13% of all glomus jugulare tumors show evidence of intracranial tumor extension. Symptoms for middle and posterior cerebral fossa can be evaluated. Obstruction of the aqueduct with hydrocephalus and compression of the ipsilateral hemisphere and the pons are signs of end-stage disease.

Diagnosis

Neuroradiology is indispensible in the diagnosis of glomus jugulare tumors and their extension and blood supply. Plain x-rays of the skull with tomographic examinations demonstrate clouding or erosion of the petrous pyramid (Fig. 2). A submental vertex view can be helpful in delineating the limits of the bone changes. Selective angiography of the external and internal carotid and the vertebral arteries demonstrate the most important vessels which supply the tumor. Angiography of the ascending pharyngeal artery is usually most informative (Fig. 3). The real extension of the tumor is seen in the postcapillary phase (Figs. 4 and 5). Sinography of the superior sagittal sinus delineates the superior level of the obstruction of the sigmoid sinus (Fig. 6). In cases with marked extension of the tumor along the internal carotid artery, orbital phlebography can be effective in demonstrating the obstruction of the cavernous sinus (Fig. 7).

Operative Technique

The principle of our operation technique is based on the knowledge that glomus jugulare tumors extend along the transbasal veins and sinuses (Fig. 8a):
1. Caudally along the jugular vein
2. Cranially along the sigmoid sinus, sometimes as far as the transverse sinus
3. Medially along the transbasilar veins to the intrapyramidal part of the internal carotid artery and to the cavernous sinus.

A skin incision is made from the ear down to the origin of the sternocleidomastoid muscle (Fig. 8b) which is cut through. The common carotid artery with its bifurcation and the internal jugular vein are dissected. All branches of the external carotid artery and the internal jugular vein are ligated. After removal of the mastoid process, the middle ear, and the labyrinth, the internal carotid artery is dissected up to its foramen, its knee, and its intrapyramidal part (Fig. 9a). The sigmoid sinus is ligated. The fibrous invagination of the internal carotid artery is removed beginning at the foramen up to the entrance into the cavernous sinus (Fig. 9b). After total petrosectomy, the tumor is removed radically, including its part in the posterior fossa (Fig. 9c). The dead space which is caused by removal of large tumors is obliterated by the sternocleidomastoid muscle which is rotated upward (Fig. 9d). In this way, infection from the eustachian tube to the posterior fossa is avoided. In addition, the muscle provides protection for the opened dura and the internal carotid artery.

Results

We have operated on nine patients with extensive glomus jugulare tumors in the described manner (six women and three men, 38-69 years of age). We had no mortality. The postoperative course was uneventful in four cases. Two patients suffered from a CSF fistula and slight meningitis. In four patients, additional cranial nerve defects occurred postoperatively, especially of the VIIth, IXth, Xth, and XIth cranial nerve. These complications required plastic surgery. The follow-up periods varied from 13 years to 9 months. No recurrence was observed, and all patients are still in full employment. These facts justify the operative treatment of glomus jugulare tumors in spite of the extremely long duration of the intervention and the knowledge that about 50% of the patients operated on have a complicated postoperative course.

Summary

Nine patients with extensive glomus jugulare tumors were operated on by means of otorhinolaryngologic-neurosurgical teamwork. Preoperative neuroradiologic examinations are indispensible in the diagnosis of these tumors, their extension, and their blood supply. The operative technique is presented. The postoperative course and the long-term results are analyzed.

References

1. CIMINO, A., FERRARA, P., MADONIA, T., RESTIVO, S.: La sindrome da paraganglioma timpano-giugulare. La Clinica O.R.L. 4, 221-289 (1971)
2. DENECKE, H.J.: Surgery of extensive glomus jugulare tumors of the ear. Rev. Laryngol. 90, 265-270 (1969)
3. FRIEDMANN, I.: Pathology of the Ear. Oxford-London-Edinburgh-Melbourne: Blackwell Scientific Publications 1974
4. GARDNER, G., COCKE, E.W., ROBERTSON, J.T., TRUMBULL, M.L., PALMER, R.E.: Combined approach surgery for removal of glomus jugulare tumors. Laryngoscope 87, 665-688 (1977)
5. GUILD, S.R.: A hitherto unrecognized structure, the glomus jugulare, in man. Anat. Rec. 79, 28-56 (1941)
6. KEMPE, L.G., VANDERARK, G.D., SMITH, D.R.: The neurosurgical treatment of glomus jugulare tumors. J. Neurosurg. 35, 59-64 (1971)
7. McMEEKIN, R.R., HARDMAN, J.M., KEMPE, L.G.: Multipe sclerosis after X-radiation: activation by treatment of metastatic glomus tumor. Arch. Otolaryngol. (Chicago) 90, 617-621 (1969)
8. PORTMANN, M.: La chirurgie des tumeurs du glomus jugulaire. Ann. Chir. 24, 1119-1127 (1970)
9. ROSENWASSER, H.: Carotid body tumor of the middle ear and mastoid. Arch. Otolaryng. 41, 64-67 (1945)
10. VALENTIN, G.: Über eine gangliöse Schwellung in der Jacobson Anastomose des Menschen. Arch. Anat. Physiol. Wissensch. Med. 287-290 (1840)

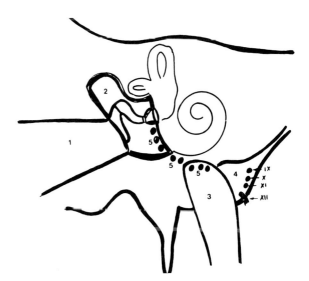

1 Auditory meatus
2 Middle ear
3 Bulb of the jugular vein
4 Jugular foramen
5 Glomic tissue

Fig. 1. Diagrammatic illustration of the distribution of glomic tissue (modified after CIMINO)

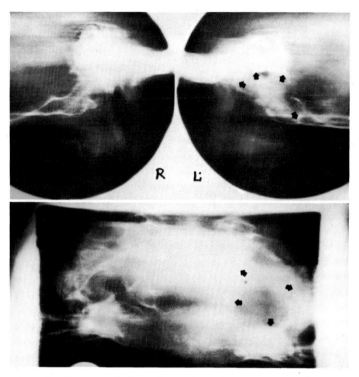

Fig. 2. *Upper right*: intact petrous pyramid; *upper left*: erosion of the petrous pyramid; *lower pane*: enlargement of the left jugular foramen (see arrows)

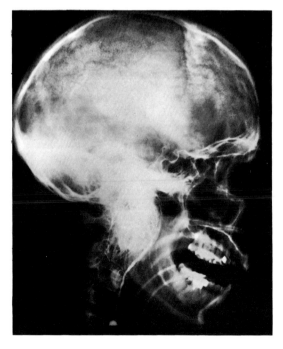

Fig. 3. Selective angiography of the ascending pharyngeal artery

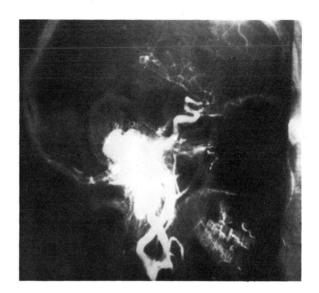

Fig. 4. Extensive glomus jugulare tumor (lateral projection)

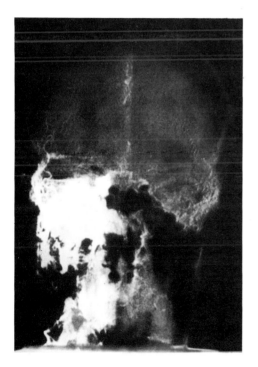

Fig. 5. Extensive glomus jugulare tumor (anteroposterior projection)

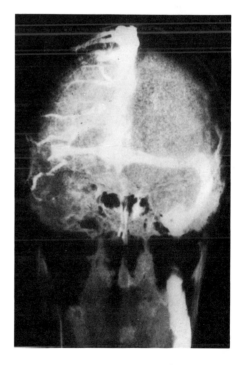

Fig. 6. Obstruction of the right sigmoid sinus by the tumor

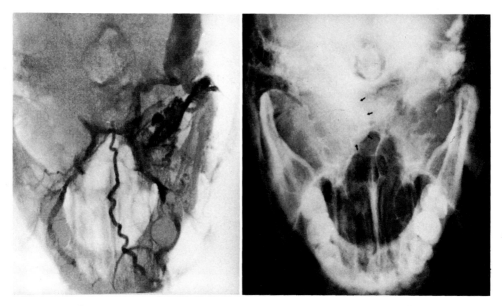

Fig. 7. *Right*: obstruction of the right cavernous sinus by the tumor; *left*: tumor in the epipharynx (see arrows)

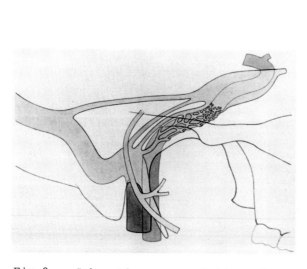

Fig. 8. *a* Schematic representation of the transbasilar veins and sinuses along which glomus jugulare tumors extend

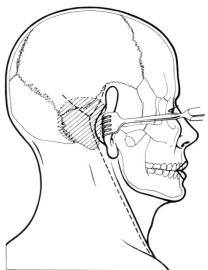

Fig. 8. *b* Skin incision

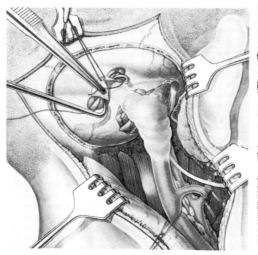

Fig. 9. *a* Preparation of the internal carotid artery and ligation of sigmoid sinus; all branches of the external carotid artery are ligated

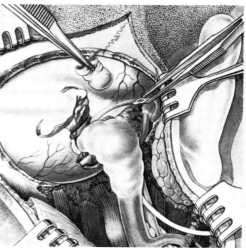

Fig. 9. *b* Dissection of the internal carotid artery up to the cavernous sinus

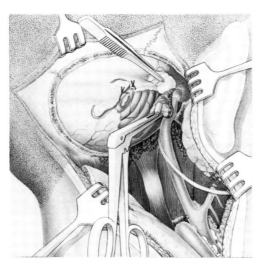

Fig. 9. *c* Resection of the tumor

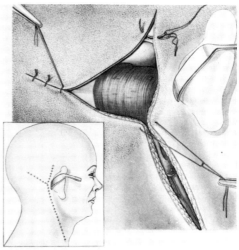

Fig. 9. *d* The dead space is obliterated by the sternocleidomastoid muscle which is rotated upward

Catamnestic Examinations of Patients With Cerebellar Tumors
H. Miltz and H.-U. Thal

We have analyzed 198 cases of infratentorial tumors on the basis of the survival time after surgical treatment. There were 49 cases of infratentorial ependymomas[1], 60% of which were male. In 50% of the patients, symptoms started well under the age of 20 years. Only a partial or subtotal extirpation of the tumors was possible in view of their close proximity to the brain stem and their invasive nature. In these tumors, the life expectancy is supposed to be poor due to CSF metastases and expected recurrences. In this group, 30% of the patients survived 3 years; at the end of 5 years, 18% were still alive, and one patient lived 11 years. Fifty-four patients with cerebral ependymomas[1] showed a better prognosis: 45% lived for 3 years, 38% were alive 5 years, and 15% lived more than 10 years after the operation (Fig. 1).

Forty-eight patients with medulloblastomas of the classic histopathologic picture were included in this study. Although postoperative radiotherapy and chemotherapy were given in selected cases, 70% of the patients died within 1 year, and none survived for more than 3 years. Our results differ from those of BOUCHARD (4), HOPE-STONE (5) and others, who reported 5-year survival rates in 27%-77% of their cases of medulloblastomas. The above difference in survival rate could be due to our definite and strict criteria of histopathologic diagnosis of medulloblastoma only in patients below 20 years of age.

The hemangioblastoma, called Lindau's disease in memory of its author (8), belongs to the group with good prognosis. In two-thirds of our 31 patients, the disease started between the 20th and 50th year of age. In 80%, we found the hemangioblastoma in the wall of a cyst and in 20% as solid mass without a cyst. This familial disease has been known for a long time, as well as its combination with several dysontogeneses like retinal angiomatosis (v. Hippel's disease) and multiple cysts in the kidneys and liver, as seen in 15% of our material. The life expectancy is more than 10 years for 80% of the patients. Thus, as in the astrocytoma of the cerebellum, a total removal of the tumor means recovery in the majority of the cases. However, in some cases of hemangioblastoma, the prognosis is somewhat poorer due to its tendency to recur. Eight of our 31 patients had to be reoperated, six patients after 2-6 years and two patients after 10 and 17 years. Two of the six patients had to be operated four times, in one patient because of repeated recurrences in the size of the cyst and in the other patient because of repeated recurrences in the size of the solid hemangioblastoma.

In the group of the cerebellar astrocytomas, the disease usually starts in childhood and adolescence. The statistically computed life expectancy of 70 patients in our series was 10 years in 90% and 20 years in 85% of the total cases. This indicates a favorable prognosis; at the moment 36 patients are alive 10-25 years after operation. Eight patients had recurrences and died within 2-4 years. Histologically, these tumors were like those of cerebral origin. KUHLENDAHL and STOCHDORPH (6, 7) prefer the nomenclature of Bergstrand tumors instead of the so-called "cere-

---

[1] Collected data of the Neurosurgical Clinics of the University Hospitals Munich, Vienna and Duesseldorf. A detailed study is in preparation.

bellar astrocytomas." BERGSTRAND (3) had pointed out the good prognosis associated with these tumors in comparison to those of cerebral astrocytomas. According to this point of view these tumors could be associated with hamartia, which is in fair agreement with the good prognosis of the dyontogenetic hemangioblastomas. ZÜLCH (9, 10) attributed these so-called astrocytomas to the polar spongioblastomas described by BAILEY and CUSHING (1) in their classification of the glioma group. A small group of cystic astrocytomas localized in the cerebral hemispheres with a nodose tumor in the wall of a large single cyst is also a type of Bergstrand tumor. We had observed seven younger patients who were operated up to 25 years ago without showing a recurrence of the tumor.

References

1. BAILEY, P., CUSHING, H.: A classification of the tumors of the glioma group on a histogenetic basis with a correlated study of prognosis. Philadelphia: J.B. Lippincott 1926
2. BARONE, B.M., ELVIDGE, R.E.: Ependymomas. A clinical survey. J. Neurosurg. 33, 428-438 (1970)
3. BERGSTRAND, H.: Über das sogenannte Astrocytom im Kleinhirn. Virchows Arch. 207, 537-548 (1932). Weiteres über sogenannte Kleinhirnastrocytome. Virchows Arch. 299, 726-739 (1937)
4. BOUCHARD, J.: Central Nervous System. IV. In: Textbook of Radiotherapy. FLETCHER, G.H. (ed.), p. 366. Philadelphia: Lea and Febiger 1973
5. HOPE-STONE, H.F.: Results of treatment of medulloblastomas. J. Neurosurg. 32, 83 (1970)
6. KUHLENDAHL, H., STOCHDORPH, O.: Über das Vorkommen des sogenannten Kleinhirnastrocytoms (Bergstrand-Tumor) im Großhirn. Beitr. Neurochir. 15, 181-185 (1968)
7. KUHLENDAHL, H., STOCHDORPH, O., HÜBNER, G.: Zur nosologischen Stellung und histologischen Herleitung des sogenannten Kleinhirnstrocytoms. Acta Neurochir. 32, 235-245 (1975)
8. LINDAU, A.: Studien über Kleinhirnzysten. Bau, Pathogenese und Beziehung zur Angiomatosis retinae. Acta Pathol. Scand. Suppl. 1, 128 (1926)
9. ZÜLCH, K.J.: On the question of cerebellar astrocytomas. Zentralbl. Neurochir. 2, 360 (1937)
10. ZÜLCH, K.J.: Über das "sogenannte" Kleinhirnastrocytom. Virchows Arch. Pathol. Anat. 307, 222-252 (1940)

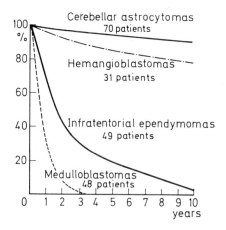

Fig. 1. Probability of postoperative life expectancy (the graphs are plotted without the early mortality up to 1 month)

Endoscopy of the Cerebellopontine Angle: Its Diagnostic and Therapeutic Possibilities

F. OPPEL, CH. ZEYTOUNTCHIAN, G. MULCH, and H.-D. KUNFT [1]

Introduction

In 1974, the otologist PROTT ([1]) was the first to report on the possibility of endoscopic examination of the cerebellopontine angle. He used a transpyramidal retrolabyrinthine approach ([4]). The first results gained from clinical application were published in 1976 ([1]). Definite areas of application for this new method have not yet been determined. From an otologic point of view, it would appear to be practical: 1) in diagnostically uncertain, non-space occupying lesions of the internal auditory canal and of the cerebellopontine angle, e.g., the differential diagnosis of intracanalicular tumors and arachnitic adhesions ([5]) if this is not possible with current methods and 2) for neurectomy of the vestibulocochlear (VIII) nerve. The method assumes additional importance in neurosurgery, because frequently tumors of the pyramidal apex and of the restricted area of the internal auditory meatus can not easily be defined by conventional neuroradiologic methods ([7]). On the other hand, cranial nerves V-XI are well-definable with various optic systems. Therefore, it is now possible to approach the trigeminal nerve surgically. Anatomic correlations make it easier to reach this particular nerve ([6]). Furthermore, for histologic evaluation, biopsies may be performed and, if necessary, small tumors could visibly be removed. It also permits a translabyrinthine enlargement of the extremely narrow endoscopic approach ([2], [3]).

Methods

Endoscopic examinations were performed on corpses of adults and, in one case, on a living subject (56 years of age, female). The mastoid is exposed by curved skin incision behind the auricle. Mastoidectomy follows exposure of the sigmoid sinus, the exterior and horizontal semicircular canal, and the endolymphatic sac. In this way, the dura of the posterior fossa can be exposed for an area of approximately 1.2 x 0.8 cm (Trautmann's triangle) (Fig. 1). After incising the dura, and sparing the endolymphatic sac, the endoscope is inserted between the posterior pyramidal surface and the cerebellum under temporary compression of the sigmoid sinus. Other than straight optics (0°) of 2.7 mm diameter, we used 30° and 70° angular optics with a diamter of 3.8 mm. The straight optic system can be inserted in combination with a coagulation electrode or microforceps. Irrigation and suction can be done by means of a corresponding shaft. For sufficient space and good visibility during the examination, the patient should be positioned such that the surgical area is uppermost. The endoscope has to be inserted very carefully since the small arachnoid vessels tear easily.

---

[1] We gratefully acknowledge the help from the Institute of Pathology, Steglitz-Clinic. We want to particularly thank Prof. Gross, Mr. Banch, and Mr. Kühne.

Results

The straight optic system initially provides a general view of the field of examination. Arachnitic adhesions of various sizes then become visible next to the posterior pyramidal surface and the cerebellum, which can be divided with a microinstrument under visual control (Fig. 2). The first cranial nerves to become visible are the vestibulocochlear, the intermedius, and the facial, sometimes together with a labyrinthine artery. Further rostral, the trigeminal nerve appears, entering the cisterna pontis from the direction of the pons. Below the trigeminal nerve, the abducens enters Dorello's canal (Fig. 3). As a constant finding, together with smaller vessels, an arachnoid membrane extends from the posteromedial trigeminus portion to the cerebellum. This might be the upper limit of the cisterna pontocerebellaris examined in detail by YASARGIL and co-workers (8).

The use of the 30°-angle optic system affords a close inspection of the posterior pyramidal surface up to the pyramidal apex, so that parts of the internal auditory meatus become visible. The trigeminal nerve is particularly well-demonstrated in its entire course from the pons exit to the entrance into Meckel's cave, spreading over the upper edge of the pyramid and tentorial fissure. Further medial, a loop of the anterior inferior cerebellar artery (AICA) becomes visible (Fig. 4). An optical differentiation of the trigeminal nerve into sensory (pars major) and motor (pars minor) portions is possible without difficulty. Section of two-thirds of the sensory branch using microforceps or a microelectrode can thus be effected visually and without risk (Figs. 5 and 6). The 70°-angle optic system lends itself mainly to the inspection of the internal auditory meatus but also permits the demonstration of the lower cranial nerve groups (IX-XI). Figure 7 shows an overall view of the area.

Discussion

Our investigations are in agreement with the results of PROTT (5) where the diagnostic applicability of endoscopy of the cerebellopontine angle is concerned. Furthermore, we were interested in the applicability of this method for the surgical approach to the trigeminal nerve. In this context, the question of unequivocally reproducible indentification of nerves arises, as well as that of differentiation of sensory and motor divisions of the trigeminal nerve and the technical management of surgical intervention. The exposure of the dura in the region of Trautmann's triangle should not present any problem to an experienced otologist.

Arachnoid adhesions and vessels may complicate the insertion of the optic system, as does a convex bulging of the posterior pyramidal surface toward the endoscope. However, using visual puncture coagulation and light pressure against the posterior pyramidal surface, the endoscope can be advanced even under unfavorable conditions. The detachment of arachnoid adhesions of various sizes can lead to minor hemorrhages and impair visibility. Once a clear view has been obtained using straight optics, it is mandatory to insert the 30°- and 70°-angle optic system for further differentiation. For purely diagnostic inquiry, the 70°-optic system has to be applied for inspection of the internal auditory meatus. Apart from that, the 30°-angle optic system is sufficient for the posterior pyramidal surface, the pyramidal apex, and for the differentiation of the divisions of the trigeminal nerve. All of this could be done easily in those cases we examined. The two-thirds resection of the sensory division - as well as its coagulation -

can only be performed in combination with the straight optic system for technical reasons. All autopsies substantiated that the motor division remained intact after endoscopic resection and that the two-thirds resection had been successful. Complications occurred with an expansive posterior pyramidal surface when the instruments veered dorsomedially and when the above-described membrane contained larger vessels.

We are in a position to substantiate the application of endoscopy of the cerebellopontine angle for differential diagnostic purposes. EHRENBERGER et al. (1) reported an endoscopically diagnosed arachnitic strangulation of the VIIIth cranial nerve as having been the cause of tympanic nerve damage in one case. In our patient, we were able to biopsy a meningeal tumor of the cerebellopontine angle growing en plaque. In this case, there existed over a period of approximately 3 1/2 years an almost stationary neurologic history without definite radiologic substantiation of a progressive space-occupying lesion.

We believe that endoscopy of the cerebellopontine angle for diagnostic purposes is indicated only in special cases. The surgical stress is relatively low. The procedure may be performed under local anesthesia. As to surgery of the trigeminal nerve, as compared to the operations performed by DANDY and FRAZIER, we recognize an advantage using the endoscopic procedure because of the smaller access and the lack of cerebral traumatization. An extension of this field of indication does not seem feasible. The endoscopic access will have to be left open for discussion.

Summary

The cerebellopontine angle is endoscopically visible using the transpyramidal retrolabyrinthine approach (Trautmann's triangle). The areas of application for this new method are not as yet definite. Its use seems to be of merit diagnostically: 1) in cases of uncertain, non-space-occupying lesions of the internal auditory canal and the cerebellopontine angle, e.g., the differential diagnosis of intracanalicular tumors and arachnitic adhesions, as well as for tumors of the pyramidal apex and internal auditory meatus region if this is not possible with otologic and neuroradiologic methods in current use and 2) therapeutically, in cases of neurectomies of the vestibulocochlear and trigeminal nerves. The endoscopic examinations were performed on corpses of adults and, in one case, on a living subject under particular consideration for possible surgery of the trigeminal nerve.

References

1. EHRENBERGER, K., INNITZER, J., KOOS, W.: Erfolgreiche Akusticusdekompression bei postarachnitischen Hörschäden. Laryngol. Rhinol. 55, 561-566 (1976)
2. GLASSCOCK, M.E., HAYS, J.W.: The translabyrinthine removal of acoustic and other cerebellopontine angle tumors. Ann. Otol., Rhinol. Laryngol. Vol. 82, 4, 415 (1973)
3. MONTGOMERY, W.W.: Surgery for acoustic neurinoma. Ann. Otol., Rhinol. Laryngol. Vol. 82, 4, 428 (1973)
4. PROTT, W.: Möglichkeiten einer Endoskopie des Kleinhirnbrückenwinkels auf transpyramidalem-retrolabyrinthärem Zugangsweg - Cisternoskopie. HNO, 22, 337-341 (1974)

5. REMBOLD, F., TÖNNIS, W.: Die Differentialdiagnose der Erkrankungen des Kleinhirnbrückenwinkels. Dtsch. Nervenheilkde. 175, 329-353 (1956)
6. SJÖQUIST, O.: Surgery of the cranial nerves. Handbuch der Neurochirurgie, Bd. VI, S. 1-57. Berlin-Heidelberg-New York: Springer 1957
7. WIRGHT, R.E., TURNER, Jr., J.S.: Positive angle myelograms without acoustic neuroma. Laryngoscope 83, 733-741 (1973)
8. YASARGIL, M.G., KASDAGLIS, K., JAIN, K.K., WEBER, H.-P.: Anatomical observations of the subarachnoid cisterns of the brain during surgery. J. Neurosurg. Vol. 44, 298-302 (1976)

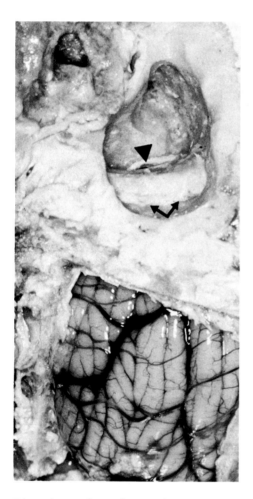

Fig. 1. Left endoscopic access as seen in relation to its anatomic topography. *Upper left*: the external auditory canal after detachment of the auricle; *below*: the cerebellum. After mastoidectomy (site partially covered by the triangular arrow), the labyrinthine block is visible below the sigmoid sinus (*double arrow*); in between lies the endoscopic access to the opened dura (*triangular arrow*)

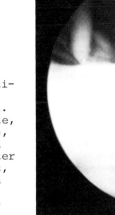

Fig. 2. Detachment of arachnitic adhesions with a microscalpel under visual control. Behind the arachnoid membrane, in the center of the picture, the facial, intermedial, and vestibulocochlear nerves enter the internal auditory meatus, with the trigeminal nerve in the background on the left. *Above:* the posterior pyramidal surface

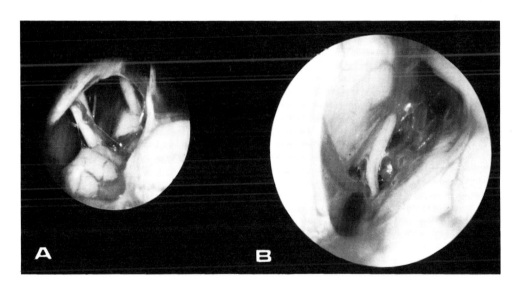

Fig. 3. *A* View (straight optics) immediately after introduction of the endoscope. On the left: the cranial nerves VII, intermedius, VIII with the labyrinthine artery; *rear right:* the vertically running n. abducens; *upper right:* the trigeminal nerve partially covered by the arachnoid membrane
B In the center of the picture is the n. abducens entering Dorello's canal (30° optics) with a labyrinthine artery running alongside on the left. On the left and in front of the facial nerve, the trigeminal nerve on the upper right. Between these two nerves, the posterior pyramidal surface above and the cerebellum below

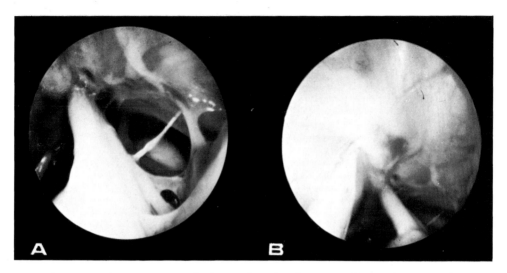

Fig. 4. *A* Entire course of the trigeminal nerve from the pons to Meckel's cave. Sensory and motor divisions are well-differentiated. From the motor division, a residual arachnoid membrane stretches to the tentorium. Below, the looped anterior inferior cerebellar artery *B* Pyramidal apex with the trigeminal nerve

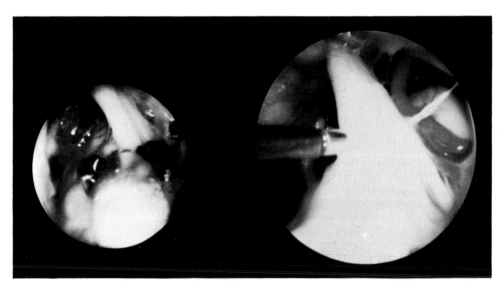

Fig. 5. Possibilities of trigeminal surgery under endoscopic view using micro-forceps or coagulation electrode. Medially, the motor division can be easily defined

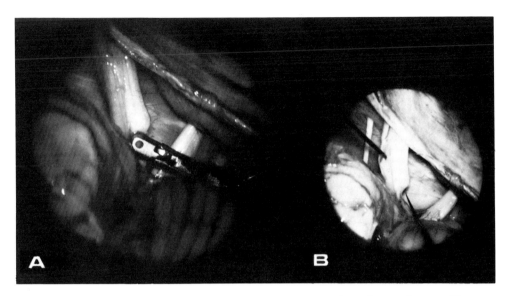

Fig. 6. Microscopic pictures at post mortem. View from above after removal of the cerebrum with section and retraction of the dura alongside the upper pyramidal edge
<u>A</u> Microforceps are easily introduced past the nerves VII, intermedius, VIII. The instrument takes hold of two-thirds of the sensory trigeminal division sparing the motor part
<u>B</u> The site after resection. The motor division is lifted with an instrument. The abducens nerve can be seen in the left background

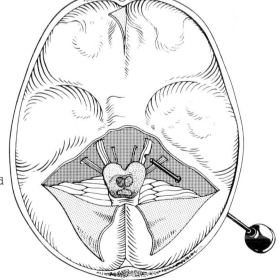

Fig. 7. Diagram of the visible area. The posterior pyramidal surface is indicated by hatched marks. From lateral to medial, cranial nerves VII, intermedius, and VIII run into the internal auditory meatus. V, VI runs into Dorello's canal. On the right, the endoscopic direction and point of trigeminal resection is indicated

Free Communications

Principles of the New WHO Classification of Brain Tumors

K. J. ZÜLCH

A correct classification of intracranial tumors and a reasonable terminology is still fundamental to create understanding between the clinician, the neuroradiologist, the neuropathologist, and the experimental neurooncologist. It seems unnecessary to emphasize the Babylonic discrepancies in terminology, and I need only point out the various systems of 1) BAILEY and CUSHING (1), which we have personally followed and modified according to modern needs (9, 10, 11, 13) and which the classification of RUBINSTEIN resembles (5), 2) the classification of KERNOHAN et al. (3) or 3) that of DEL RIO HORTEGA (4). Our endeavors to unify the various systems led to an International Symposium in Cologne in 1961 (15) and to the classification meeting with the Spanish school in Bilbao in 1967.

Yet these efforts have failed. We personally made further attempts to proliferate an international system by adopting the terminology of the Unio internationalis Contra Cancrum (UICC) in our "Histological Atlas" (12) and also later in the "Atlas of Gross Neurosurgical Pathology" (14).

However, this UICC classification of the tumors of the human body (8) was never accepted. Then, fortunately, the WHO approached Dr. Rubinstein and myself to help activate a system of collaborative institutions for a classification of brain tumors, paralleling similar previous successful actions for the wider classification of tumors of the other organs of the body (so-called "Blue Books" of the WHO). We designed a preliminary classification. A "reference center" was chosen - which we had the honor to have in Cologne (see scheme on p. 280) in our institute - and this had to work together with "collaborational centers" in the USA (2), Belgium, England, Japan, Mexico, Poland, Russia, and Switzerland.

Interesting cases were selected by the reference center, and there was a feedback by returning diagnoses and comments. The mutual discussions ended with two 1-week symposia in Geneva in 1974 and 1976. In the latter symposium, we agreed on a final classification, which was a compromise in only a few points. We all believed that this final classification was universally acceptable. It will probably appear in 1978 as a Blue Book on the histologic classification of tumors of the nervous system.

What is now basic in this classification?

1. It is well-defined on easily recognizable morphologic characteristics.

2. It gives biologic information by "grading" similar to the attempts formerly made by BAILEY and CUSHING (1) and later in a more simplified way by the 1-4 grading of malignancy. However, not every tumor group will have four subtypes of different malignancy. On the contrary, each tumor has only one or two grades of malignancy, which are not exactly in terms of survival times. However, I had the impression that they correspond to the definitions I previously made (14).

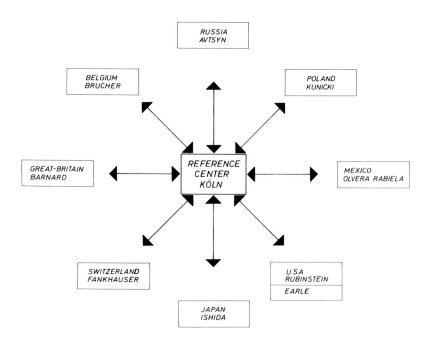

3. This classification could not solve some of the open problems of interpretation, such as that of the correct position of the monstruous cell tumors, where two interpretations will still be possible in the future: a monstrocellular sarcoma or a giant cell glioblastoma; similarly, whether pineal tumors are true two-cell anisomorphous "pinealocytomas" or "germinomas," and wheter these two exist and can be distinguished from one another also remains open.

4. In most tumor entities, the process of "malignization" or "dedifferentiation" is accounted for by the term "anaplastic" transformation.

I will now briefly discuss the majority of the well-accepted and some of the arbitrary tumor entities. The *astrocytic* tumors will be subdivided into the customary three groups: fibrillary, protoplasmic, and gemistocytic. The isolation of a special subtype in the astrocytic tumors under the designation of "pilocytic astrocytoma" is new and agreed upon by all. This entity corresponds to the old "polar spongioblastoma" of BAILEY and CUSHING's and of our classification. Important is that it was recognized as a very benign glioma, which has its predilection site in the midline and is characterized by Rosenthal fibers and granulated bodies. New is the biologic separation from the other astrocytomas. The ventricular tumor of tuberous sclerosis is correctly included as subependymal giant cell astrocytoma. The astroblastoma still remained a matter of discussion. This dubious subgroup should be restricted to pure neoplasms with astrocytic cells arranged in a particular pattern, e.g., with perivascular arrangement of these elements having thick processes containing fibers. The formation of morphologically somewhat similar astroblastic structures - such as is sometimes seen in glioblastomas and other tumors - will not include such tumors in the group of astrocytic tumors.

In the *oligendroglial* tumors, apart from the conventional oligodendroglioma, a subgroup of mixed oligoastrocytomas is foreseen, since very many of these tumors are actually mixtures of oligodendroglial and astrocytic cells. The anaplastic oligodendroglioma, described and emphasized by our institute since 1955 (11) as the "polymorphous" oligodendroglioma, is characterized by multinucleated giant cells, usually of the Langhans type, however with abundant necrotic zones, proliferated vessels, and other features of anaplasia.

Among the *ependymal* tumors, the typical ventricular tumor is foreseen as is the myxopapillary variant in the cauda equina. The latter is well-recognized as a subgroup. The anaplastic type of ependymomas is commonly found in youth as large extraventricular calcified and cystic tumors as described in 1937 (7).

Among the *chorioid plexus papillomas*, again, besides the conventional tumor, only the rare anaplastic (malignant, polymorphous) variant has to be mentioned.

Interesting is the classification of the *pineal gland tumors*, where we have: 1) the pinealocytoma, a more benign, not very common tumor of *isomorphous* pattern, and 2) the "anisomorphous two-cell type" pattern pinealocytoma, which has an architecture similar to that of the germinoma. Personally, I hold that these pineal gland tumors can be characterized both the histochemical (PAS negative) and metallic methods (positive in Girolami's impregnation). It can thus be distinguished from the germinomas in the same region, which, apart from polynucleated (Langhans) cells, show the opposite staining qualities. Therefore, the two-cell type or anisomorphous pinealoma can be classified twofold either as a pinealocytoma or as a germinoma. On the other hand, the pineoblastoma is a malignant variant similar to the medulloblastoma.

Among the *neuronal tumors*, it only seems interesting to call attention to the neuroblastoma, which is probably a rare tumor with a tendency to form pseudorosettes similar to medulloblastoma and, moreover, real Homer-Wright rosettes.

In the *glioblastoma multiforme* group, a "dualistic" classification similar to that of pineal gland tumors is possible. Here, two subgroups merit consideration: 1) the giant cell glioblastoma, which has already been mentioned in the differential diagnosis to the monstrocellular sarcoma and 2) the glioblastoma with a sarcomatous component or mixed glioblastoma and sarcoma. Again, we personally believe that two types of different tumors can be morphologically distinguished in subgroup 1.

Among the *medulloblastomas*, a "desmoplastic" variant (5) is included which corresponds to the former "circumscribed cerebellar arachnoidal sarcoma" of FOERSTER and GAGEL (2). Exceedingly rare tumors are the *"medulloepithelioma"* and the *"primitive polar spongioblastoma,"* both sufficiently characterized by reports in the world literature.

The study group recommended that "gliomatosis cerebri" be more fully characterized by the cell type observed, in which case it may correspond to terms like "astrocytomatosis" or "oligodendrogliomatosis." The biologic behavior of these tumors has not yet been sufficiently worked out.

The former well-known term neurinoma now appears as *neurilemmoma*, a compromise in order to avoid the term "schwannoma;" proper names, the group felt, should be excluded from the tumor terminology. Here, as in most other tumors, synonyms are included in brackets, e.g., schwannoma and neurinoma. The anaplastic variant of neurilemmoma is likewise mentioned, as is also the "anaplastic" dedifferentiation of the *neurofibroma* for which the synonyms "neurofibrosarcoma" and "neurogenic sarcoma" exists.

In the large *meningioma* group, three rarer variants have to be particularly discussed: 1) the angiomatous meningioma, when the tumor contains numerous large and small vascular channels, 2) the hemangioblastic form, when it is histologically indistinguishable from the Lindau tumor of the cerebellum, being, however, well-encapsulated and not invasive, and, finally, 3) the hemangiopericytic group, which again is indistinguishable from the hemangiopericytoma elsewhere in the body, but, as the former, encapsulated and not invasive.

A rare form of mengioma is the "anaplastic" type which may lead to sarcomatous degeneration and develop into a frank fibroblastic sarcoma of the meninges. Therefore, two groups of *real meningeal sarcomas* are mentioned: 1) the fibrosarcoma, the malignant counterpart to the meningioma, and 2) a rare polymorphic cell sarcoma which may develop from a meningioma. Both are characterized by their tendency to infiltrate and by their malignancy. Moreover, the well-known "primary" *meningeal sarcomatosis* exists as a group which, together with a secondary carcinomatosis and seeding of tumors such as the medulloblastoma and the pinealocytoma, originate diffuse metastases into the arachnoid space.

I will skip the xantomatous and melanotic tumors and come to the primary malignant *lymphomas*, for which a very complex classification has been worked out. However, only the "periadventitial" sarcomatous proliferation and the "reticular sarcomas" (of lower malignancy) will be mentioned, the latter not so uncommon in the spinal epidural space.

We have already mentioned the *hemangioblastoma* as a benign yet infiltrating tumor originated from the blood vessels. In this group of angiomatous tumors one also finds the *monstrocellular* sarcoma with reticular fiber production, which has been mentioned in the differential diagnosis to the giant cell glioblastoma. Probably an important group may be that of the *germ cell tumors*, where the "germinoma" of the pineal gland has already been mentioned. As concerns the morphology of this tumor, apart from the two-cell pattern of large epithelial and small lymphoid cells, multinucleated giant cells (Langhans type) also have to be emphasized as a very important characteristic, as well as the positive reaction of most cells to PAS stains.

Teratomas, *craniopharyngiomas*, *epidermoid* and *dermoid* cysts, the *ependymal colloid cysts* of the third ventricle, lipomas and choristomas, hamartomas, and the so-called nasal gliomas exist as entities, as also do the vascular malformations, where the traditional subgrouping is continued.

The tumors of the *pituitary gland* are not fully discussed in the new classification, since this is the topic of another group of histologists, working on the endocrine organ tumors. However, in our terminology nothing has changed in the subgroups.

Finally, for completion, we may mention the *vascular malformations* and the *local extensions* of tumors into the brain and spinal cord. Metastatic and unclassified tumors complete the table of entities.

Even when the histologic descriptions are not too extensive in the forthcoming new Blue Book of the WHO, they at least seem to be sufficient for differential diagnosis, particularly since they are supplemented by a large series of color photographs and slides. Moreover, larger books in the world literature, such as the AFIP volume by RUBINSTEIN (5) on brain tumors, the publication of Dr. RUSSEL and RUBINSTEIN (6), my two books, the "Atlas of the Histology of Brain Tumors" (12) and "Atlas of Gross Neurosurgical Pathology" (14) supported by my little tumor book "Brain Tumors, Their Biology and Pathology" (9, 11, 13) which will soon appear as a revised and enlarged edition, may help to characterize the tumor groups of the WHO classification.

In conclusion, I think that the World Health Organization has created an excellent piece of work which, as a manual, is a good tool to provide the neurosurgeon, the neurologist, the neuroradiologist, the neuropathologist, and the general pathologist with a classification which will be understood world-wide, if he - as we hope - decides to use it.

References

1. BAILEY, P., CUSHING, H.: A Classification of the Tumors of the Glioma Group on a Histiogenetic Basis with a Correlated Study of Prognosis. Philadelphia: J.B. Lippincott 1926

2. FOERSTER, O., GAGEL, O.: Das umschriebene Arachnoidalsarkom des Kleinhirns. Z. Neurol. 164, 565-580 (1939)

3. KERNOHAN, J.W., MABON, R.F., SVIEN, H.J., ADSON, A.W.: A simplified classification of the gliomas. Proc. Staff Meet. Mayo Clin. 24, 71-75 (1949)

4. RIO-HORTEGA, P. del: Nomenclatura y clasification de los tumores del sistema nervioso. Buenos Aires: Lopez & Etchefoyen 1945

5. RUBINSTEIN, L.J.: Atlas of Tumor Pathology. Tumors of the Central Nervous System. II. Series, Fasc. 6. Washington, Armed Forces Institute of Pathology (AFIP), 1972

6. RUSSELL, D.S., RUBINSTEIN, L.J.: Pathology of Tumours of the Nervous System, 3rd ed. London: E. Arnold 1971

7. TÖNNIS, W., ZÜLCH, K.J.: Das Ependymom der Großhirnhemisphären im Jugendalter. Zentralbl. Neurochir. 2, 141-164 (1937)

8. UNIO INTERNATIONALIS CONTRA CANCRUM: Illustrated Tumor Nomenclature. Berlin-Heidelberg-New York: Springer 1965/1969

9. ZÜLCH, K.J.: Die Hirngeschwülste in biologischer und morphologischer Darstellung, 3. Aufl. Leipzig: Joh. Ambr. Barth 1958

10. ZÜLCH, K.J.: Biologie und Pathologie der Hirngeschwulste. Handbuch der Neurochirurgie. Bd. III. Berlin-Göttingen-Heidelberg: Springer 1956

11. ZÜLCH, K.J.: Brain Tumors. Their Biology and Pathology, 2nd ed. New York: Springer 1965

12. ZÜLCH, K.J.: Atlas of the Histology of Brain Tumors. Berlin-Heidelberg-New York: Springer 1971

13. ZÜLCH, K.J.: Tumori Cerebrali. Biologia e Patologia. Translated by A. Ferrara and D. Batolo. Padova: Piccin Editore 1974
14. ZÜLCH, K.J.: Atlas of Gross Neurosurgical Pathology. Berlin-Heidelberg-New York: Springer 1975
15. ZÜLCH, K.J., WOOLF, A.L.: Classification of Brain Tumors. Report of the 1st International Symposium at Cologne 1961. Acta Neurochir. Suppl. X. Wien: Springer 1964

Objective Characterization of Proliferation and Malignancy in Human Brain Tumors

W. Heienbrock, M. Roters, and W. A. Linden

Introduction

Histologic diagnosis of proliferation tendency and malignancy is - at least in certain cases - difficult and somewhat arbitrary. Objective parameters may be obtained by flow cytometric DNA measurements. The DNA content of individual cells varies during the division cycle according to a fixed schedule. Flow cytometric DNA determinations of cell suspensions yield DNA distribution patterns, DNA histograms (3, 4, 6). From a computer analysis, the fractions of cells in the various phases of the cell cycle are obtained (1, 2). This is illustrated in Figure 1. DNA content and chromosome set of the cell cycle phases G_1 (prereplicative phase), S (DNA synthesis phase), and G_2+M (premitotic and mitotic phase) are shown together with the corresponding idealized DNA histogram. In normal proliferative tissue, the cell populations contain a high fraction of G_1 (or better nonproliferating G_0) cells and a low fraction of S and (G_2+M) cells. During the S phase, the DNA content is doubled, implicating that the (G_2+M) cells have twice the DNA content (4C) of the G_1 cells (2C). The peak position (e.g., 2C...4C) are denominated as ploidy stages. These ploidy stages permit a judgement on the malignancy of a tumor tissue.

Results and Discussion

Since no methods for the preparation of representative cell suspensions from human tumors had been available, we made several preparations of each brain tumor and developed a standard method which may be applied for all solid human tumors (7). A total of 70 tumors was analyzed by flow cytometry.

Our measurements revealed that in benign brain tumors only a relatively small fraction of cells are in the (G_2+M) phase, corresponding to a small proliferation tendency. On the contrary, in medulloblastomas and glioblastomas, significantly higher fractions of (G_2+M) cells were observed. This is demonstrated in Figure 2. In the upper part (2A) a typical DNA histogram of a mengioma is given. The lower part shows the histogram of a medulloblastoma (2B). As compared to the meningioma histogram, we notice an appreciable increase in the second peak and a shift of both peaks to the right in the glioblastoma histogram, indicating increased malignancy.

Table 1 contains the significant cytokinetic parameters for the judgement of proliferation tendency and malignancy for normal brain tissue, meningiomas, and glioblastomas/medulloblastomas. Malignant glioblastomas greatly differ from the more bonign meningiomas by both the mean fraction of cells in G_2+M and the ploidy stages. The fractions of cells in G_2+M are about 0% in normal brain tissue, 1,3% in benign, and 22.1% in malignant brain tumors. In mengiomas, we normally observed ploidy stages of 2C or 2C...4C, while in malignant tumors, practically all ploidy stages from 2C over 2.5C to 8C were found. Cells in ploidy stage 8C represent a third peak of cells which have been generated by endomitosis. Comparable results have been reported by HOSHINO (5).

Table 1. Fraction of cells in (G_2+M) phase (mean ± SE) and ploidy stages in normal brain tissue, meningiomas, and glioblastomas/medulloblastomas

	Normal brain tissue	Meningioma	Glio/medulloblastoma
G_2+M fraction (%)	0	1.3 ± 1.6	22.1 ± 5.5
Range of ploidy	2C	2C	2C, 2.5C, 3C...8C
		2C...4C	
		[2.5C...5C	
		4C...8C]	

Among the 17 meningiomas, we found two exceptions: one meningioma with the ploidy stages 2.5C...5C and another with the ploidy stages 4C...8C. The first case deserves a more detailed discussion. Additionally to the higher ploidy stages as an indication of increased malignancy, this tumors also revealed a relatively high fraction of cells in G_2+M as a sign of increased cell proliferation. Histologically, apart from some atypical nuclei, there were no signs of malignant degeneration. On the other hand, the peculiar flow cytometric findings are reflected by a remarkable clinical evolution: the patient had undergone surgery for a frontal meningioma 30 years prior and had been free of complaints since then. Now, following a history of only 3 months of headache, a very extensive recurrence infiltrating the base of the skull was observed and removed by surgery. Thus, the rapid tumor progression is in good correlation with the high proliferation tendency found by flow cytometry. Another exception was found in the group of histologically verified glioblastomas. It was a case with normal DNA distribution. The patient was a child who has so far survived surgery in very good condition for more than 18 months.

Both cases may be taken as examples that histology supplemented by flow cytometry may result in a better correlation with the clinical progression. Of course, it is still too early to discuss the definite value of the flow cytometric DNA measurements for tumor diagnosis and tumor therapy. The aim of this paper is to point out that, with the advent of flow cytometry, the histologic criteria can be supplemented by objective cytokinetic paramets which, in doubtful cases, might furnish clearer indications for postoperative irradiation or chemotherapy.

Summary

Flow cytometric DNA measurements provide objective parameters for the diagnosis of proliferation tendency and malignancy as a supplement to histologic criteria. The fraction of tumor cells in the (G_2+M) phase of the cell cycle was taken as an indication of cell proliferation and the ploidy stages of DNA content as a criterium for the judgement of malignancy. In our material, consisting of 70 human brain tumors, the benign tumors revealed only a small proliferation tendency which, on the contrary, was quite pronounced in malignant tumors. The latter also showed a striking shift of the ploidy stages to higher DNA values. These findings are discussed and correlated to the clinical course in several cases.

References

1. BAISCH, H., GÖHDE, W., LINDEN, W.A.: Analysis of PCP-Data to Determine the Fraction of Cells in the Various Phases of Cell Cycle. Radiat. Environ. Biophys. 12, 31-39 (1975)

2. BECK, H.-P.: Proliferationskinetische Untersuchungen an Zellkulturen und menschlichen Tumoren. Flußzytometrische und autoradiographische Experimente und Entwicklung neuer Auswerteverfahren. Thesis. Universität Hamburg 1977

3. VAN DILLA, M.A., TRUJILLO, T.T., MULLANEY, P.F., COULTER, J.R.: Cell Microfluorometry: A Method for Rapid Fluorescence Measurement. Science 163, 1213-1214 (1969)

4. GÖHDE, W., DITTRICH, W.: Impulsfluorometrie - ein neuartiges Durchflußverfahren zur ultraschnellen Mengenbestimmung von Zellinhaltsstoffen. Acta Histochem. Suppl. X, 429-437 (1971)

5. HOSHINO, T., NOMURA, K., WILSON, C.B.: Nuclear DNA distribution of human brain tumor cells, as determined by flow cytometry. Abstract, 6. World Congress of Neurosurgery, June 1977 in Sao Paulo, Brasilien

6. KAMENTSKY, L.A., MELAMED, M.R., DERMAN, H.: Spectrophotometer: New Instrument for Ultrarapid Cell Analysis. Science 150, 630-631 (1965)

7. ROTERS, M., LINDEN, W.A., HEIENBROK, W.: Comparison of three different methods for the preparation of human tumors for flow cytometry. European Press Medikon (1977). Ghent, Belgium (In press)

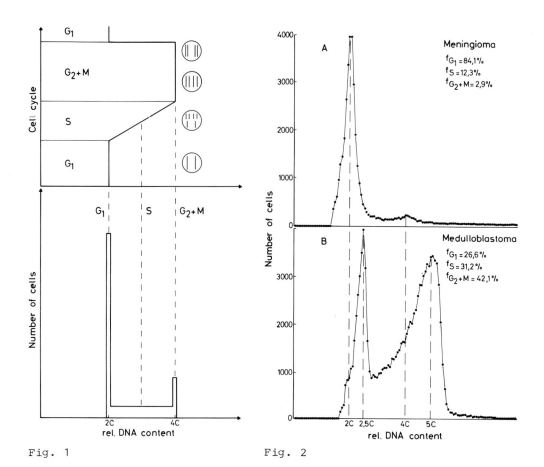

Fig. 1   Fig. 2

Fig. 1. Schematic presentation of DNA content of the cell cycle phases G_1 (prereplicative phase), S (DNA synthesis phase), and G_2+M (premitotic and mitotic phase), together with the chromosome sets and the corresponding DNA distribution pattern (DNA histogram). In this euploid DNA distribution, G_1 cells have a DNA content of 2C, (G_2+M) cells a DNA content of 4C

Fig. 2. 2A is a typical DNA histogram of a meningioma (2C...4C), 2B a DNA histogram of a medulloblastoma, which reveals an increased fraction of cells in the (G_2+M) phase and a peak shift to a higher DNA content (2.5C...5C...), f_{G_1}... gives the fraction of cells in the phases of the cell cycle

Chemotherapy of Brain Tumors – Experimental Results

H. D. MENNEL and J. SZYMÁS

A combination of three chemotherapeutically active substances, i.e., adriamycin, epipodophyllotoxine, and lomustine, has been found to be active in malignant brain tumors by POUILLARD et al. (1). Epipodophyllotoxine as a single agent was equally effective in a series of human brain tumors, although this substance does not cross the blood-brain barrier to a significant extent. On the other hand, good results have been described with the nitrosourea derivatives lomustine and carmustine both in human and in experimental brain tumors.

We first investigated the effectiveness of the single agents in the treatment of intracerebrally transplanted tumors. Our model is derived from neoplasms induced with alkylating agents in BD-IX rats. For these experiements, the carcinostatic compounds were tested in the line G-XII, which is now in the 20th intracerebrally grafted passage.

Transplantation tumors derived from neoplasms originally induced in the brain of experimental animals by resorptive carcinogens took a characteristic course when transplanted repeatedly. Three stages can be observed. In the first passages, the original morphology is mostly preserved. The second stage is characterized by changing morphologic features; gliomas as well as repetitive patterns, thought to be indicative of ependymomas, were found regardless of the original morphology. The final stage is reached at about the 12th passage. Then, a low differentiated glioma is seen which is rich in mitosis and is of high malignancy. Investigations of the vascular architecture of these tumors proved their similarity to human glioblastoma multiforme. The localization, however, is mostly in the ventricular system (Fig. 1.).

The "simplified" pattern which occurs after 12 passages is equally documented by the stable induction time of about 3 weeks for transplanted tumors. Growth characteristics of these tumors, their in vitro behavior and vascular architecture, have been reported elsewhere. We first investigated the effectiveness of adriamycin on this model. Our experience with this substance as a single agent in four experiental arrangements proved that adriamycin did not increase the survival time of experimental animals. Since other experimental and clinical data of its effectiveness are lacking, the carcinostatic activity of this substance in brain tumors seems doubtful.

Epipodophyllotoxine, on the other hand, has been described to act in human brain tumors (2). This substance is lipophilic. However, an accumulation of this substance in the brain following systematic application has not been shown. In our model, epipodophyllotoxine as a single agent was equally ineffective. The toxicity of this substance has, furthermore, been high, so that control animals had longer survival times than treated rats. Therefore, we investigated a combination of epipodophyllotoxine and lomustine. This combination led to a significant increase in the life span of the treated animals only if epipodophyllotoxine had been given first. The effect, however, was weaker than after the application of lomustine alone. The toxicity of this substance partly limited its growth-inhibiting effect. In our view, the effectiveness of these substances in the treatment of brain tumors is not yet completely established; confirmed experimental results are still lacking. In contrast, lomustine as a single agent significantly increased the life span. Lomustine is one of the widely investigated urea derivatives considered to be more or less effective in the treatment of brain tumors. Our investigations were performed with different concentrations and application forms. All groups had a significantly higher life span than the controls (Fig. 2). Higher doses, of course, are more effective; in addition, we found indications that the single application gives better results than repeated doses. The relationship of dose, number of injections, and time of application will be further investigated.

Alterations at the histologic and cytologic levels only occurred in animals treated with lomustine. Extensive necroses and necrobiotic changes in single cells, lack of mitoses, and occassionally occurrence of giant cells were met.

In conclusion, it seems that the effect of the combination of the three substances in human brain tumors is mainly due to the role of the alkylating urea. A better result of the combination as compared to the monotherapy with lomustine was not observed. The consequences for human brain tumor chemotherapy should be discussed based on these results.

References

1. POUILLARD, P., MATHE, G.: Treatments of malignant gliomas and brain metastases in adults with a combination of adriamycin, VM 26 and CCNU. Cancer 38, 1919-1916 (1976)
2. SLANSKY, B.D., MANN-KAPLAN, R.S., REYNOLDS, Jr., A.E., ROSENBLUM, M.L., WALKER, M.D.: 4'-Demethyl-epipodophyllotoxin-β-D-thenylidene-glucoside (PTG) in the treatment of malignant intracranial neoplasms. Cancer 33, 460 (1974)

Fig. 2. Effect of CCNU in intracerebrally transplanted gliomas in rats. Dashed lines: treated animals. Solid lines: controls. The percentage figures give the overall increase in life span in the single experiments

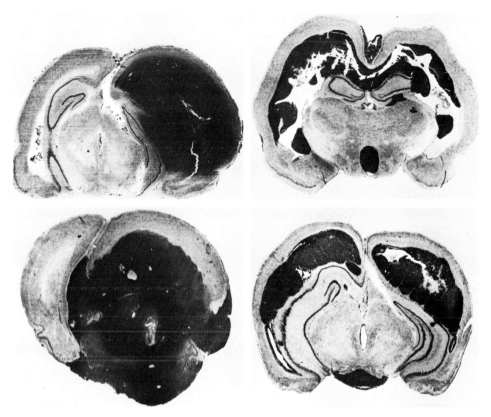

Fig. 1. Different localization patterns of intracerebrally transplanted gliomas in rats

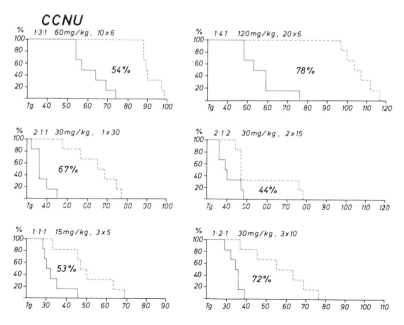

Chemotherapy of Brain Tumors
J. N. Petrovici and H.-W. Ilsen

Introduction

The nitrosourea compounds have been shown to be effective against transplantable brain tumors in animals and to lead to an increased survival time. The clinical effectiveness of these drugs has also been reported (2, 3, 4). POUILLART et al. (1) reported the results of employing combinations of agents rather than single modality therapy. Their patients with malignant brain gliomas received adriamycin followed by VM 26 (4'-dimethyl-epipodophyllotoxin-D-thenylidene glucoside) and CCNU (lomustine, 1-(2-chloroethyl)-3-cyclohexyl-1-nitrosourea). Adriamycin is supposed to have a synchronizing effect on tumor cell growth and, thus, to enhance the cytolytic effect of CCNU and VM 26. Such combination chemotherapy has been shown to be effective in both prolonging survival time and decreasing morbidity of patients with malignant gliomas (1).

Material and Methods

This series comprises 27 patients (20 male and 7 female) aged 26-75 years. Twenty-one patients suffered from malignant gliomas (malignancy degree III or IV) and six from semibenign gliomas (malignancy degree II). Nine patients received chemotherapy after surgery, while in 18 patients the brain tumor was considered to be inoperable; in these latter cases, the nature of the tumor was established neuroradiologically and/or by postmortem examination. The patients were divided into two groups: 11 patients with increased intracranial pressure and/or severe neurologic deficit and 16 patients without signs of increased intracranial pressure and with mild neurologic symptoms. The patients received a combined therapy consisting of adriamycin (40 mg/m^2 1 day), VM 26 (60 mg/m^2 2 days), and CCNU (60 mg/m^2 2 days). Each cycle of treatment lasted 5 days and was restarted only after an average interval of 4 weeks in order to allow hematologic recovery. Further medication consisted, when necessary, of anticonvulsive drugs, dexamethasone and chlorpromazine, to prevent gastrointestinal disturbances. In three patients, chemotherapy was used in conjunction with radiotherapy.

Results

1. Clinical Response (Table 1)

A good clinical response with an improvement in neurologic symptoms and a neuroradiologic reduction of the tumor size (Figs. 1 and 2) was observed in ten patients, nine of whom had malignant gliomas and one a semibenign glioma. Three patients of this group were able to resume work. Twelve patients (eight with malignant gliomas, four with semibenign gliomas) showed a fair response with only mild or no clinical improvement but with a better clinical course than could have been expected without any therapy. There was no response in five patients (four with malignant and one with semibenign gliomas).

Table 1. Clinical response after combined chemotherapy of brain tumors

	Malignant	Semibenign	Total
Good response	9	1	10
Fair response	8	4	12
No response	4	1	5

2. Survival Time (Table 2)

Patients with malignant gliomas and with increased intracranial pressure and/or severe neurologic deficit had an average survival time of 96 days in the chemotherapy-and-surgery group and 151 days with chemotherapy alone. Two patients are still living. The number of patients in each group was too low and the individual variation too great to permit statistical analysis. The survival time was increased (202 days in the chemotherapy-and-surgery group, 181 days with chemotherapy alone) in patients having a good general condition, i.e., without increased intracranial pressure and with moderate neurologic symptoms. In this group, four patients are still alive. As expected, the survival period in patients with semibenign gliomas was longer than in those with malignant tumors.

3. Side-Effects

Eighteen of 28 patients showed reversible loss of hair. Bone marrow depression with white blood cell counts under 2000/mm^3 often occurred between the therapy cycles but was reversible. In one case, chemotherapy was stopped because of leukopenia.

Discussion

Patients with malignant gliomas and without signs of increased intracranial pressure had an average survival time of 6-7 months. This is in agreement with the results of POUILLART et al. (1). Since in untreated patients a survival time of 3-4 months can be expected, this form of chemotherapy provides a further prolongation of 3-4 months survival. Individual clinical response seems to be unpredictable. A small number of patients showed no response, but in the majority chemotherapy was followed by an impressive clinical improvement lasting over a period of several months, during which time some were able to return to work. Considering the ineffectiveness of all previous efforts in treating malignant brain tumors, our results suggest that further clinical studies on the therapeutic value of the nitrosourea compounds are justified.

Summary

Twenty-one patients suffering from malignant gliomas and six patients suffering from semibenign gliomas received a combination chemotherapy consisting of adriamycin, VM 26, and CCNU. Ten patients showed a good clinical response with improvement of neurologic symptoms and with neuroradiologic reduction of the tumor. Eleven patients showed a fair response, and in five patients no response was observed. The patients with malignant gliomas and without preceding surgery had an average

Table 2. Survival time (days) after combined chemotherapy

		Malignant gliomas				Semibenign gliomas		
	No.	Still alive	$\bar{x}$	Range	No.	Still alive	$\bar{x}$	Range
With increased intra-cranial pressure								
After surgery	4	1	96	71–148	–			
Without surgery	7	1	151	34–333	–			
Without increased intra-cranial pressure								
After surgery	4	2	185	91–262	1	1	207	
Without surgery	6	2	202	56–351	5	4	319	178–501

survival time of 151 days when signs of increased intracranial pressure were observed before commencing chemotherapy and of 202 days when there were no signs of increased intracranial pressure.

References

1. POUILLART, P., MATHE, G., POISSON, M., BUGE, A., JUGUENIN, P., GAUTIER, H., MORIN, P., THY, H.T., LHERITIER, J., PARROT, R.: Essai de traitement des glioblastomes de l'adulte et des metastases cerebrales par l'association d'adriamycine, de VM 26 et de CCNU. Presse Med. 5, 1571-1576 (1976)
2. ROSENBLUM, M.L., REYNOLDS, A.F., SMITH, K.A., RUMACK, B.H., WALKER, M.D.: CCNU (2-(2-Chloroethyl)-3-cyclohexyl-1-nitrosourea; NSC-79037) in the treatment of malignant brain tumors. J. Neurosurg. 39, 306-314 (1973)
3. WALKER, M.D., WEISS, H.D.: Chemotherapy in the treatment of malignant brain tumors. In: Advances in Neurology. FRIEDLANDER, W.J. (ed.), Vol. 13. New York: Raven Press 1975
4. WILSON, C.B., BOLDREY, E.B., ENOT, K.J.: 1-3-bis (2-chloroethyl)-1-nitrosourea (NSC-409962) in the treatment of malignant brain tumor. Cancer Chemother. Rep. 54, 273-281 (1970)

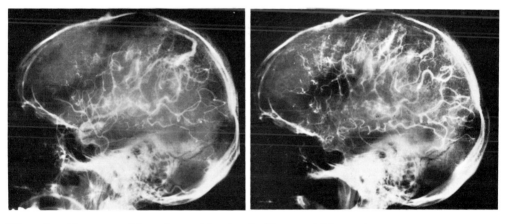

Fig. 1. 49-year-old male patient. Left carotid angiogram.
Left: Parietal malignant glioma with pathologic vessels
Right: Reduction of tumor mass and involution of tumor vessels after 4 months chemotherapy

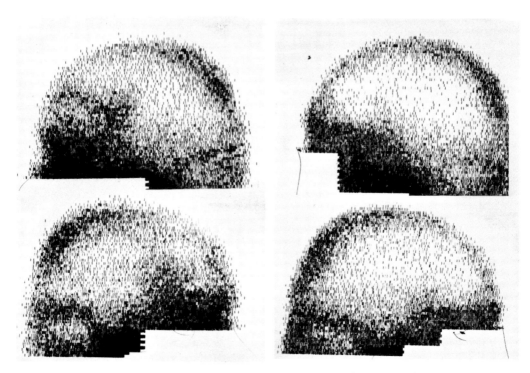

Fig. 2. 53-year-old male patient. Brain scan.
Left: Frontal pathologic accumulation of radioisotope indicating a callosal tumor
Right: Almost normal scan finding after 5 months chemotherapy

Agenesis of the Perisylvian Region (Temporal Lobe Agenesis): Neurologic Symptoms and Therapy

E. MARKAKIS, R. HEYER, L. STÖPPLER, and J. TAEGERT

The first signs of sylvian depression in embryogenesis may be detected at the end of the 2nd intrauterine month and become more apparent as a sylvian groove at the end of the 3rd month. The temporal operculum grows more effectively in the anterior two-thirds and reaches the sylvian fissure in the 4th month. At the same time, the frontoparietal operculum becomes evident and gradually extends backward to meet the anterior part of the temporal operculum. These changes occur in the later half of the 5th month (2). As the growth energy of the temporal operculum is more intense than that of the frontoparietal, it follows that, when the opercula meet in the 6th intrauterine month, there is more of the sylvian area covered by the temporal than by the frontoparietal operculum.

The present syndrome, herein called "temporal lobe agenesis" (7, 8, 9, 10) is considered to be a disturbance of this cerebral embryogenesis, especially of the frontoparietal region, and becomes evident during the last 3 months of fetal life (1, 5, 11). Arachnoid cysts are found in this hypoplastic region, sometimes with space-occupying character (1, 11).

Seventy cases of agenesis of the frontotemporal area with arachnoid cysts overlying this region are reported prior to 1970 (10, 11). The diagnosis was made during surgery in most cases. The patients were operated on under the tentative diagnosis of a space-occupying lesion such as subdural hematoma, external hydrocephalus, porencephaly, intracerebral hematoma, or tumor.

Until the syndrome of temporal lobe agenesis was completely understood, the following synonyms were used: cystic pseudotumor cerebri (11), meningitis serosa circumscripta (11), relapsing juvenile subdural hematoma (3), subarachnoid pouch (7), cerebral arachnoid cyst (11, 12), chronic subarachnoid cyst (13), and temporal lobe agenesis syndrome (10).

The external appearance of the patients is characterized by face and skull asymmetries with depression or elevation of the eyebrow. Sometimes, other congenital anomalies, such as broad oculofacial malformations, may occur. Other frequent symptoms are: skull and face asymmetries, localized bulging of the head, enlargement of the skull, exophthalmus, strabism, hydrocephalic findings, convulsive seizures, and retarded psychomotor development. In some cases, transillumination can be positive as in cases of external hydrocephalus (1). The EEG may show focal abnormalities, slow waves or low voltage (4), over the region of the lesion. In patients with increased intracranial pressure, papilledema and unspecific neurologic signs can be found.

The typical radiologic signs are: rounded and enlarged cranial vault, thinned cranial bone over the lesion, displacement of the sagittal sinus groove, elevated sphenoid ridge, and depressed and elongated floor of the middle fossa (1, 6, 10, 11). Carotid angiography shows nonspecific signs of a great space-occupying lesion, the temporal area being poor in vessels, and sometimes hydrocephalic findings.

Pneumencephalography or ventriculography demonstrates dilatation, deformity, or displacement of the ventricles. Sometimes, as a result of the brain stem shifting, an obstruction of the aqueduct occurs and leads to a hydrocephalus occlusus. Computerized tomography demonstrates a hypodense region in the perisylvian area (Fig. 1).

In cases with a space-occupying arachnoid cyst or subdural hematoma, the CT scan diagnosis may be difficult.

The summary of the clinical signs in our ten patients (Fig. 2) demonstrates that:
1. As in the literature (relation 4:1 or 5:1), the male sex dominates (9:1).
2. The perisylvian agenesis was left-sided except in one case.
3. There is a high incidence of left-handed or ambidextrous patients.
4. The arachnoid cysts were always localized in the temporal region. In three cases, they were frontotemporal; in another case, the whole frontotemporoparietal region was occupied by a huge arachnoid cyst of 280 ml volume.
5. Five patients decompensated after a slight trauma, four of them with subdural hematoma. The rest showed an increased frequency of convulsive seizures, deterioration of EEG findings, or general clinical signs of increased intracranial pressure.

The psychoneurologic investigation (at the earliest 6 months after operation) showed that right-handed patients always have pathologic findings, especially in the visual constructive capacity, speech, reading, perimetry, audiogram, and dichotic listening. The left-handed are free of such symptoms (Fig. 3). In a 2-year-old boy with a preoperative right-sided hemiparesis and postoperative neurologic defects, we assume a so-called paretic left-handedness.

Operative treatment consists in resection of the cyst and cyst walls, communication to the basal subarachnoid space, and sometimes, implantation of an Ommaya reservoir with the catheter in the cyst cavity (Fig. 4).

Summary

The syndrome of temporal lobe agenesis represents an embryogenetic hypoplasia of the whole perisylvian region, and not only of the temporal lobe, in accordance with the surface anatomy of cerebrum at the 5th-6th month of fetal life. It is accompanied by space-occupying arachnoid cysts. The left-sided agenesis and the male sex are predominant. Many patients are left-handed or ambidextrous. If the patients become left-handed or ambidextrous, there are only slight or no neurologic defects. Convulsive disorders are frequent. Cerebral decompensation or subdural hematoma after slight trauma may occur and are not unusual.

References

1. ANDERSON, F.M., LANDING, B.H.: Cerebral arachnoid cysts in infants. J. Pediatr. 69, 88-96 (1966)

2. CUNNINGHAM, D.J.: Contributions to the surface anatomy of the cerebral hemispheres. Cunningham Memoirs, R. Irish Acad. Dublin, 7, 1-358 (1892)

3. DAVIDOFF, L.M., DYKE, C.G.: Relapsing juvenile chronic subdural hematoma. A clinical and roentgenological study. Bull. Neurol. Inst. New York, 7, 95-111 (1938)
4. DE SANCTIS, A.G., GREEN, M., LARKIN, V.: Porencephaly. J. Pediatr. 22, 673-689 (1943)
5. GRUSS, P., AUER-DOINET, G.: Zur Genese der temporalen Arachnoidalzysten. Neuropaediatrie 5, 175-180 (1974)
6. HARDMAN, J.: Asymmetry of the skull in relation to subdural collections of fluid. Br. J. Radiol. 12, 455-461 (1939)
7. KARVOUNIS, P.C., CHIU, J.C., PARSA, K., GILBERT, S.: Agenesis of temporal lobe and arachnoid cyst. New York J. Med. 70, 2349-2353 (1970)
8. ROBINSON, R.G.: Intracranial collections of fluid with local bulging of the skull. J. Neurosurg. 12, 345-353 (1955)
9. ROBINSON, R.G.: Local bulging of the skull and external hydrocephalus due to cerebral agenesis. Br. J. Radiol. 31, 691-700 (1958)
10. ROBINSON, R.G.: The temporal lobe agenesis syndrom. Brain 87, 87-106 (1964)
11. STARKMAN, S.P., BROWN, T.C., LINELL, E.A.: Cerebral arachnoid cysts. J. Neuropathol. Exp. Neurol. 17, 484-500 (1958)
12. TIBERIN, P., GRUSZKIEWICZ, J.: Chronic arachnoidal cysts of the middle cranial fossa and their relation to trauma. J. Neurol. Neurosurg. Psychiatry 24, 86-91 (1961)
13. TÖRMÄ, T., HEISKANEN, O.: Chronic subarachnoidal cysts in the middle cranial fossa. Acta Neurol. Scand. 38, 166-170 (1962)

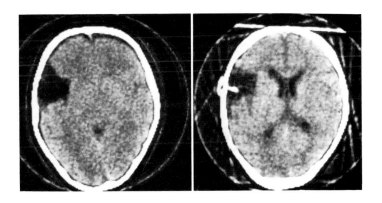

Fig. 1. Perisylvian agenesis in CT scan
Left: Before operation
Right: After operation with Ommaya reservoir

Age yrs.	Sex M	Sex F	Side of Agenesis R	Side of Agenesis L	Handedness R	Handedness L	Cause of Admission: Seizures EEG	Decomp. aft. Traum	Neurol. Signs	Papill-edema	Hydro-cephalus	Localisation of Arachn. Cyst: frontal	tempor	parietal
12	●		●		●			○	○	○			○	
5	●			●		●		○		○	○	○	○	
6	●			●	●	●		○		○	○		○	
44		●		●	●		○		○		○		○	
33	●			●	●		○		○				○	
2	●			●		●	○		○				○	
12	●			●	●	●	○					○	○	○
7	●			●	●				○			○	○	
42	●			●	●		○	○	○			○	○	
9	●			●	●	●		○	○	○			○	

Fig. 2. Clinical signs in ten patients with perisylvian agenesis

Handedness R	Handedness L	Side of Agenesis R	Side of Agenesis L	Postoperat. Pathological Findings: Audiogr. Deficits R	Audiogr. Deficits L	Speech	Reading	Dichotic Listen. R	Dichotic Listen. L	Perimetry	Visual Construct. Capacity
●		●			●		●	●			●
●			●			●			●		●
●			●					●		●	
●			●			●					●
	●		●								
●	●		●								
●	●		●								
	●		●			●			●		

Fig. 3. Postoperative pathologic findings in eight patients

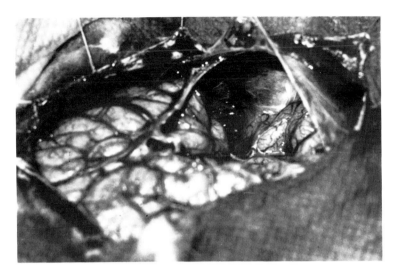

Fig. 4. Left-sided agenesis of the perisylvian area (operative picture)

Interhemispheric Subdural Empyema
G. Graef

The clinical importance of subdural empyema lies not in its absolute
frequency but rather in the acute, life-threatening character of this
disease. The most common causes of subdural empyema are otorhinologic
infections (2, 5, 13, 18). In spite of combined surgical and antibiotic
therapy, mortality rates between 30% and 40% have been reported by
some authors (1, 3, 4, 9, 18), even in the last decade.

Subdural empyema is most often located over the cerebral convexity,
although empyemas in the interhemispheric fissure are not unusual (1, 2,
3, 5, 7, 10, 11, 12, 13, 15, 16, 17). An interhemispheric empyema can
be either combined with a convexity empyema or isolated. It develops
preferably from infections of the paranasal sinuses. According to some
authors (1, 3, 5, 12), interhemispheric empyemas constitute 25%-40%
of all subdural empyemas.

A classic evidence of the interhemispheric empyema is the "falx syndrome" as described by KEITH (7) and LIST (10, 11). This comprises
monoparesis of the contralateral leg or ascending hemiparesis as well
as pronounced focal seizures in the contralateral leg. Paraparesis
results if the empyema spreads under the falx to the opposite side of
the interhemispheric fissure.

The pathognomonic angiographic sign of the interhemispheric empyema
(6, 8, 14, 15, 16, 17) is the demonstration of a parafalcine avascular
area on the anteroposterior view: the branches of the anterior cerebral artery are displaced away from the falx or, in case of bilateral
filling, the anterior cerebral arteries are separated from each other.
This parafalcine avascular area remains visible in the capillary
phase. Sometimes, the avascular area is surrounded by a stain of curly
vessels as a sign of hyperemia and inflammatory reaction. However, not
all interhemispheric empyemas can be demonstrated angiographically
(5, 12). This might be explained by the fact that most of the patients
are seriously ill, lying in the recumbent position. The pus in the
interhemispheric fissures can then sink to the occipital area, and the
characteristic displacement of the anterior cerebral artery is no
longer demonstrable.

We found 19 subdural empyemas in our own records covering the period
from 1955-1977. Thirteen of these cases have been documented since 1970.
Otorhinologic infections were the source of 15 of these empyemas, while
five others had different origins. Three of six patients (50%) died in
the period of 1955-1969, and 5 of 13 patients (38.4%) died in the period
1970-1977. The overall mortality rate is 42%! In 15 cases, the empyemas
were located over the cerebral convexity unilaterally; in one case
bilateral convexity empyemas were found. In one case, a convexity and
an interhemispheric empyema were associated. Isolated empyemas of the
interhemispheric fissure were found in two cases.

All 3 cases of interhemispheric empyema occurred in adolescents, between
14 and 16 years of age, with purulent infections of the paranasal
sinuses. Interhemispheric empyemas accounted for only 16% of the 19 subdural empyemas but constituted one-third of the nine empyemas resulting
from rhinologic infection!

In the first case (1955), a subdural empyema over the left cerebral convexity was demonstrated angiographically and treated by means of craniotomy and drainage. After temporary improvement, the patient's condition deteriorated despite massive antibiotic therapy, and the patient died. Postmortem examination revealed an extensive empyema on the left side of the interhemispheric space. The second patient (1969) exhibited right-sided hemiparesis, most pronounced in the leg. The angiogram (Fig. 1a and b) revealed the typical picture of an interhemispheric empyema on the left side. The empyema was evacuated through burr holes, and the patient recovered after local and systemic antibiotic therapy.

The third patient (1977) manifested a left-sided hemiparesis, most pronounced in the leg. The right carotid angiogram (Fig. 2a and b) showed only a small avascular area lateral to the upper border of the falx on the anteroposterior view, while the lateral projection demonstrated curly hyperemic vessels. However, only computerized tomography showed the full extent of the empyema, which reached the parieto-occipital area of the interhemispheric space (Fig. 3). The illustration reproduces (A) the upper slices of the computerized tomogram, where the empyema appears as a stripe of low density on the right side of the falx. Following enhancement with contrast medium, the surrounding area of hyperemic inflammatory reaction is clearly demonstrated. The empyema was drained through a single accurately placed burr hole, and the patient recovered after local and systemic antibiotic therapy. The lower part of the illustration (B) shows the follow-up study 4 weeks later.

Computerized tomography served as a valuable complement to angiography for the diagnosis and treatment of subdural interhemispheric empyema. This is true in cases in which angiography cannot provide definitive information. CT scan revealed the full extent of the empyema and allowed precise therapy with the most limited surgical intervention.

References

1. BHANDARI, Y.S., SARKARI, N.B.S.: Subdural empyema. J. Neurosurg. 32, 35-39 (1970)
2. COURVILLE, C.B., Subdural empyema secondary to purulent frontal sinusitis. Arch. Otolaryngol. 39, 211-230 (1944)
3. FARMER, T.W., WISE, G.R.: Subdural empyema in infants, children and adults. Neurology 23/3, 254-261 (1973)
4. HENSELL, V., ZIMMERMANN, D.: Zur Diagnostik und Therapie des subduralen Empyems. Zentralbl. Neurochir. 32, 129-147 (1971)
5. HITCHCOCK, E., ANDREADIS, A.: Subdural empyema: A review of 29 cases. J. Neurol. Neurosurg. Psychiatry 27, 422-434 (1964)
6. ISFORT, A.: Angiographische Befunde beim Hämatom und Empyem im Interhemisphärenspalt. Fortschr. Geb. Röntgenstr. Nukl. Med. 107, 127-130 (1967)
7. KEITH, W.S.: Subdural empyema. J. Neurosurg. 6, 127-139 (1949)
8. KRASEMANN, P.H.: Isolierte Empyeme im Interhemisphärenspalt. Zentralbl. Neurochir. 30, 291-298 (1969)
9. LEBEAU, J., CREISSARD, P., HARISPE, L., REDONDO, A.: Surgical treatment of brain abscess and subdural empyema. J. Neurosurg. 38/2, 198-203
10. LIST, C.F.: Interhemispheral subdural suppuration. J. Neurosurg. 7, 313-324 (1950)

11. LIST, C.F.: Diagnosis and treatment of acute subdural empyema. Neurology 5, 663-670 (1955)
12. MORITZ, R., SZDZUY, D., MÖSER, E.: Zur Problematik des angiographischen Nachweises von Subduralempyemen im Interhemisphärenspalt. Zentralbl. Neurochir. 37, 111-118 (1976)
13. SCHILLER, F., CAIRNS, H., RUSSELL, D.S.: Treatment of purulent pachymeningitis and subdural suppuration with special reference to penicillin. J. Neurol. Neurosurg. Psychiatry 11, 143-182 (1948)
14. SEGALL, H.D., RUMBAUGH, C.L., BERGERON, R.T., TEAL, J.S.: Neuroradiology in infections of the brain and meninges. Surg. Neurol. 1, 178-186 (1963)
15. TORRES, H., YARZAGARAY, L., WEST, Ch.: Subdural empyema, angiographic and clinical considerations. Neurochirurgia (Stuttg.) 13,6, 201-210 (1970)
16. VERDURA, J., WHITE, R.J., RESNIKOFF, S., BROWN, H.: Interhemispheric subdural empyema: angiographic diagnosis and surgical treatment. Surg. Neurol. 3, 89-92 (1975)
17. WILKINS, R.H., GOREE, J.A.: Interhemispheric subdural empyema: angiographic appearance. J. Neurosurg. 32, 459-462 (1970)
18. WOODHALL, B.: Osteomyelitis and epi-, extra- and subdural abscesses. Clin. Neurosurg. 14, 239-255 (1967)

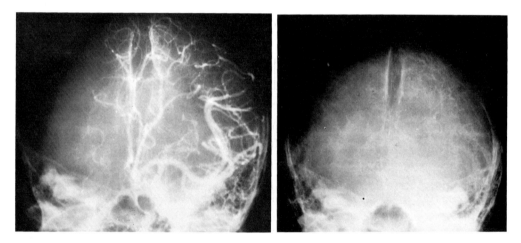

Fig. 1. Pathognomonic angiographic findings in interhemispheric subdural empyema (case 2)
Left: Arterial phase
Right: Capillary phase

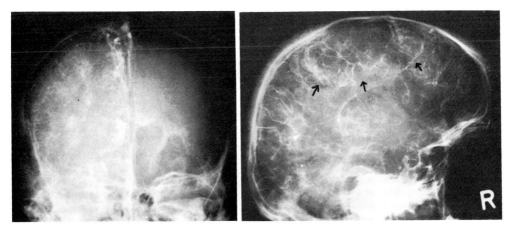

Fig. 2. Angiographic findings in interhemispheric subdural empyema (case 3)
Left: Only small parafalcine avascular area in the a.p. view
Right: Curly vessels in the surrounding area in the lateral view

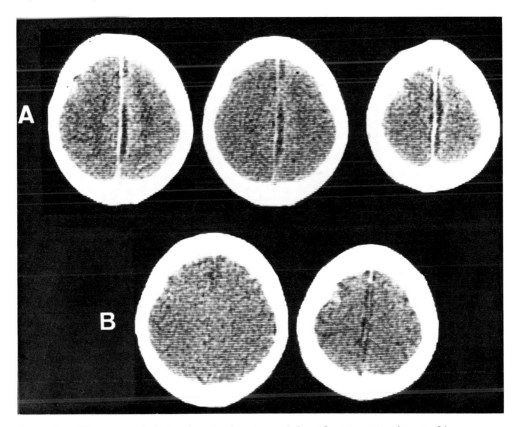

Fig. 3. CT scan of interhemispheric subdural empyema (case 3)
A Preoperative study
B Follow-up study

A Case of Intraventricular Hydatid Cyst

J. KRÜGER, A. RITZ, and W. INGUNZA

Hydatid disease is caused by the *Echinococcus granulosus* of the canine tapeworm. The normal cycle is: dog as worm carrier and definitive host and sheep as echinococcus carrier and intermediate host. Man is an accidental echinococcus carrier (28).

The adult tape-worm is at most 6 mm long and lives about 5 months. Eggs deposited by the dog feces are ingested by grazing cattle, in particular by sheep. In the intestines, the embryo hatches out, passes through the intestinal wall, and reaches the liver via the portal vein, possibly also reaching the lungs and the general circulation as well as other organs. Here, the embryo develops into the *Taenia echinococcus* with surrounding cysts which can reach the size of a man's head. In addition, the tenia is capable of agamous reproduction, so that an internal cyst can harbor hundreds of teniae or several daughter cysts can develop from a mother cyst. If the infected organs reach the dog's intestines, then a tapeworm can develop from each taenia (36). Man becomes infected by close contact with the contaminated dogs, which contain the eggs everywhere, including the coat and around the muzzle. Children who grow up in rural areas are particularly susceptible (24).

In 1550, PARANOLI first mentioned the echinococcus in the human brain. He found it in the corpus callosum of a deceased epileptic. Between 1855 and 1860 LEUCKHARDT and KÜCHENMEISTER outlined the life cycle (31), and since the end of the last century, exact reports exist on the disease - mostly single accounts (16, 26, 5, 27, 19, 8, 17, 33, 1). GIERLICH, in 1902, was the first to report on a successfully operated hydatid cyst in the brain (15). Most of the cases have been described by BIANCHI SAUS et al. (7), a total of 107 patients. Geographically, the disease is spread over countries with sheep raising, in particular Australia (35, 13). New Zealand (38, South America (3), North Africa (39, 9, 40), South Africa (12, 32), India (6, 29), Turkey (24), Southern Europe (4, 34, 10), and in Germany, Friesland, Mecklenburg, and Pommern (15, 30).

Infestation of the brain is observed in 1% (23)-7% (34), mostly single cysts, particularly in the right frontal and temporal regions. However, intraventricular and infratentorial cysts have also been reported (7, 24). Organs other than the brain are infested only seldom (14).

Clinical symptoms - with an anamnesis lasting from years (21) to a few hours (37) - are usually restricted to intracranial hypertension with headache, nausea, and vomiting in spite of a general well-being (1). According to BIANCHI SAUS et al. (7) 70% of the patients have clinical or electroencephalographic signs of epilepsy (18). Focal attacks correspond to the location of the cyst and were seen in 95% of the cases by BIANCHI SAUS et al.

Additionally to the general signs of chronic intracranial hypertension, x-rays reveal space-occupying lesions without involvement of the blood vessels (12). Air studies by "cystography" (4, 25) have been abandoned because of the danger of dissemination. With the aid of computerized tomography (CT) it is possible to demonstrate the cysts without risks.

Intraventricular cysts, however, cannot be clearly defined due to their thin capsule, in particular when further daughter cysts are present (Fig. 1).

The only treatment is surgery. The best method of approach is that described by ARAÑA-IÑIGUEZ and SAN JULIAN in 1955 (3), whereby the brain tissue above the cyst is widely exposed. By the injection of saline through a thin tube, the cyst is mobilized and removed intact, if necessary by lowering the head and shaking. One must avoid rupturing the cyst so as to prevent dissemination of the teniae. If this is achieved, the prognosis is good. ARSENI and SAMITCA (4), who produced the mobilized cyst by jugular compression or by awakening the patient, reported that following intraoperative rupture of the cyst, only one out of four patients survived. KAYA and others (24) described 15 operated cysts, of which eight ruptured. Four of the latter patients died, the other four had to be operated on repeatedly - up to four times. However, they recovered completely over a period of observation from 2-5 years. This survival rate of 50% following intraoperative puncture of the cyst was also mentioned by CARRERA and others (11). The success of treatment with cystostatica (22) is uncertain, in our case this form of therapy was unsuccessful.

Case Report

A 6-year-old Turkish boy was admitted in May, 1976 with signs of cerebral compression and the diagnosis, confirmed by angiography, of an avascular space-occupying lesion in the right frontal region. Because of the short anamnesis of only 3 weeks (increasing headache, vomiting, and hemiparesis on the left), a malignant tumor was first suspected. The operation was performed immediately. Following reflection of the osteoplastic flap in the right frontal region and small brain resection, one arrived at a smoothly defined milky-white cyst at a depth of about 5 mm. It was punctured, 100 ml of watery fluid extracted, and then removed from the right anterior horn. The cyst had a diameter of 9 cm, so that in the beginning it appeared too large to be removed without puncture. Histology confirmed a hydatid cyst (Dr. SCHOBER, Max-Planck-Institut für Hirnforschung, Frankfurt/Main).

Fluctuating fever resulted after the operation. All in all, the boy made a quick recovery and could be discharged without any neurologic symptoms 3 weeks later. Eleven months later, the child was readmitted, somnolent, with headache, nausea, and vomiting, as well as a left-sided hemiparesis. Now CT revealed daughter cysts, not only intraventricular but also intracerebral in the right frontotemporal region (Fig. 1). At the second operation, nine daughter cysts were removed from both the lateral and the third ventricle, as well as from the right frontal region. The cysts were 1-5 cm in diameter. Once again, the child made a complete recovery.

A third operation was performed at the end of July, 1977, and this time a cyst with a diameter of 5 cm, located in the right temporobasal region (Fig. 2), and four further cysts in the third ventricle were removed. At present, the child is still under hospital care.

Discussion

According to the case reports contained in the literature - in particular those from ARAÑA-IÑIGUEZ (2, 3) and KAYA et al. (24) - the prognosis of cerebral hydatid cysts following surgery is not as poor as we thought up to now (20). When these cysts, which are nearly always solitary, are removed intact, the patient generally makes a complete recovery (1).

The relatively high percentage of workers from Southern European countries, especially from Turkey, should always lead us to consider the possibility of hydatid disease, particularly in the case of a child from this group of inhabitants, admitted with a cystic brain tumor. Here also, the exact anamnesis is very important (after the first operation, we found out that our patient had close contact with an infected dog in Instanbul). Possibly the puncturing of the cyst in our case could have been avoided, if an exact case history had been obtained with the aid of an interpreter and a preoperative CT.

Conclusion

The case of a 6-year-old Turkish boy is reported, who initially underwent an emergency operation since a malignant tumor in the right frontal region was suspected. A hydatid cyst was, however, found and punctured. Recurrences resulted which required two further operations within a period of 16 months.

References

1. ANDERSON, M., BICKERSTAFF, E.R., HAMILTON, J.G.: Cerebral hydatid disease in Britain. J. Neurol. Neurosurg. Psychiatry 38, 1104-1108 (1975)
2. ARAÑA-IÑIGUEZ, R., GURRI, J.: Echinococcosis of the Nervous System. Revue Neurol. 20, 187-191 (1962)
3. ARAÑA-IÑIGUEZ, R., SAN JULIAN, J.: Hydatid Cysts of the Brain. J. Neurosurg. 12, 323-355 (1955)
4. ARSENI, C., SAMITCA, D.C.: Cranial and cerebral hydatid disease. Acta Psychiat. K.B.H. 32, 389-398 (1957)
5. AYRES, C.M., DAVEY, L.M., GERMAN, W.J.: Cerebral Hydatidosis. J. Neurosurg. 20, 371-377 (1963)
6. BALASUBRAMANIAM, V., RAMANNJAN, P.B., RAMAMURTHI, B.: Hydatid Disease of the Nervous System. Neurol. India, 18, Suppl. 1, 92-95 (1970)
7. BIANCHI SAUS, A., GAUDIN, E.S., DE MARABAL, M.P., ARAÑA-IÑIGUEZ, R.: Hydatid Cyst of the Brain as an Epileptogenic Factor. Act. Neurol. Lat. Am. 19, 78-88 (1973)
8. BONIS, G., STURM, K.W.: Echinococcus alveolaris im Gehirn. Med. Klin. 64, 891-893 (1969)
9. BORNE, G.: Un cas de Kyste Hydatique cérébral intraventriculaire. Bull. Soc. Pathol. Exot. 57, 28-32 (1964)
10. CARCASSONNE, M., AUBRESPY, P., DOR, V., CHOUX, M.: Hydatid Cysts in Childhood. Prog. Pediatr. Surg. 5, 1-35 (1973)
11. CARREA, R., DOWLING, E.J., GUEVARA, J.: Surgical Treatment of Hydatid Cysts of the Central Nervous System in the Pediatric Age (Dowling's Technique). Childs Brain 1, 4-21 (1975)
12. DANZIGER, J., BLOCH, S.: Tapeworm Cyst Infestations of the Brain. Clin. Radiol. 26, 141-148 (1975)

13. DEW, H.R.: Primary cerebral hydatid disease. Aust. N.Z.J. Surg. 24, 161-171 (1955)
14. FEICHTER, G.E., BÜCKING, H., MOLL, A.: Ungewöhnliche Echinokokkuserkrankung mit Befall von Herz und Gehirn. Münch. Med. Wochenschr. 116, 2073-2076 (1974)
15. FISCHER, W.: Die parasitären Erkrankungen des ZNS und seiner Hüllen. In: Handbuch der speziellen pathologischen Anatomie und Histologie, Bd. XIII/3. UEHLINGER, E. (Hrsg.), S. 372-412. Berlin-Heidelberg-New York: Springer 1955
16. FLEMING, N.B.B., BURNY, G.W.: A case of primary Hydatid Disease of the Brain. Lancet 2, 1186-1189 (1919)
17. FORTUNA, A., GIOFFRE, R.: Cisti da echinococco solitaria soprasellare. Riv. Neurol. 40, 465-472 (1970)
18. FUSTER, B., CASTELLS, C., GASTAUD, H.: The electroencephalographic study of hydatid cysts of the brain EEG. Clin. Neurophysiol. 7, 415-421 (1955)
19. GEIGER, L.E.: Hydatid Cyst of the Brain. J. Neurosurg. 23, 446-449 (1965)
20. GERLACH, J., JANSEN, H.P., KOOS, W., KRAUS, H.: Pädiatrische Neurochirurgie. Stuttgart: Georg Thieme 1967
21. JACKSON, H.: Infestation with Particular Reference to Hydatid Cysts of the Brain. Proc. R. Soc. Med. 57, 15-22 (1964)
22. JAKOWIDIS, Th., TZAMALUKAS, G.: Beitrag zur chirurgisch-cystostatischen Behandlung bei der multiplen Bauch- und Leberechinococcose. Chirurg 46, 558-561 (1975)
23. KATZ, A.M., PEN, C.-T.: Echinococcus disease in the USA. Am. J. Med. 25, 759-770 (1958)
24. KAYA, U., ÖZDEN, B., TÜRKER, K., TARCAN, B.: Intracranial hydatid cysts. Study of 17 cases. J. Neurosurg. 42, 580-584 (1975)
25. KING, T.T., COUCH, R.S.C.: The Diagnosis of Cerebral Hydatid Disease. Clin. Radiol. 12, 190-193 (1961)
26. LANGMAID, C., ROGERS, L.: Intracranial Hydatids. Brain 63, 184-190 (1943)
27. MASSON, R., ALLEGRE, G., ROCHET, M., COTTE, F.: Récidive d'un kyste hydatique du cerveau. Rev. Otoneuroophtalmol. 38, 54-57 (1966)
28. MATTHES, D., MATTHES, C.: Plagegeister des Menschen. Schmarotzer in und an uns. Stuttgart: Frauenklin. Verlagshandlung 1974
29. NATARAJAN, M.: Surgical Removal of a Hydatid Cyst of the Brain. Int. Surg. 60, 292-293 (1975)
30. NITSCHE, W.: Echinokokkose. Z. Allg. Med. 52, 1592-1603 (1976)
31. OLIVE, J.I., ANGULO-RIVERO, P.: Cysticercosis of the Nervous System. J. Neurosurg. 19, 635-640 (1962)
32. ORMAN, D.N., LE ROUX, P.A.T.: Cerebral Hydatid Disease: A radiological Review. S.A. Med. J. 42, 1048-1051 (1968)
33. PAP, Z., EMÖDY, J.: Diagnostizierte primäre Gehirn-Echinokokken-Zyste aufgrund von Augensymptomen. Klin. Monatsbl. Augenheilkd. 157, 87-92 (1970)
34. PHILIPPOV, Ph.: Klinik und Behandlung des Gehirnechinokokkus. Beitr. Neurochir. 13, 192-197 (1966)

35. PHILLIPS, G.: Primary Cerebral Hydatid Cysts. J. Neurol. Neurosurg. Psychiatry 11, 44-52 (1948)
36. PIEKARSKI, G.: Medizinische Parasitologie. Berlin-Heidelberg-New York: Springer 1973
37. RHODES, P.L.: Unusual Case of Hydatid Cyst of the Brain. Br. Med. J. 2, 739 (1954)
38. ROBINSON, R.G.: Hydatid Disease Affecting the Nervous System. Annu. R. Coll. Surgeons 26, 145-156 (1960)
39. SAMIY, E., FAZL, A.J.: Cranial and intracranial hydatidosis. J. Neurosurg. 22, 425-433 (1965)
40. SLIM, M.S., KHAYAT, G., NASR, A.T., JIDEJIAN, Y.D.: Hydatid Disease in Childhood. J. Pediatr. Surg. 6, 440-448 (1971)

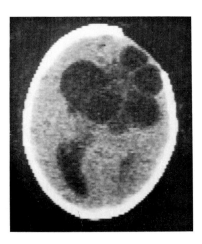 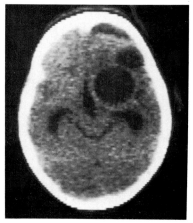

Fig. 1   Fig. 2

Fig. 1. Computerized tomography: several hydatid cysts in the ventricular system and right frontal and temporal lobe 11 months after the first operation of a punctured cyst in the right ventricle (courtesy of Prof. Dr. med. H. Hacker, Department of Neuroradiology, University Clinic at Frankfurt a.M.)

Fig. 2. Same patient 2 months later: another cyst with a diameter of 5 cm is seen in the right temporobasal region (courtesy of Prof. Dr. med. H. Hacker, Department of Neuroradiology, University Clinic at Frankfurt/Main)

Benign Osteoblastoma of the Skull With Secondary Aneurysmal Bone Cyst Formation, With Special Reference to the Differential Diagnosis of Osteogenic Sarcoma

D. Voth, P. Gutjahr, and J. Spranger

Modern oncology provides a real chance for permanent cure even in patients with osteogenic sarcoma, by means of radical surgery and high-dose methotrexate as chemotherapy. The latter, however, may cause severe and even life-threatening side-effects. Keeping this in mind, it seems necessary to report on an 8 4/12-year-old girl with benign osteoblastoma of the skull which can be mistaken for an osteogenic sarcoma but does not require the same aggressive treatment.

History

Painless and an apparently rapidly growing right frontal swelling was noticed by an 8 4/12-year-old girl after a minor trauma. She was operated on for a suspected hematoma, but on surgery a friable, intensely bleeding bone tumor was found. The diagnosis of osteogenic sarcoma was established after cautious curettement.

On admission to our hospital, the child was in good condition and neurologically normal. Radical surgery was initially refused by the mother, and radiotherapy which seemed to be of little help would have had severe side-effects; aggressive combination chemotherapy with high-dose methotrexate and citrovorum factor rescue was instituted. Three cycles of chemotherapy were given, during which severe myelosuppressive, hepatotoxic, and gastrointestinal side-effects occurred. Since the tumor evidently did not respond and continued growing, the mother finally consented to a radical operation. The tumor had not infiltrated the meninges and was subtotally removed. Twenty-one months later, the right frontal lobe and the ventricles are at their regular place and there has been no recurrence.

Diagnosis

Benign neoblastoma of the skull with aneurysmal bone cyst formation was diagnosed. The differential diagnosis must include giant cell tumor, osteoid osteoma, osteogenic fibroma, fibrous dysplasia, aneurysmal bone cyst, and osteogenic sarcoma.

Discussion

Benign osteoblastoma is the widely accepted designation for a rare bone tumor (1%-2% of primary bone tumors) that occurs predominantly in the 2nd and 3rd decades of life and shows a definite predilection for males. Almost half of the tumors affect the vertebral column. Cranial location is unusual. The term giant osteoid osteoma, used synonymously, indicates the similarity to osteoid osteoma, at the same time respecting the difference in size of the average tumor.

Clinically, long-lasting local pain (several months to several years) is the cardinal symptom in these slowly developing tumors. Local swelling may be observed, when the overlying soft tissue forms only a thin layer.

Radiologic findings are not characteristic, lytic lesions may be more or less well-circumscribed and do not always suggest a benign tumor. The central nidus is supposed to be larger than in ordinary osteoid osteomas. Occasionally, a thin layer of bone beneath an expanded periosteum gives the appearance of an aneurysmal bone cyst.

Gross pathology is supposed to be characteristic when a well-circumscribed greyish-red or brownish hemorrhagic granular and friable tumor with variable degrees of calcification is found. Tumors up to 10 cm diameter have been reported.

Microscopically, some of the tumors show only slight osteoid formation and many giant cells in an abundance of connective tissue (early lesions), whereas, in others, considerable calcification may be present (older lesions). Less mature lesions may contain numerous mitoses in rapidly proliferating cells, suggesting osteogenic sarcoma.

The presence of blood vessels in almost all of the benign osteoblastomas and the occasional features of an aneurysmal bone cyst in parts of the tumors raise the question of an etiologic relationship between these two lesions or of the vascular origin of benign osteoblastomas.

The *prognosis* is good after complete surgical excision, and even after subtotal removal, e.g., by curettement, cure may be achieved, which raises the question of the true neoplastic nature of benign osteoblastoma, the more so since even a few untreated patients have been found asymptomatic after several years. Development of malignancies at the primary site of a benign osteoblastoma usually can be related to preceding radiotherapy, which is of little help in these benign lesions.

Development of an osteoblastoma in the skull of an 8-year-old girl is unusual. An even more important reason for presenting the case is - in our opinion - to recognize the disease entity of benign osteoblastoma as such and to be aware of the possibility of mistaking it for osteogenic sarcoma, which then may lead to most aggressive combined modality therapy of current oncology as in our case, with all the possible severe and potentially life-threatening early and late side-effects.

References

1. AEGERTER, E., KIRKPATRICK, J.A.: Orthopedic Diseases. 4th ed. Philadelphia-London-Toronto: Saunders 1975
2. DAHLIN, D.C.: Bone Tumors. 2nd ed. Springfield, Ill.: Thomas 1973
3. VON RONNEN, J.R.: Osteoblastoma spinous process of C-2. Skeletal Radiol. $\underline{1}$, 61 (1976)
4. ROSEN, G., TAN, C., SANMANEECHAI, A., BEATTIE, Jr., E.J., MARCOVE, R., MURPHY, M.L.: The rationale for multiple drug chemotherapy in the treatment of osteogenic sarcoma. Cancer $\underline{35}$, 936 (1975)

EEG-Changes With Acute Secondary Mesencephalic Lesions Accompanied by Disturbances of Consciousness

A. GRIMMER

A group of 69 patients with disturbances of consciousness caused by supratentorial space-occupying lesions was studied. We are interested in the question of whether there was a significant correlation between EEG changes and neurologically defined altered states of consciousness.

Most of the patients sustained head injuries. The concept of PLUM and POSNER (4) served as a basis for the neurologic coma classification, taking into account a rostrocaudal deterioration: 1) early diencephalic stage (we called it early stage of mesencephalic syndrome, MHS I), 2) late diencephalic stage (middle stage of the mesencephalic syndrome, MHS II), 3) midbrain-upper pons stage (late stage of the mesencephalic syndrome, MHS III), and 4) lower pons-upper medulla stage (bulbar syndrome, BHS).

In order to also include the very early phases of a mesencephalic syndrome, we have enlarged - according to a proposal by JOUVET (3) - the concept of PLUM and POSNER as follows: first prodromal phase with a "positive waking reaction" (arousable to verbal commands) and second prodromal phase with a "positive waking reactivity" (arousable to pain stimuli only) (Table 1).

Electroencephalographic semiology included the following categories: morphology, rhythms, amplitudes, topography, symmetry, periodicity, continuation of the bioelectric activity, and finally, reactivity (1, 2).

In the following, we shall discuss only the investigations on reactivity. In order to determine whether or not the bioelectric activity over the hemispheres was able to produce changes in rhythms and/or amplitudes by application of stimuli, we stimulated the patients with painful pricks on the extremities and in the face; a series of acoustic stimuli followed. One hundred and fifty-two out of 190 single EEG investigations were performed under the program of stimulation (Table 2).

We differentiated the following modalities of reactivity:
1. Blocking reaction of δ-, θ-, and of superimposed α-rhythms.
2. Activating reaction of δ-rhythms and of α- and θ-rhythms (Fig. 1-3).

How do the modalities of reactivity distribute themselves among the various stages of the mesencephalic syndrome and the prodromal phases? We evaluated each modality of reactivity in a single EEG tracing. (For instance, in the same tracing, θ-rhythms could be activated by acoustic stimulation and blocked by painful pricks, etc.) (Table 3).

The following conclusions can be made:
1. The efficacy of stimulation decreases as the disturbances of consciousness worsen.
2. In the early phases of the comatose stage, several modalities of reactivity appear; in the late stage of the mesencephalic syndrome (MHS III) we observed only one modality in a single EEG record.
3. Most of the modalities of reactivity are of the activating type; the number of activating reactions decreases as the coma becomes

Table 1. The mesencephalic syndrome and its prodromal phases (including only the states of reactivity). Acute secondary mesencephalic syndrome (modality of reactivity)

1st prodromal phase	2nd prodromal phase	Early stage of MHS (I)	Middle stage of MHS (II)	Late stage of MHS (III)	BHS
Positive waking reaction	Negative waking reaction	Negative	Negative	Negative	Negative
Arousability positive	Arousability positive	Negative	Negative	Negative	Negative
Orientation reaction positive/negative	Negative/positive	Negative	Negative	Negative	Negative
AL – facial-vocal-reaction possible	AL – facial-vocal-reaction possible	Negative	Negative	Negative	Negative
AL – strong, directed defence reaction	AL – directed, non-directed defence reaction	Nondirected defence reaction, homolateral	– occasional turning of head; flexion and/or extension synergy	– bilateral extension synergy	– Extension synergy reduced but still possible; vegetative reaction
Beginning hemisphere semiology	Pronounced hemisphere semiology	Hemisphere semiology	Hemisphere semiology	Hemisphere semiology still possible	Spinal automatisms

Table 2. Number of EEG investigations in the various stages of the mesencephalic syndrome and its prodromal phases

		Stimulation		
		Without	With	Total
Prodromal phases	I	12	35	47
	II	3	20	23
MHS	I	6	31	37
	II	4	17	21
	III	9	44	53
BHS		4	5	9
		38	152	190

deeper. The number of blocking reactions, however, increases as the coma worsens.

Which pattern of reactivity - symmetric or asymmetric - appears in the various comatose stages, correlated with previous symmetric and asymmetric tracings (Table 4)? The following conclusions can be drawn:
1. In asymmetric tracings, a focus is rather activated than blocked.
2. In asymmetric tracings, only a few symmetric reactivities appear. Blocking reactions occur more frequently over the less damaged hemisphere, activating reactions more frequently over the more damaged hemishere.
3. In symmetric EEG tracings, the most frequent pattern of reactivity is a symmetric one (both blocking and activating reactions).

Summary

None of the various stages of the mesencephalic syndrome and its prodromal phases demonstrates a characteristic form of reactivity. In all comatose stages, the activating reactions are overwhelming. While the disturbances of consciousness progress, the activating reactions decrease; the blocking reactions, however, increase. In symmetric EEG tracings, asymmetric reactivity is most frequently observed (activating reactions over the more damaged hemisphere, blocking reactions over the less damaged hemisphere). In all stages of coma and in symmetric tracings, nearly all forms of reactivity are symmetric.

Table 3. Modalities of reactivity in the various stages of the mesencephalic syndrome and its prodromal phases

		Reactivity/ Stimulation	Blocking reaction of			Activation reaction of	
			Polymorph Delta	(Super-imposed) Theta	(Super-imposed) Alpha	Monomorph frontal right Delta	Central Alpha Theta
Prodromal phases	I	33/35	1	0	3	27	8	39
	II	17/20	1	1	2	12	6	22
MHS	I	23/31	4	2	2	13	3	24
	II	11/17	1	1	1	9	1	13
	III	14/44	3	2	1	8	0	14
BHS		(2)/5	0	0	(1)	0	(1)	(2)

Table 4. Asymmetric and symmetric reactivities in asymmetric and symmetric EEG tracings in the various stages of the mesencephalic syndrome and its prodromal phases

		Prodromal phases			MHS			BHS
		I	II	I	II	III	
Asymmetric	Focus - blocked by stimulation	1	0	0	0	0	0	1
	Focus - activated by stimulation	7	3	1	1	1	0	13
	Blocking reactions over more damaged hemisphere	0	0	1	0	0	0	1
	Blocking reactions over less damaged hemisphere	1	1	1	0	2	0	5
	Activating reactions over more damaged hemisphere	4	3	3	0	1	0	11
	Activating reactions over less damaged hemisphere	2	1	2	0	1	0	6
	Bilateral blocking and activating reactions	4	3	3	6	1	(1)	17
Symmetric	Blocking reactions unilateral	0	1	0	0	0	0	1
	Blocking reactions bilateral	2	1	3	1	3	0	10
	Activating reactions unilateral	3	1	1	0	2	0	7
	Activating reactions bilateral	15	8	9	5	3	(1)	40

References

1. ARFEL, G., Introduction to Clinical and EEG Studies in Coma. In: Handbook of Electroencephalography and Clinical Neurophysiology, Vol. 12; Clinical EEG, II: Altered States of Consciousness, Coma, Cerebral Death. REMOND, A. (ed.)
2. FISCHGOLD, H., MATHIS, P.: Obnubilations, comas et stupeurs, Etudes électroencephalographiques. Electroencephalography and Clinical Neurophysiology. Suppl. 11. Paris: Masson & Cie. 1959
3. JOUVET, M.: Coma and other disorders of Consciousness. In: Handbook of Clinical Neurology, Vol. 3: Disorders of Higher Nervous Activity. VINKEN, P.J., BRUYN, G.W. (eds.)
4. PLUM, F., POSNER, J.B.: Diagnosis of Stupor and Coma, 2nd ed. Contemorary Neurology Series. Philadelphia: F.A. Davis Company 1972

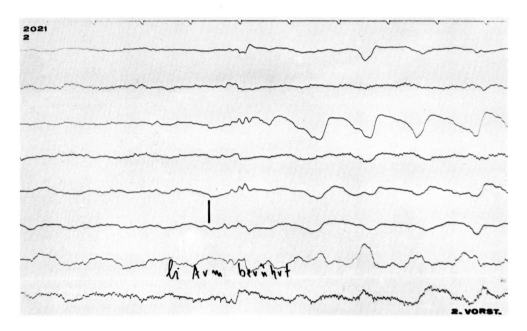

Fig. 1. Example of an activating reaction of δ-rhythms (second prodromal phase) more pronounced over the more damaged hemisphere and elicitated by a touch

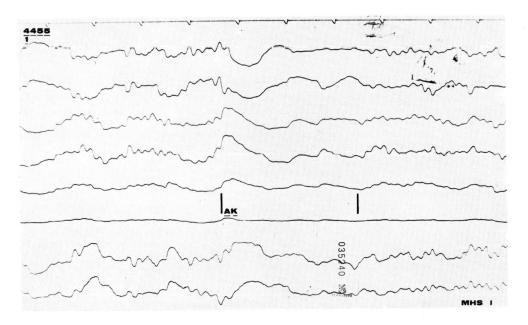

Fig. 2. Example of a symmetric blocking reaction of superimposed
θ-rhythms (middle stage of the mesencephalic syndrome) simultaneous
with an acoustic stimulus

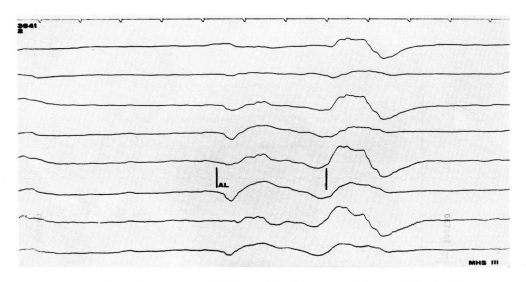

Fig. 3. Example of an asymmetric activating reaction of δ-rhythms
(late stage of the mesencephalic syndrome) elicited by a painful
prick

Value of Measuring the Cranial Circumference
R. MÜKE

Despite critical comments, it is still a common practice, especially among pediatricians, to take the circumference of the cranium as reference for intracranial volume. The skull development curve of HARNAK-HEIERLI, with the 3% and 97% percentiles, wherein the circumference of every child's head is marked as an index for its volume, is well-known. There are several reasons for doing so. First, there are relationships between circumference and volume, but the question is what are they and are they constant? The other reason is that measuring the circumference is not invading, not expansive, can be performed by everybody and, thus, is especially valuable in follow-up studies, as opposed to many other diagnostic aids, such as electroencephalography, echoencephalography, diaphanoscopy, pneumencephalography, or computerized tomography.

As early as 1862, WELKER emphasized that there can be differences in volume up to 150 cm^3 in normally sized and configured heads with equal circumference. We obtained similar results in a study on 76 infant skulls (13) where, among other parameters, we measured circumference and volume. One example: skull A, with a circumference of 42.8 cm has a volume of 880 cm^3, while skull B has a circumference of 41.8 cm, i.e. 1 cm less, but a volume of 1150 cm^3, more than 270 cm^3 more. Thus, there may be differences in volume of more than 20% as related to the circumference in normal skulls.

Several authors have, therefore, looked for different parameters for measuring the intracranial volume. There were suggestions that the volume be calculated from straight lines (1, 2, 3, 4, 5, 7, 8, 10, 11, 12, 16) as well as straight lines and planes (6, 9, 13, 14, 15, 17) from skull x-rays. Lately, the possibility of measuring intracranial volume by analyzing stereoscopic x-rays by biophotogrammetry or by computerized tomography was added. We examined all these possibilities looking for a simple and practicable method that would be sufficiently accurate. We think we found this method by taking the product of the maximum biparietal diameter and the planimetric medial sagittal plane. It provides an accuracy of about 3% (14). The measurements were made on 20 macerated adult and 76 infant skulls. With this method, the volume can be calculated as follows:

$V = 0.5156 \cdot (D \cdot F) + 46.55.$

In order to find out whether one of intracranial volumes as measured by this method deviates from the standard volumes as related to age, we calculated the volume in 156 Hamburgian children of different ages by the described method, and took the results to draw a curve of age-dependent intracranial volume development with corresponding percentiles, comparable to the circumference development curve. Simultaneously, head circumference was measured in these children. These curves showed a relatively good correlation, despite the above-mentioned considerable individual deviations in single cases. All children had a normal head circumference. A second random test gave the same result. Patients with normal cranial circumference almost always have a normal intracranial volume as measured by the above-mentioned method.

The situation is different in pathologically configured skulls. Here more discrepancies are evident. The same circumference can be measured in skulls with volumes that differe by a factor of 1:2.

Case 1: microcephalic, circumference 41.6 cm; volume 560 cm^3
Case 2: microcephalic, circumference 41.0 cm; volume 891 cm^3
Case 3: macrocephalic, circumference 59.5 cm; volume 1217 cm^3
Case 4: macrocephalic, circumference 62.0 cm; volume 2445 cm^3

For further illustration, we calculated intracranial volume in 25 children with an increased skull circumference and in 26 children with a reduced circumference with the help of our method and marked the results on a normal volume development curve (Fig. 1). The positions in the volume development curve were then compared with the corresponding points on the circumference development curve of the same children (Fig. 2). It became evident that the points on the volume development curve differ much more from each other than the corresponding points on the circumference development curve, and furthermore, that macrocephalics or microcephalics by circumference do not have to be macro- or microcephalic by volume. Comparison of both figures shows that five macrocephalics by circumference and 13 microcephalics by circumference have volumes within the normal range. Even though this is a pilot study (the volume development curve has to be stabilized by more cases), the tendency is obvious that measuring the circumference gives a good reference for the intracranial volume in normally developed skulls, but becomes unreliable in skulls with pathologic configuration. Therefore, in cases where a pathologic shape of the skull is suspected, we suggest evaluation of the D · F values in addition to measuring the circumference. The D · F volume determination is more time-consuming than measuring the circumference but can, nevertheless, be performed everywhere. In this way, it would be possible to gather more date with both methods and also to limit more interfering and expensive examinations. Our study indicates that the measurement of head circumference alone permits no definite conclusion as to skull development.

References

1. AUSTIN, J.H.M., GOODING, Ch.A.: Roentgengraphic measurement of skull size in children. Pediatr. Radiol. 99, 641-646 (1971)

2. BERNARD, J., LICHTENBERG, R.: Evaluation radiographique de la cranienne de l'enfant. J. Radiol. Electrol. 43, 877 (1962)

3. BRAY, P.F., SHIELDS, W.D., WOLCOTT, G.J., MACKEN, J.A.: Occipitofrontal head circumference - an accurate measure of intracranial volume. J. Pediatr. 75, 303-305 (1969)

4. CRONQUIST, S.: Roentgenologic evaluation of cranial size in children. Acta Radiol. 7, 98-111 (1968)

5. DEKABAN, A., LIEBERMANN, J.E.: Calculation of cranial capacity from linear dimensions. Anat. Rec. 150, 215-220 (1964)

6. FUCHS, G., BAYER, O.: Eine radiologische Methode zur Bestimmung der Schädelkapazität. Radiol. Austria 8, 51-55 (1955)

7. GORDON, I.R.A.: Measurement of cranial capacity in children. Br. J. Radiol. 39, 377-381 (1966)

8. GRADZKI, J., PZYMSKI, K., MULAREK, O.: Proba oceny wielkosci i ksztaltu czaszak maloglowiowych metoda rentgenometryczna. A trial of assessment of the size and shape of microcephalic skulls by the roentgenometric method. Neurol. Neurochir. Psychiatr. Pol. T. VIII, Nr. 4, 541-546 (1973)

9. KAUFMANN, B., SHULMAN, A.: A method of intracranial calculation. Invest. Radiol. 7, 533-538 (1972)

10. KOIVISTO, E., PYKÖNEN, L., WEGLIUS, C.: A method for roentgenologic measurements from spot fluorograms (its application to skull capacity determination). Am. J. Roentgenol. 84, 96-98 (1960)

11. McKINNON, I.L.: The estimation of skull capacity from roentegenological measurements. Am. J. Roentgenol. 76, 303-310 (1956)

12. MENICHINI, G., RUIU, A.: On the radiological evaluation of the cranial capacity in infants. Minerva Pediatr. 12, 1358-1363 (1960)

13. MÜKE, R.: Neue Gesichtspunkte zur Pathogenese und Therapie der Kraniosynostose. Acta Neurochir. 26, 191-250, 293-326 (1972)

14. MÜKE, R., HOMANN, G., KELLNER, H.: Untersuchungen zur Schädelvolumenbestimmung. Fortschr. Röntgenstr. 125, 3, 219-225 (1976)

15. NEUERT, W.I.A.: Zur Bestimmung des Schädelinhaltes am Lebenden mit Hilfe von Röntgenbildern. Z. Morphol. Anthropol. 29, 261-287 (1931)

16. SCHMID, F., FILTHUT, I.: Angewandte Schädelmetrik. Monatsschr. Kinderheilkd. 109, 299-301 (1961)
    Grundlagen der radiologischen Schädelmetrik. Monatsschr. Kinderheilkd. 109, 292-296 (1961)

17. WEINMEISTER, G., INKE, G.: Die Bestimmung der Schädelkapazität aus der lateralen Röntgenaufnahme bei Vertretern der drei Großrassen. Gegenbauers Morphol. Jahrb. 112, 19-81 (1968)

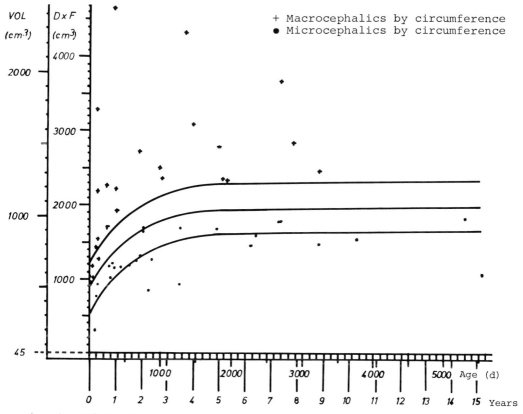

Fig. 1. Volume development curve

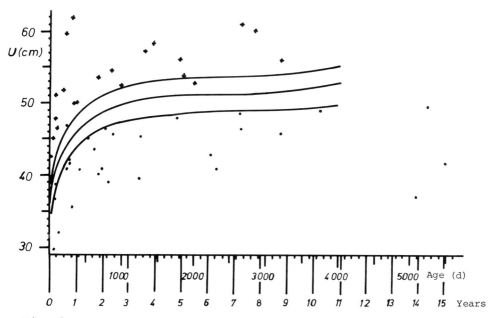

Fig. 2. Circumference development curve

Neurosurgical-ENT Treatment of Lesions of the Base of the Skull
M. SAMII and W. DRAF

Space-occupying lesions of the base of the skull offer special problems for the following reasons:
1. They are relatively rare.
2. Diagnosis in the early stages is difficult, because the symptoms are uncharacteristic and can involve various other medical fields.
3. They lie in a surgical area, so that the optimal diagnosis and operative treatment can only be performed with the close cooperation of affiliated specialities. Working in a combined ENT and neurosurgical team in a number of cases, we were able to gather experience in the diagnosis of new growths and expand operative techniques (Table 1). The acoustic neuroma and tumors of the glomus jugulare are intentionally not considered here.

Increasing diminution of the sense of smell, dull headache deep behind the eyes, epistaxis, trigeminal irritation, and orbital symptoms should lead to the suspicion of a tumor in the area of the anterior and middle cranial fossa. Neoplasms in the posterior region of the skull base, especially at the jugular foramen, present a clinical picture (not unusually) of a one-sided vocal cord paralysis. With larger tumors, there are disorders of swallowing with deviation of the soft palate to the healthy side as a result of a complete glossopharygeal and vagus paralysis. On occasion, an accessory lesion and a unilateral hypoglossus paralysis with articulation disorders can be seen.

If the mastoid process and the petrous bone are involved, an air conduction deafness, by perforation into the internal auditory meatus, loss of bone conduction, tinnitus, a vestibular deficit, and a facial nerve paralysis add to the clinical picture. Brain pressure symptoms as signs of intracranial space occupation were not observed even in large tumors.

Diagnosis

The exact estimation of the extent of the process and details of the type of lesion are obtained from the conventional x-rays and with the aid of special neuroradiologic investigations (Table 2). Computerized tomography has, in the last 2 years, found an important role in the

Table 1. Space-occupying lesions of the skull base (No. of patients)

Anterior cranial fossa	1 Carcinoma of ethmoid cells and frontal sinus (left)
Middle and posterior cranial fossa	1 Aneurysm of internal carotid artery
	3 Neurinomas of jugular foramen
	1 Neurofibromatosis v. Recklinghausen
	6

Table 2. Neuroradiologic methods of examination

1. Tomography
2. Vasography
   Carotid artery
   Vertebral artery
   Jugular vein
3. Computerized tomography
4. Contrast radiograph of basal cisterns

diagnosis of tumors of the base of the skull. Because of the bone covering, negative findings may not definitely mean that an intracranial tumor can be excluded. In such cases, the positive and negative contrast medium examination of the intracranial CSF pathways must not be omitted.

Indications for Operation

The indication for operating on malignant lesions is given only when a radical extirpation of the growth is possible. Moreover, the relationship between prognosis of the illness on the one hand and the postoperative quality of life for the patient on the other hand must be weighed one against the other. However, even with extensive benign tumors, through the combined work of the otolaryngologist and neurosurgeon, reorganizational advancements regarding the maintenance of function or functional reconstruction of sense organs and cranial nerves can be achieved. With this policy, one would, for example, in neurinomas, which, although they grow very slowly, are increasingly destructive, be able to decide on a date for operation while the clinical symptoms are still discrete. It must be made clear to the patient that further cranial nerve loss and destruction due to the tumor can only be avoided, if at all possible, by early surgical intervention.

Operative Procedure

The basic principles for the combined approach to the base of the skull anteriorly has been described by BOENNINGHAUS (2), DEROME (8), GUGGENHEIM and KLEITSCH (13), KETCHAM (15-17), KREKORIAN and KEMPE (18), LITTLEWOOD and MAISELS (19), ZEHM (23) and other authors.

Case 1

The patient was a 55-year-old female with an extensive, predominantly left-sided ethmoid and frontal sinus carcinoma spreading to the anterior cranial fossa. The extent of the tumor in the area of the left anterior fossa was ascertained by means of computerized tomography. The tumor was totally removed in one stage by a combined intracranial-transfacial approach. After a bifrontal craniotomy, the tumor adhered to the dura but did not perforate it. A wide excision of the dura from the anterior cranial fossa to the wing of the sphenoid bone and the planum sphenoidale was made. Resection of the cranial border of the tumor and the entire base of the skull, including the lamina cribrosa on the left intracranially, was undertaken. After this, transfacial resection of the left upper facial skeleton, including orbital contents was performed. The skull vault and skull base were reconstructed with Palacos-R. The dural defect was sealed by a pedicle flap from the galea. The synthetic material was covered from behind by the skin of the upper lid. Normal recovery ensued. The patient was discharged 3 weeks postoperatively and later treated with a prosthesis.

A clearly defined description of the middle and posterior fossae of the skull has been given by ARENA (1), CONLEY, GRUNERT (12), FISCH (10), REHN (21), and ZEHM (23). DENECKE (5-7) gives, today as in the past, useful advice on operative techniques. WULLSTEIN and WULLSTEIN (22) have reported on the current position of surgery of ear tumors. Entry to the middle and posterior fossae of the skull follows after turning down a flap of the sternomastoid muscle from above and behind (Table 3, Fig. 1). It can be widened according to necessity by the temporary splitting of the mandible (21) with elevation of the accompanying part of the joint, by a tangential resection of the ascending ramus of the lower jaw, including the condyloid process, followed by removal of the styloid process and possibly of the tip of the mastoid, so that the internal carotid artery can be isolated with the necessary caution. In the case of lesions in the jugular foramen, the dissection and eventually the resection of the jugular bulb, after tying off the sigmoid sinus, either with double suturing or clipping, is necessary. By this means, it is possible to expose the IXth, Xth, and XIth cranial nerves clearly in the anterior compartment of the jugular foramen and therefore in extensive tumors to save them. Here are three examples:

Case 2

The patient was a 79-year-old female with increased difficulties in swallowing and breathing which developed within a few days. She was transfered to our clinic due to suspected right peritonsillar abscess. A pulsing protrusion in the area of the right wall of the pharynx was observed. The angiogram showed a large aneurysm of the internal carotid artery. The aneurysm was exposed by temporary resection of the lower jaw (Fig. 2). Owing to marked redundancy of the artery, it was possible, after removal of the aneurysm, to perform an end-to-end anastomosis.

Case 3

The patient was a 49-year-old male with swallowing disorders and indistinct speech resulting from a right-sided hypoglossal paresis and obvious protrusion of the tonsillar region. There was an extensive tumor in the infratemporal area with destruction of the pyramid of the petrous bone. The carotid angiogram showed considerable extracranial expansion of the tumor with forward displacement of the internal carotid artery. Pneumoencephalotomography showed an intracranial extension of the tumor in the right cerebellopontine angle with obstruction in the area of the cerebellopontine cistern. The entire tumor was exposed and removed exclusively from behind and without resection of parts of the skull base.

Table 3. Possibilities of improving the posterioinferior approach to the middle and posterior cranial fossa

1. Temporary splitting of mandible
2. Tangential resection of ascending ramus of mandible
3. Amputation of styloid process
4. Removal of mastoid tip
5. Resection of jugular bulb after ligature of sigmoid sinus

Case 4

The patient was a 15-year-old youth. The first symptom was hoarseness due to a right-sided vocal cord paralysis. Three years later, a left bone conduction hearing loss with tinnitus and paresis of the left marginal branch of the facial nerve were diagnosed. Radiologically, an extensive tumor from the jugular foramen extending widely into the petrous bone was observed. Computer tomography (Fig. 3.) showed the tumor extending to the cerebellopontine angle. A combined approach to the tumor was made from the mastoid to the neck. The tumor perforated the mastoid part of the exposed facial nerve. Total removal of the tumor was undertaken after ligature of the sigmoid sinus and extirpation of the jugular bulb, preserving the accessory and vagus nerves. Six days postoperatively, the facial nerve paralysis was completely recovered. Histologically, this was a neuroma.

The last two cases are, as isolated schwannomas in the area of the jugular foramen, especially rare. In the available literature, there are only five of these tumors described to date. In our experience, we can state, in conclusion, that through diagnosis and, when indicated, operative team work between the otolaryngologist and the neurosurgeon, using microsurgical operative techniques, significant advances regarding the maintenance and restoration of function are possible in the surgery of the base of the skull. From this point of view, endeavors must be made in this area in the case of slowly growing benign new growth to make an early diagnosis and perform the earliest possible operation, thus promoting the chances of preserving the remaining undamaged blood vessels and nerves.

Summary

Adequate tumor surgery on the base of the skull is difficult and hazardous due to the close connection with vital blood vessels and nerves. An account is given here of the experience which was gained in six rare cases, working in a combined ENT and neurosurgical team. In particular, the surgical approach to lesions of the anterior, middle, and posterior cranial fossa is discussed. Based on diagnostics and, when indicated, operative teamwork between the otolaryngologist and the neurosurgeon, using microsurgical operative techniques, significant advances regarding the maintenance and restoration of function are possible in the surgery of the base of the skull.

References

1. ARENA, S.: Tumour Surgery of the Temporal Bone. Laryngoscope 84, 645 (1974)

2. BOENNINGHAUS, H.-G.: Rhinochirurgische Aufgaben bei der Chirurgie des an die Schädelbasis angrenzenden Gesichtsschädels. Arch. Otorhinolaryngol. 207, 1-228 (Kongreßbericht 1974)

3. CHAMPY, COUSSIEU, P., DANY, A., DESPROGES-GOTTERON, R.: Neurome du trou déchiré postérieur. Rev. Laryngol. (Bordeaux) 85, 1034-1036 (1964)

4. COLUMELLA, NICOLA and DELZANO: zit. n. CHAMPY

5. DENECKE, H.J.: Die oto-rhino-laryngologische Operationen. In: Allgemeine und spezielle Operationslehre, Bd. V. Begr. v. M. KIRSCHNER. Berlin-Heidelberg-New York: Springer 1953

6. DENECKE, H.J.: Operationstechnische Probleme bei der Entfernung großer Neurinome im Bereich von Felsenbeinpyramide, N. facialis, Pharynx, Gefäßscheide, Ösophagusund und Zunge. HNO 8, 343 (1959/60)

7. DENECKE, H.J.: Diskussionsbemerkung Nobel Symposion 10, p. 294. Stockholm: Almquist & Wiksell 1969

8. DEROME, P.: Les tumeurs sphéno-ethmoidales. Neurochir. 18, Suppl. 1 (1972)

9. DRAF, W.: Schallempfindungsschwerhörigkeit beim Foramen jugulare-Neurinom. Vortrag 60. Versammlung der Vereinigung Südw. dtsch. HNO-Ärzte, Baden-Baden, 1976

10. FISCH, U.: Chirurgie im inneren Gehörgang und an benachbarten Strukturen. In: Kopf- und Halschirurgie, Bd. 3: Ohrregion. NAUMANN, H.H. (Hrsg.). Stuttgart: Georg Thieme 1976

11. GACEK, R.R.: Schwannoma of the jugular foramen. Ann. Otol. 85, 215-224 (1976)

12. GRUNERT, K.A.: Die operative Ausräumung des Bulbus venae jugularis (Bulbusoperation). Arch. Ohrenheilkd. 36, 71 (1894)

13. GUGGENHEIM, P., KLEITSCH, W.P.: Combined craniotomy-rhinotomy for ethmoid cancer. Ann. Otol. 76, 105 (1967)

14. KERN, E.: Chirurgische Behandlung maligner Weichteiltumoren. Dtsch. Ärztebl. 74, 1757 (1977)

15. KETCHAM, A.S., HAMMOND, W.G., CHRETIEN, P., VAN BUREN, J.M.: Treatment of advanced cancer of the ehtmoid sinuses. Nobel Symposium 10, p. 327. Stockholm: Almquist & Wiksel 1969

16. KETCHAM, A.S., HOYE, R.C., VAN BUREN, J.M., JOHNSON, R.H., SMITH, R.R.: Complications of intra-cranial facial resection for tumours of the paranasal sinuses. Am. J. Surg. 112, 591 (1966)

17. KETCHAM, A.S., WILKINS, R.H., VAN BUREN, J.M., SMITH, R.R.: A combined intracranial facial approach to the paranasal sinuses. Am. J. Surg. 106, 699 (1963)

18. KREKORIAN, E.A., KEMPE, L.G.: The combined otolaryngology-neurosurgery approach to extensive benign tumors. Laryngoscope 79, 2086 (1969)

19. LITTLEWOOD, M., MAISELS, D.: Reconstructive surgery in the intracranial approach to facial malignant disease. Proc. Soc. Med. 63, 681 (1970)

20. MIEHLKE, A.: Diskussionsbemerkung zu DRAF. 48. Jahresvers. d. Dtsch. Ges. f. HNO-Heilkd., Kopf- u. Halschirurgie, Bad Reichenhall 1977. Arch. Otorhinolaryngol. 216 (2), 1977 (In press)

21. REHN, Ed.: Die Freilegung der A. carotis interna in ihrem oberen Halsteil. Zentralbl. Chir. 17 (1919)

22. WULLSTEIN, H.L., WULLSTEIN, S.R.: Chirurgie der Tumoren des Mittelohres. In: Kopf- und Halschirurgie, Bd. 3: Ohrregion. NAUMANN, H.H. (Hrsg.). Stuttgart: Georg Thieme 1976

23. ZEHM, S.: The surgical approach to the external part of the base of the skull related to the anterior and middle cranial fossa. Nobel Symposium 10, p. 321. Stockholm: Almquist & Wiksell 1969

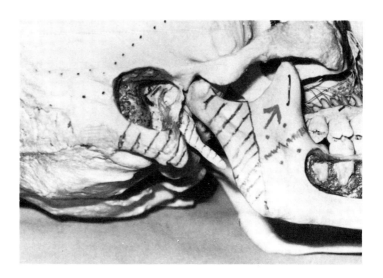

Fig. 1. Possibilities of improving the posteroinferior approach to the middle and posterior cranial fossa, demonstrated on skull specimen. *Hatched area*: the possibilities of bone removal. The arrow shows the direction of retraction of the proximal part of the mandible after temporary splitting

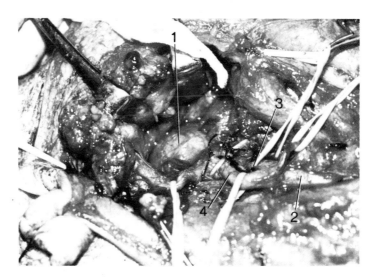

Fig. 2. Case 2: exposure of a large internal carotid artery aneurysm after temporary splitting of the mandible and removal of the styloid process (*1* aneurysm; *2* common carotid artery; *3* internal carotid artery; *4* external carotid artery)

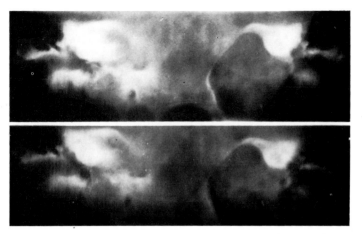

Fig. 3. Case 4: tomography of petrous bones (anteroposterior). Extensive destruction (*sharp margins*) of left pyramid and jugular foramen as far as the internal auditory meatus

Increase in Intracranial Pressure

Elucidation and Histologic Technique: An Aid in Determining Pathologic Changes in Bones as Exemplified by Hydrocephalus in the C57 Black Murine Strain

M. HOLZGRAEFE and O. SPOERRI

Introduction

Within the C57 black murine strain, a repeated appearance of hydrocephalus was observed during genetic experimentation (6). This strain belongs to 1 of the 14 known murine strains which have congenital hydrocephalus (1). It has been proposed (5) that the cause of hydrocephalus is a premature ossification of the skull base. Within the mouse family "ch," it has been proved (3, 4) that ossification of the base of the skull during embryonic development caused the formation of hydrocephalus. This observation contrasts sharply to the case of the C57 variety. Within the framework of a more extensive project, we would like to clarify to what degree a disorder in the development of the skull can be considered to be the cause of hydrocephalus in the C57 black murine strain. In addition to the radiologic technique, the histologic and elucidation technique proved especially useful in the hydrocephalic skull.

Materials and Methods

1. Elucidation

In this study, a modified elucidation technique was chosen (2). Following evisceration, the heads of the mice are placed in pure alcohol for 24 h, for the same length of time in pure acetone, and then dried for 48 h under normal atmospheric conditions. This causes shrinking of the tissues. The specimens are then placed in a 1% potassium hydroxide solution until a satisfactory elucidation of the bone and cartilaginous parts of the skull have taken place. At this point, the skull is dyed with 1% alizarin red 5 solution and then placed in a mixture of 1% potassium hydroxide and glycerin (1:1). The soft tissues hereby, loose their color making it possible to observe the red-colored bones through the transparent soft parts. The specimens are stored in a mixture of 1% potassium hydroxide and glycerin (1:5).

Twelve mouse skulls were studied. A series of nonhydrocephalic skulls from 1 to 100-day-old animals were observed, and the results were compared to those obtained from the observation of hydrocephalic animals.

2. Histology

Twenty-five animals were anesthetized with ether and perfused with 10% formalin. Following decalcification of the bone, the heads were embedded in paraffin. Ten micron serial sections were cut and stained using azan, gallocyanin, and hematoxylin and eosin techniques.

Results

1. *Elucidation*

a) *The Nonhydrocephalic Skull*

The individual parts of the cranium and the base of the skull are already recognizable at the age of 1 day. An ossified connection of the individual bone elements of the skull does not yet exist. In this phase of development, these elements are largest in the region of the os occipitale and the os interparietale. In the frontal and nasal regions, they are least developed. The skull of a 5-day-old mouse displays the same conditions, with the exception of a general increase in the size of the skull. In the 10-day-old mouse, the desmal ossification of the cranial vault has progressed and the individual skull bones have moved almost completely together, separated only by a narrow gap. In comparison, the skull of a 5-day-old mouse is relatively smaller. In the skull of a 20-day-old mouse, these sutures appear closed to the naked eye. Between the 20th and 60th day, the only change in the skull observed is an increase in volumen. In the period between the 60th and 200th day, no change in form or volume of the skull of a normal mouse is to be found.

b) *The Hydrocephalic Skull*

The 30-day-old mouse (C57 black) with extreme hydrocephalus, the youngest hydrocephalic animal in this series, displays a clearly visible deformation of the cranial vault when compared to an equally old nonhydrocephalic specimen. The cranial vault is especially protruding in the region of the os interparietale and the ossa parietalia. The fissure between the ossa parietalia and the fissure between the os interparietale and the ossa parietalia are 3-4 mm dehiscent. The sutura occipitalis-interparietalis, the sutura occipitalis-parietalis, and the sutura parietalis-frontalis are in comparison split very slightly apart. The remaining fissures, as far as can be ascertained through the elucidation technique, are not affected by the intracranial, hydrocephalic rise in pressure (Figs. 1 and 2).

2. *Histology*

a) *Normal Base of Skull*

There are two synchondroses of the base of the skull in which the longitudinal growth of the head takes place, in the synchondrosis occipito basissphenoidalis and the synchondrosis basissphenoidalis-parasphenoidalis (Fig. 3). The longitudinal growth of the skull is completed at age 40-60 days. Later, only thickening of the bone takes place due to appositional formation of bone.

b) *Normal Cranial Suture*

The following cranial sutures were studied histologically: sutura interparietalis-parietalis, interparietalis. At gross examination, these sutures have a dentate appearance which gives them the technical term sutura serrata. The os occipitale and os parietale, however, are connected through a sutura squamosa. All cranial sutures show the same morphologic substrate; firmly anchored to the bone, there is a dense mass of short connective tissue structures connecting opposite bones.

Due to osteoblastic activity, this syndesmosis gradually narrows and finally is converted into the synostosis. The sutures of the base of the skull are built differently. They close earlier than the sutures of the vault. Continued increased intracranial pressure induces loosening of these sutures. This could be observed even in old hydrocephalic animals. Predehiscence of the basal sutures could be seen in no case.

c) The Base of the Skull of the Hydrocephalic Mouse

The base of the skull of the 20-, 40-, 60-, and 120-day-old hydrocephalic mouse was examined. Apart from all other elements of cartilage, the synchondrosis of the 20-day-old hydrocephalic mouse contains young cartilaginous cells still capable of cell division. In the 40- and 60-day-old hydrocephalic animal, these young cells are found less frequently. In the 120-day-old hydrocephalic mouse, the synchondrosis contains less young cartilaginous cells.

d) Cranial Sutures in the Hydrocephalic Mouse

The described cranial suture consists of stretched connective tissue connecting two opposite bones. This connective tissue is formed by dermal wrapping of the diploe, i.e., the periosteum and endosteum. The periosteal contribution to the connective tissue of the suture is higher than the endosteal.

Discussion

With the aid of the elucidation and histologic techniques, this study has attempted to clarify whether within the C57 black murine strain a disorder similar to that previously described in the "ch" murine strain (2, 3) would appear in the development of the skull. In contrast to the "ch" variety (2, 3), the C57 black strain developed hydrocephalus only in the 4th-6th week. The elucidation technique made it possible to identify all parts of the skull. The growth of the skull base is normal even in the hydrocephalic specimen. A physiologic separation of the cranial fissures is present up to the age of 20 days. The closing of the sutures depends on the growth of the underlying brain. Since the development of the parieto-occipital brain is completed later, the parieto-occipital area is delayed with respect to the sutures when compared to the frontal parts of the skull. In the hydrocephalic animal, the influence of a rise in the intracranial pressure is, therfore, especially apparent in the os interparietale and the regions of the ossa parietalia. The earlier the hydrocephalus develops, the more the cranial vault tends to assume a spheric shape due to persisting rise in pressure.

The pathologic alterations in the skull as described are secondary. They are thought to be due to abnormal increase of the surface of the brain. The cause of hydrocephalus in the C57 black murine strain remains unclear.

Summary

An elucidation technique is described which permits identification of all parts of the mouse skull. Both bone and cartilage can be easily observed. The hydrocephalic C57 black murine strain showed a deformation of the cranial vault at the region of the os interparietale and the ossa parietalia. The fissures between the bones were dehiscent by 3-4 mm. The remaining fissures were not influenced by the intracranial hydrocephalic rise in pressure. The synchondroses of the base of the skull in which longitudinal growth is taking place are not affected by hydrocephalus. The normal as well as the dehiscent sutures of the vault are endosteal and periosteal structures. Ossification of dehiscent sutures does not seem to take place.

References

1. BUDWEG, A.: Klinische Beobachtungen und histologische Untersuchungen des Ventrikelsystems an einer hydrocephalen Linie des Mausstammes C 57 Bl. Dissertation, Georg-August-University of Göttingen, Göttingen 1972
2. FALLER, E.: Die Entwicklung der makroskopischen anatomischen Präparierkunst von Galen bis zur Neuzeit. Acta Anat. 4, 88-89 (1947/48)
3. GRÜNEBERG, H.: Congenital hydrocephalus in the mouse, a case of spurious pleiotropism. J. Genet. 45, 1-21 (1942a)
4. GRÜNEBERG, H.: The new mutant genes in the house mouse. J. Genet. 45, 22-29 (1943b)
5. TARASZEWSKA, A., ZALESKA, Z.: Congenital hydrocephalus in mice of strains BN and C 57 Bl. Pol. Med. J. 9, 187-195 (1970)
6. THEILER, K.: Personal communication, 1971

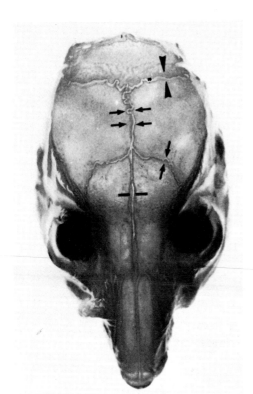

Fig. 1. Mouse C57B1, normal; elucidation of the skull and staining of the bones with alizarin red S. Note that the sutures of the cranial vault are closed (x 4)

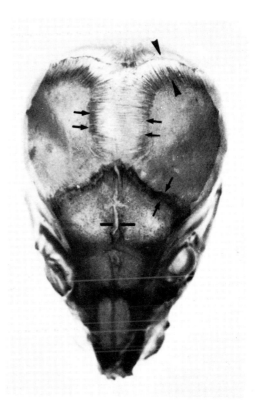

Fig. 2. Mouse C57B1, hydrocephalic; elucidation of the skull and staining of the bones with alizarin red S. Note extreme enlargement of the sutura parieto-parietalis (⇉ ⇇) and of the sutura parietalis-interparietalis (▶ ◀). There is only minimal dehiscence between sutura parietalis-frontalis (→ ←) and sutura interfrontalis (— —) (x 4)

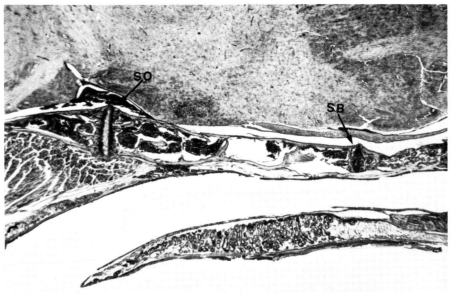

Fig. 3. Mouse C57B1, normal; sagittal section of base of skull. Synchondroses occipitalis-sphenoidalis (SO) and basissphenoidalis-praesphenoidalis (SB) (gallocyanin stain; x 18)

Comparison of the Effects of Osmotherapeutic Agents, Hyperventilation, and Tromethamine (THAM) on Brain Pressure and Electric Activity of the Brain in Experimental and Clinical Brain Edema

O. E. Knoblich, M. Gaab, U. Fuhrmeister, F. Herrmann, K. Dietrich, and P. Gruss

Introduction

In the presence of brain edema, intracranial pressure (ICP) is raised by the space-occupying swelling of the brain (14), whereas cerebral perfusion pressure is reduced and the pH of the brain tissue falls (3). There is, consequently, a disturbance of autoregulation. In patients with severe craniocerebral injuries, in addition to agents used to lower brain pressure osmotically, buffers acting on acidosis and hyperventilation (HV) were tested. For comparison, 11 cats were observed under the same treatment after cryogenic brain edema.

Materials and Methods

In 30 patients, epidural pressure (EP) on the operated side was measured continuously (12) and the EEG continuously recorded with bilateral bipolar fronto-occipital silver electrodes. The power intensity was calculated by means of a computer (Intertechnique Plurimat S, FFT) in δ- (1-3.5 Hz), ϑ- (4-7.5 Hz), α- (8-13.5 Hz), and total frequency range (1-25 Hz). Through multiplication factors, the same sign scale was obtained for the power (arbitrary units) of all frequency ranges. For comparison, we induced a standardized cryogenic trauma to the brain (with acetone-dry cooled copper stamp of 2 cm diameter, cooling time 5 min at -75°C (14)) following right parietal trepanation in 35 anesthetized ($N_2O:O_2$, 3:1) cats under controlled artifical respiration. The bone defect was subsequently closed with a Palacos graft. Epidural pressure (7) was measured over both hemispheres (rEP; lEP). CSF pressure of the left lateral ventricle (VP) was recorded by means of a catheter. In addition, 80 rats were decapitated following a right-sided cryogenic trauma to the brain and the water content of the brain determined in separate hemispheres (as loss of weight after freeze-drying until constant weight). Of these, 24 animals were treated with THAM.

Results

1. Investigations in Craniocerebral Trauma

a) Brain Pressure and EEG Before Treatment

All brain pressures rose rapidly after experimental trauma. Peak pressure and steepness of rise vary from animal to animal. The EEG power immediately decreases post-traumatically.

b) Mannitol[1], Sorbitol[2] (Four Animals, Fig. 1a and b)

Osmotherapy with 20% mannitol or 40% sorbitol rapidly lowers ICP, more markedly if the higher osmolality sorbitol is used. The EEG power improves toward the end of the therapy but only over the nontraumatized left hemisphere.

---

1 1310 mosmol/kg, 50 ml.
2 3200 mosmol/kg, 40 ml.

c) Hyperventilation (Four Animals, Fig. 2a and b)

If HV is performed early after trauma, brain pressure decreases rapidly. The EEG power increases moderately at the beginning of therapy (↓ Fig. 2a). If HV is begun after a massive rise in brain pressure (VP 50 mm Hg) (↓ Fig. 2b), there is only a slight fall of ICP. The EEG power is improved by HV only over the left noninjured hemisphere.

d) THAM Treatment (Three Cats, Fig. 3a; 90 Rats, Fig. 3b)

There is a very steep fall of all brain pressures upon i.v. infusion of 5-7 mmol/kg THAM. The pressure difference between rEP and lEP is thereby abolished. THAM leads to an increase in the EEG power on both sides (↓ Fig. 3a), especially in the α-band. The rats treated with THAM show a lower water content in both hemispheres than control animals (Fig. 3b) in the left hemisphere even after 24 h.

2. Clinical Investigations

a) Mannisorb[3] (Nine Patients, Fig. 4: Patients 1 and 2)

When mannisorb (100-200 ml, 3000 mmol/kg) is infused i.v. in the presence of postoperatively raised ICP, there is a reduction in brain pressure. Serum osmolality increases by 20 mosmol/kg while blood pressure (aP) increases. In both patients, EEG power of the left operated side was lower than over the opposite hemisphere. There is a slight increase in intensity (more pronounced on the right side) only toward the end of the osmotherapy (Fig. 4: patient 1). With further rise in ICP, 1 h after therapy, the power deteriorated, especially over the left (operated) hemisphere. Occasionally, there is a decrease in EEG intensitiv during therapy (Fig. 4: patient 2) which is more pronounced over the damaged side.

b) THAM Treatment (Four Patients, Fig. 5: Patients 3 and 4)

When THAM (4-5 mmol/kg) is infused i.v., brain pressure falls rapidly. Even after 1 h, ICP is still lower than its initial value (Fig. 5: patient 3). In some cases, brain pressure remains low for hours (Fig. 5: patient 4). Arterial pressure is stable. EEG power increases markedly only after the end of THAM administration. In patient 3 (Fig. 5), power improved practically only on the right (nonoperated) side. In patient 4 (Fig. 5), there is an impressive bilateral increase in the α-power.

Discussion

The frequency of post-traumatic brain edema varies between 20% and 80% according to earlier studies (10, 13, 15). A development within the first 24 h is stated to be rare (10, 12, 15). Even in our standardized cryogenic brain edema, a rise in ICP is not observed in all cases. Furthermore, the peak pressure reached varies from animal to animal. Since various pathologic processes are acting, the development of brain edema does not follow rigid rules (11, 15). A rise in ICP is observed in only 13 of 30 patients (ca. 50%) investigated after severe craniocerebral injury. A latency is rare. Since patients with severe craniocerebral injuries are endangered by an elevation of intracranial pressure, this must be constantly checked. A reduction of ICP as well as a therapeutic effect can be seen and related to the EEG computer evaluation (6, 8).

---

3 Mannitol 15%, sorbitol 30%.

The osmotic effect of 20% mannitol, as compared to 40% sorbitol, is moderate. Only at a serum osmolality difference of more than 20 mmol/kg is a lowering of ICP to be expected (14). Because of the disturbed blood-brain barrier, lowering of ICP over the injured hemisphere is less marked. The EEG improvement limited to the left side and appearing only toward the end of therapy, the pronounced fall in brain pressure, and the increase in systemic pressure point to a hemodynamic cause for the effect on EEG (21).

At an osmolality similar to that of 40% sorbitol, mannisorb leads to a fall in brain pressure. The effect on the EEG is more pronounced on the nonoperated side in consequence of the improvement in circulation. Because of the disturbed blood-brain barrier (rebound effect (16)), a deterioration in bioelectric activity can occur.

HV leads to a lowering in ICP by vasoconstriction (20). A prerequisite is that autoregulation is preserved (2, 4). Since autoregulation is disturbed in the presence of brain edema (15), ICP is reduced only slightly. Thus, improvement of the EEG is dependent on lactate buffering and on ganglion cell activation.

THAM leads to an immediate buffering of fixing acids (17, 19). The acidosis arising in the vessel wall is thereby improved. The responsiveness of the catecholamine-sensitive vascular receptors is stated to be restored (1). This effect can be detected even in the presence of pronounced vasoparalysis. In the cryogenic lesion experiments, rEP is particularly lowered over the damaged hemisphere. Due to THAM distribution in tissue fluid (17, 19) and to its reduced concentration in the vessel wall, its effect on ICP lasts only a short time. EEG recovery lasts much longer. A buffering of the acidotic glial metabolism should be assumed (9). The good improvement in the α-region is probably explained by an adrenergic activation of ganglion cells independent of perfusion pressure.

Treatment of brain edema should not be restricted to application of a single drug. The objective must be to lower ICP and to improve tissue acidosis. Osmotherapeutic agents remove fluid from nonedematous brain tissue and decrease brain pressure. However, the metabolic disorder and the vasoparalysis are not directly influenced. When inducing HV arterial pCO_2 should be lowered at 20-25 mm Hg. Forced HV leads to further tissue hypoxia (5) through vasoconstriction. THAM markedly can improve disturbed autoregulation. The effect on brain pressure is pronounced. The improvement in glial metabolism and the marked activation of ganglion cells persists for a long time. It therefore appears reasonable to use THAM in addition to other measures.

Summary

Treatment of brain edema should lower intracranial pressure and improve the acidotic tissue metabolism. Epidural pressure was measured in patients with craniocerebral trauma. EEG was recorded at constant intervals and evaluated with the aid of a computer (FFT). The effects of osmotherapy, hyperventilation, and THAM were appraised. For comparison, 11 cats were also examined under the same treatment after a standardized cryogenic injury to the brain. In addition, water content in the brain was assessed in 24 rats following cryogenic injury and THAM treatment. Osmotherapy lowers ICP but improves the EEG only for a short time. HV leads to a lowering of intracranial pressure only in areas with intact cerebrovascular regulation. THAM reduces the uptake of water by the brain and improves vasoparalysis directly. Lowering of ICP is usually short-lasting, whereas the recovery of bioelectric activity persists for a long time.

References

1. AKIOKA, T., OTA, K., MATSUMOTO, A., IWATSUKI, K., DOI, A., OKAO, S., NINOMIYA, K., NISHIMOTO, A.: The effect of THAM on Acute Intracranial Hypertension. An Experimental and Clinical Study. In: Intracranial Pressure III. BEKS, J. et al. (eds.), p. 219. Berlin-Heidelberg-New York: Springer 1976
2. DECKER, D.P., VRIES, J.K., YOUNG, H.F., WARD, J.D.: Controlled Cerebral Perfusion Pressure and Ventilation in Human Mechanical Brain Injury: Prevention of Progressive Brain Swelling. In: Intracranial Pressure II. LUNDBERG, N. et al. (eds.). Berlin-Heidelberg-New York: Springer 1975
3. BRUCE, D.A., VAPALATHI, M., SCHUTZ, H., LANGFITT, T.W.: RCBF, $CMBRO_2$ and Intracranial Pressure Following a Local Cold Injury of the Cortex. In: Intracranial Pressure. BROCK, M. et al. (eds.), p. 85. Berlin-Heidelberg-New York: Springer 1972
4. CHRISTENSEN, M.St., PAULSON, O.B., OLESEN, J., ALEXANDER, S.C., SHINHØJ, E., DAM, W.H., LASSEN, N.A.: Cerebral Apoplexy (Stroke) Treated With or Without Prolonged Artificial Hyperventilation: 1. Cerebral Circulation, Clinical Course and Cause of Death. Stroke $\underline{4}$, 568-619 (1973)
5. CZERNICKI, Z., JURKIEWICZ, J., KUNICKI, A.: The Effect of Hypocapnia on Normal and Increased Intracranial Pressure in Cats and Rabbits. In: Intracranial Pressure II. LUNDBERG, N. et al. (eds), p. 471. Berlin-Heidelberg-New York: Springer 1975
6. DE ROUGEMENT, J., BURGE, M., BENBID, A.L.: L'enregistrement de la pression intracrânienne dans la surveillance des traumatismes crâniens en période aigue. Observations sur nor prémiers résultats. Neurochir. $\underline{19}$, 125-134 (1973)
7. DIETRICH, K., GAAB, M., KNOBLICH, O.E., SCHUPP, J., OTT, B.: A New Miniaturized System for Monitoring the Epidural Pressure in Children and Adults. Neuropädiatrie $\underline{8}$, 21-28 (1976)
8. DOLCE, G., KÜNKEL, H.: CEAN. Computerized EEG Analysis. Stuttgart: Fischer 1975
9. EWERBECK, H., HAGER, J., WELTE, W.: Tris-Pufferbehandlung schwerer Verbrennungen bei Kindern zur Vermeidung von Hirndauerschäden. Dtsch. Med. Wochenschr. $\underline{91}$, 1333-1338 (1966)
10. FIESCHI, C., BEDUSCHI, A., AGNOLI, A.: Regional Cerebral Blood Flow and Intraventricular Pressure in Acute Brain Injury. Eur. Neurol. $\underline{8}$, 192-199 (1972)
11. FLEISCHER, A.S., PAYNE, N., TINDALL, G.: Continous Monitoring of Intracranial Pressure in Severe Closed Head Injury without Mass Lesions. Surg. Neurol. $\underline{6}$, 31-34 (1976)
12. GAAB, M., KNOBLICH, O.E., DIETRICH, K., GRUSS, P.: Miniaturized Methods of Monitoring Intracranial Pressure in Craniocerebral Trauma Before and After Operation. This volume, pp. 5-11
13. GRUSS, P., JESCHKE, R.: Besonderheiten beim Epiduralhämatom im Säuglings- und Kleinkindesalter. Klin. Pädiatr. $\underline{187}$, 281-284 (1975)

14. KNOBLICH, O.E., SCHUPP, J., DIETRICH, K., FUHRMEISTER, U., GRUSS, P.: Wirkung unterschiedlicher Osmo- und Onkotherapie auf Hirndruck und elektrische Hirnaktivität beim experimentellen Hirnödem. (Be published)

15. GOBIET, W.: Monitoring of Intracranial Pressure in Patients with Severe Head Injury. Neurochirurgia $\underline{20}$, 35-47 (1977)

16. GUISADO, R., ARIEFE, A.J., TOURTELLOTTE, W.W., MASSRY, S.O.: Efficacy of Glycerol in the Treatment of Cerebral Edema. Neurology $\underline{24}$, 390 (1974)

17. HENSCHLER, D.: Trispuffer (THAM) als Therapeutikum. Dtsch. Med. Wochenschr. $\underline{88}$, 1328-1331 (1963)

18. HESS, O.: Tierexperimentelle Untersuchungen zur Therapie des Hirnödems. Drug. Res. $\underline{17}$, 931-934 (1967)

19. NAHAS, G.G.: The Clinical Pharmacology of THAM. Clin. Pharmacol. Ther. $\underline{4}$, 784-803 (1963)

20. PAULSON, O.B., OLESEN, J., CHRISTENSEN, M.St.: Restoration of Autoregulation of Cerebral Blood Flow by Hypocapnia. Neurology $\underline{22}$, 286-293 (1972)

21. SCHMITT, K., SCHMALZ, H.: Zur Blutvolumenänderung nach Osmo-Onkotherapie. Anästhesist $\underline{16}$, 201-204 (1967)

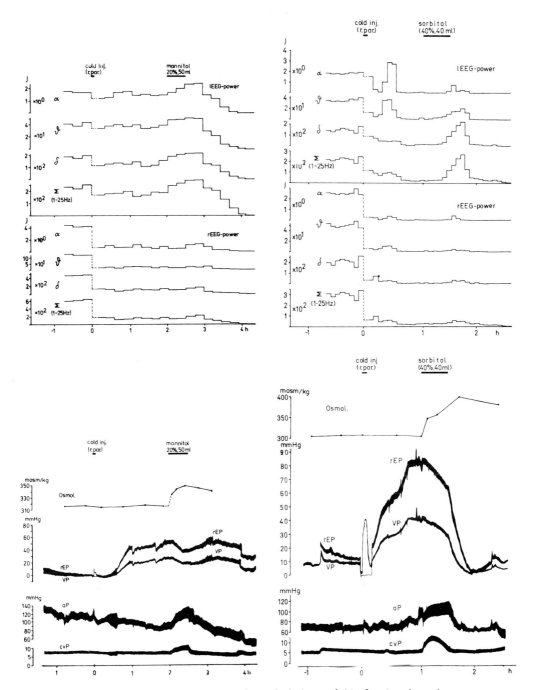

Fig. 1. Infusion of 20% mannitol and 40% sorbitol. A rise in serum osmolality leads to a fall in brain pressures (particularly 40% sorbitol). EEG improvement (above all in the lower frequencies) occurs almost only over the left (undamaged) hemisphere. Despite high osmolality, ICP increases again

cold inj.: cold injury; *r.par.*: right parietal; *VP*: ventricular pressure; *rEP*: right epidural pressure; *aP*: arterial blood pressure; *cvP*: central venous pressure; *osmol*: serum osmolality; *I*: EEG power intensity

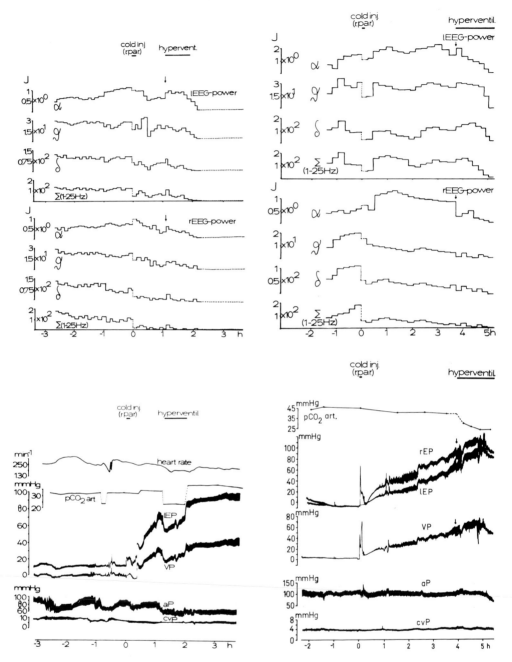

Fig. 2. Hyperventilation 1 h and 4 h following cryogenic injury to the brain: 4 h after injury only slight lowering of brain pressure ( ). Hyperventilation (↓) improves EEG for only a short time over the left hemisphere, especially in the lower frequency regions. With falling perfusion pressure (aP - VP < 50 mm Hg), zero line on both sides lEP: left epidural pressure; other symbols as in Figure 1

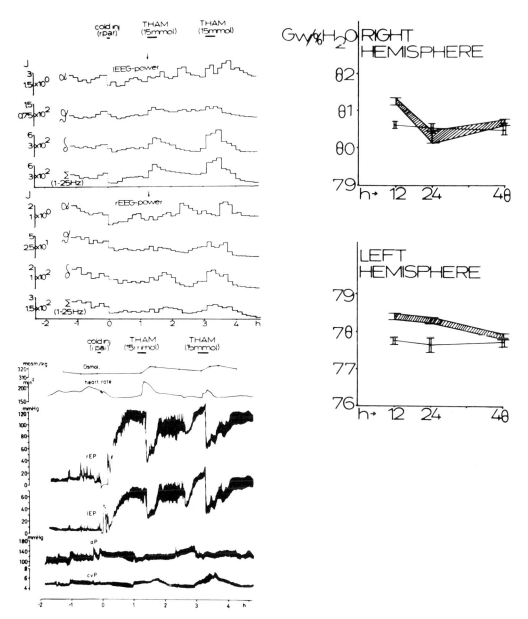

Fig. 3. Infusion of THAM in cats. Brain water content in rats after cryogenic injury to the brain (copper stamp 4 mm diameter, cooling time 4 min at -73°C, closed skull) and treatment with THAM. At the beginning of infusion there is an immediate fall in brain pressure, whereas ICP rises again even during therapy. Improvement of the EEG, especially in the α-region. Rats treated with THAM (1 h after injury, 7 mmol/kg, 30 min i.v.): II————x and 26 x̄ (12 h after cryogenic injury to the brain 14, after 24 h 10, after 48 h 10 animals). Control animals I———— and grey x̄ + 26 x̄ (12 h after cryogenic injury to the brain 14, after 24 h 14, after 48 h 18 animals) and 10 animals without cryogenic injury to the brain and without therapy (right hemisphere 77.15 ± 0.46; (26), left hemisphere 77.65 ± 0.50; (26) GW/% H_2O). Symbols as in Figures 1 and 2

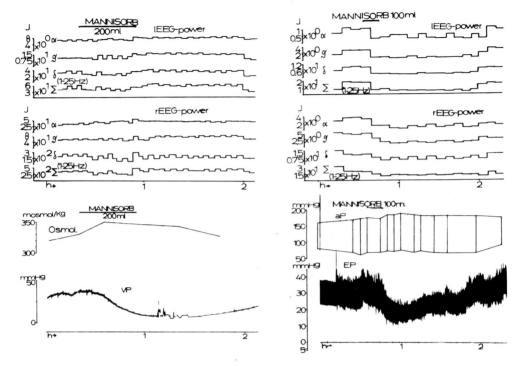

Fig. 4. Clinical treatment with mannisorb (15% mannitol, 30% sorbitol). Marked reduction of brain pressure with rise of serum osmolality. Rise if ICP again after 30 min. Slight increase in EEG power on both sides. In patient 2, decrease of the EEG intensity despite pronounced lowering of brain pressure
EP: epidural pressure over the left side operated in each case;
aP: determined by auscultation. Symbols as in Figures 1 and 2

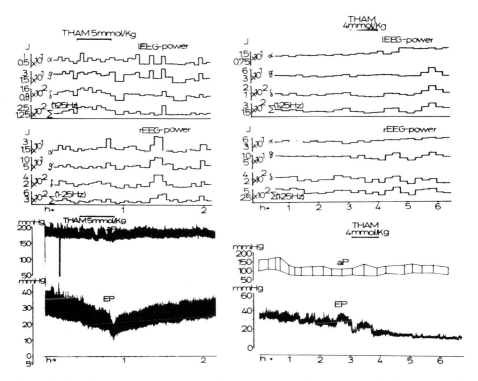

Fig. 5. Clinical investigation under THAM. Patients 3 and 4 were both operated on the left side. THAM reduces ICP quickly and markedly, the effect persisting for a long time in patient 4. Increase in EEG power more pronounced on the right side. Marked bilateral increase in the α-band in patient 4. aP determined by auscultation in patient 4. Symbols as in Figures 1 and 2

Chronomorphology of Brain Death

R. Schröder

Morphologic analysis of the brain death syndrome is associated with considerable difficulties, documented in the literature by the different interpretations of the findings. The cause is that, after death of the whole organism, lesions can be found in the brain which originate in different phases of the disease. They should be classified into:
1) primary lesions, which are the cause of the consecutive, irreversible and lethal brain edema, 2) lesions which arise during the phase of increase of intracranial pressure to the level of systemic blood pressure, and 3) late changes developing during complete ischemia of the brain. This overlapping of several lesions results in unsolved problems because the identifiable anoxic injuries can be attributed to all phases of the disease. Only the analysis of a sufficiently large number of cases under chronologic points of view, i.e., the morphologic evaluation of the findings in their particular relation to the duration of the clinical syndrome of dissociated brain death, may be of help. In this way, only the relationship of the histologic changes to complete brain ischemia is recognizable.

This study is based on 100 cases of brain death (duration from 2 h to 6 days following the onset of total failure of the cerebral functions). The diagnosis included apnea and isoelectric EEG, with occasionally preserved spinal reactions. In part of the cases, cerebral ischemia was directly proved by angiography.

It becomes apparent that, despite total ischemic infarction of the brain, a necrosis does not develop. We shall restrict ourselves to the study of the most sensitive cells, the neurons. Figure 1 shows a giant cell of Betz after a 3-day brain death syndrome. The nucleus reveals the usual bubble-like picture with a large, intensively colored nucleolus and preserved Nissl substance. This can be seen very often. In contrast to this, in the presence of *local* infarction, neuronal necrosis appears after only 5 h (own unpublished results) with hyperchromatic structureless nucleus and homogen eosinophilic cytoplasm without Nissl substance. Here, a fundamental difference exists between the complete ischemic situation of brain death on the one hand and the focal infarction on the other, where, at least in the marginal zone, circulation is intact. Evidently the cause of this is the necessity of preserved circulation and diffusion for the development of the necrosis, which is not the case in complete ischemia. Therefore, this condition equals the postmortal one, in which the cellular picture is likewise preserved for a long time, although cell death had occurred long ago.

That the cells are really dead in total cerebral infarction is proved by very rare cases in which, despite massive increase of intracranial pressure, there is a temporary recirculation. Two such cases have been reported by FUCHS and SCHNEIDER (1). In our material, we also have one observation. The dead tissue is infiltrated by granulocytes from the brain surface in the manner of a symptomatic meningeocephalitis, which resembles the inflammatory reaction of focal lesions. Another proof of the death of the whole brain tissue are the know demarcations in the border zones of intracranial circulation in the fasciculus opticus and the spinal cord. In these areas, a very early decrease in coloration of the myelin can be seen, the limit of which lies in the optic foramen nerve (Fig. 2), in the upper cervical segments C1-3. This is a time-related intravital reaction (Table 1). In the optic nerve, the demarcation is seen regularly 8 h following loss of the last cerebral function. This can also be seen in the spinal cord. However, here the beginning of such changes seems to be more irregular. Some cases exhibit the demarcation in the optic nerve but not in the cervical cord. This indicates temporal differences in onset of circulatory stop between supra- and infratentorial space, as known from clinical observations. Further studies are necessary in order to determine the maximal possible time difference.

Total ischemic infarction of the brain, as found in cases with brain death syndrome, is not characterized by the development of necrosis, in contrast to the occasionally accepted opinion (2, for instance). On the contrary, complete ischemia prevents its appearance. Therefore, the anoxic lesions frequently seen in these cases must originate prior to the cerebral circulatory arrest.

Table 1. Demarcation as shown by decreased myelin coloration (+) in relation to the duration of the brain death syndrome: comparison between optic nerve and upper spinal cord

Cases	Duration (hours)	Optic nerve	Cervical nerve
210/77	3	-	-
300/75	5	-	-
517/74	8	+	+
340/77	8	+	-
108/76	9	+	-
297/75	4-13	+	-
63/76	9-13	+	+
498/75	12	+	+
180/75	13	+	+
48/76	13	+	+
497/75	14	+	+
261/75	14	+	+

References

1. FUCHS, E.C., SCHNEIDER, H.: Terminal vascular lesions in the dying brain after recirculation. Proc. VIIth Int. Congr. Neuropath., Vol. II, pp. 561-564. Amsterdam: Excerta Medica 1975
2. INGVAR, D.H.: Brain death - total brain infarction. Acta Anaesthesiol. Scand., Suppl. 45, 129-140 (1971)

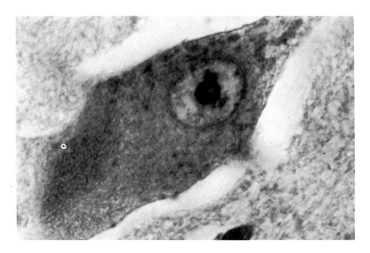

Fig. 1. Preserved structure of a Betz cell 3 days after total ischemic infarction of the brain (hematoxylin and eosin stain, x 1280)

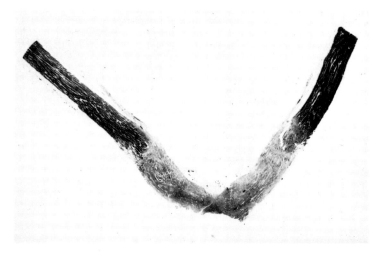

Fig. 2. Horizontal section through chiasma and optic nerves with demarcation as shown by decreased myelin coloration (Klüver-Barrera, x 2.6)

Intensive Therapy

Catheterization of the Superior Vena Cava With the ALPHA System
R. Nessler

During the past years, catheterization of the superior vena cava has become more and more important in emergency cases and long-term infusion therapy. On the basis of more than 3,000 caval catheterizations, the Alpha System (manufacturer: STERIMED GmbH, 6600 Saarbrücken, FRG) has been developed. The Alpha system represents the "indirect" technique of caval catheterization. That means that the cannula is inserted into the vein, e.g., innominate vein (Fig. 1), internal jugular vein (Fig. 2), subclavian vein, and the mandrin is removed. Then, an elastic plastic guide of high stability (Fig. 3) is inserted through the cannula with gentle rotational movements, the flexible tip first. Afterward, the cannula is removed along the guide. The catheter (Fig. 4) is then introduced into the vein along the plastic guide with gentle rotational movements.

The integrated plastic guide allows the use of catheters of optimum flexibility and high tissue tolerance. The "direct" catheter-through-cannula or catheter-through-needle technique mainly used up to now runs the risk of complications such as cutting and breaking off, knotting, and false positions of the catheter. False positions are caused by deficiency of guidance stability of the flexible catheter. A catheter cannot be flexible and gentle as well as stable in guidance at the same time.

The use of the Alpha system (indirect method) guarantees minimum risk at catheterization of the internal jugular, the innominate, and the subclavian veins.

The advantages are as follows:
1. Quick and safe catheterization. The duration of catheterization (very important in emergency cases) is shortened by the exact guidance of the catheter over the plastic guide. As compared with the "direct" method; nonexistence of false position of the catheter tip.
2. No risk of puncture-caused bleedings. The tapping hole is very small (puncture cannular with small lumen causing only slight puncture trauma).
3. The risk of the catheter being cut or damaged (the so-called catheter embolism) - as is possible in the case of a catheter-through-needle system - can be positively excluded. By leading the catheter along the plastic guide, damages by knotting or cutting off are avoided.
4. Due to the standard length of the catheter, cardiac embarrasment or even heart perforation through the intracardiac position of the catheter tip are avoided.
5. Recatheterization along the plastic guide is possible at any time without new puncture.

6. By use of the Alpha system, the tapping hole is completely occluded by the catheter; therefore, there is less risk of infection for the subcutaneous and the perivascular tissue. The small tapping hole of the puncture cannula and an adequate catheter diameter reduce the risk of infection and thrombosis.
7. High success rate of 95% at innominate vein puncture and 92% at internal jugular vein puncture.

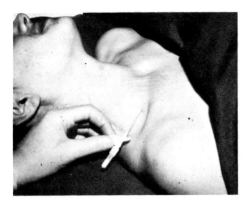

Fig. 1. Puncture site and direction of cannula for the puncture of the innominate vein

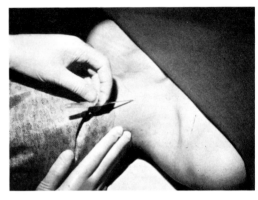

Fig. 2. Puncture site and direction of cannula for the internal jugular vein puncture

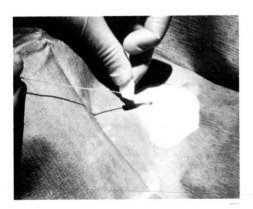

Fig. 3. Puncture cannula after removal of the guide. The plastic guide is introduced into the vein (internal jugular vein)

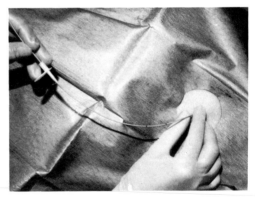

Fig. 4. The catheter is advanced into the internal jugular vein along the plastic guide

Vascular Surgery

Operative Treatment of Giant Basal Intracranial Aneurysms
W. WALTER and H. ALTENBURG

At the previous meeting of the German Neurosurgical Society in Berlin (1976), we reported on the problems associated with the operative treatment of large basal intra- and suprasellar aneurysms, reporting the diagnostic and therapeutic procedure we employ (1). In the meantime, we have acquired more experience with the treatment of these "giant" aneurysms which are a challenge to every neurosurgeon (2, 3, 7, 8, 11, 12, 13).

Studying the numerous methods of treatment proposed by various authors, we first encountered the promising experiences of American and French neurosurgeons and neuroradiologists (4, 5, 9, 10), as well as a paper by the neurosurgical clinic in Homburg (6) and, most of all, the papers by SERBINENKO in Moscow (14). These authors reported the successful use of the Fogarty catheter in neurosurgery, mainly in the treatment of carotid-cavernous sinus fistulas. The principle of this method appeared to be transferable to the therapy of giant basal aneurysms of the internal carotid artery.

In our patients, the space-occupying effect of the aneurysm led to symptoms comparable to those of a suprasellar pituitary adenoma (Fig. 1), so that there was unilateral amaurosis and increasing loss of vision on the other eye as well. The patients were desperate and demanded active treatment.

The following procedure was decided upon: following adequate angiography (Figs. 2 and 3), the internal carotid artery was dissected in the neck under local anesthesia so that a Fogarty catheter could be introduced and advanced under fluoroscopic control as far as the origin of the suspected aneurysm. During the operation, the aneurysm was visualized again and the balloon at the tip of the catheter inflated. Following the injection of contrast medium, it was seen that the vessel was completely occluded. The patients tolerated this well. Postoperative x-ray control showed the position of the dye-filled balloon. By means of a contralateral and vertebral control angiography, an adequate collateral circulation and the absence of the aneurysm could be documented a few days later. Furthermore, the attempt to thrombose the aneurysm was also successful. At a second procedure, a week later, a craniotomy was performed with the goal of removing the space-occupying aneurysm itself.

In summarizing our limited experience, we want to emphasize the importance of the diagnostic and therapeutic measures and stress that this is a method of treatment for large basal space-occupying intracranial aneurysms. Improvement in catheter material will hopefully open new perspectives in the near future.

References

1. ALTENBURG, H., STÖWSAND, D., WALTER, W.: The use of the Fogarty catheter method in the treatment of carotid-cavernous sinus fistulas and giant basal sack-shaped aneurysms. Annual Meeting of the German Neurosurgical Society, Berlin, 1976

2. BENEDETTI, A., CURRI, D., CARBONIN, C., RUBINI, L.: On the radical treatment of a large carotid-opthalmic aneurysm. Case report. J. Neurosurg. Sci. 19, 176-180 (1975)

3. BULL, J.: Massive aneurysms at the base of the brain. Brain 92, 535-570 (1969)

4. DEBRUN, G., LACOUR, P., CARON, J.P., HURTH, M., COMOY, J., KERAVEL, Y.: Inflatable and released balloon technique experimentation in dog - application in man. Neuroradiology 9, 267-271 (1975)

5. FLEISCHER, A.S., BERG, D.J.: Balloon occlusion and embolization of an internal and external carotid-cavernous fistula. Surg. Neurol 7, 145-148 (1977)

6. HERRMANN, H.-D., FISCHER, D., LOEW, F.: Experiences with intraluminal occlusion with the Fogarty catheter in the treatment of carotid-cavernous sinus fistulas and other lesions at the base of the skull. Acta Neurochir. 32, 35-54 (1975)

7. MAXWELL, R.E., CHOU, S.N.: Aneurysmal tumors of the basifrontal region. J. Neurosurg. 46, 438-445 (1977)

8. MORLEY, T.P., BARR, H.W.K.: Giant intracranial aneurysms: diagnosis, course and management. Clin. Neurosurg. 16, 73-94 (1969)

9. PICARD, L., LEPOIRE, J., MONTAUT, J., HEPNER, H., ROLAND, J., GUYONNAUD, J.C., JACOB, F., ANDRE, J.M.: Endarterial occlusion of carotid-cavernous sinus fistulas using a balloon tipped catheter. Neuroradiology 8, 5-10 (1974)

10. PROLO, D.J., BURRES, K.P., HANBERY, J.W.: Balloon occlusion of carotid-cavernous fistula: introduction of a new catheter. Surg-Neurol. 7, 209-214 (1977)

11. SARWAR, M., BATNITZKY, S., SCHECHTER, M.M.: Tumerous aneurysms. Neuroradiology 12, 79-97 (1976)

12. SELKER, R.G., WOLFSON, S.K., MAROON, J.C., STEICHEN, F.M.: Preferential cerebral hypothermia with elective cardiac arrest: resection of "giant" aneurysm. Surg. Neurol. 6, 173-179 (1976)

13. SENGUPTA, R.P., GRYSPEERDT, G.L., HANKINSON, J.: Carotid-opthalmic aneurysms. J. Neurol. Neurosurg. Psychiatry 39, 837-853 (1976)

14. SERBINENKO, F.A.: Balloon catheterization and occlusion of major cerebral vessels. J. Neurosurg. 41, 125-145 (1974)

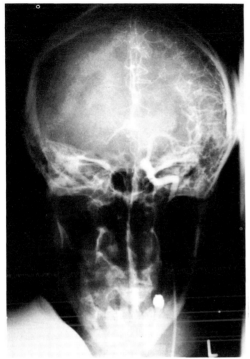

Fig. 1

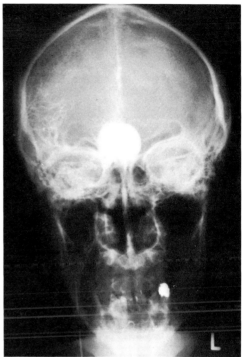

Fig. 2

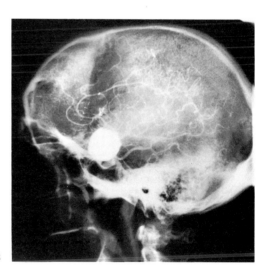

Fig. 3

Fig. 1. Carotid angiogram showing a suprasellar mass (same patient as in Figs. 2 and 3!)

Figs. 2 and 3. Frontal and lateral carotid angiogram showing the giant aneurysm of the right internal carotid artery

Therapeutic Embolization of the External Carotid Artery

V. OLTEANU-NERBE, H. INGRISCH, F. MARGUTH, and H. STEINHOFF

Since the pioneer work of BROOKS (1) therapeutic embolization has been applied to various craniocerebral and vertebromedullar (7, 15) vascular and tumoral lesions (3, 4, 11). Artificial embolization was used mostly for the treatment of internal carotid-cavernous sinus fistulas (16) and in cases of inoperable cerebral arteriovenous malformations (12, 18). Following the introduction of superselective catheterization of the branches of the external carotid artery (6, 14), a new application of the embolization procedures seems to be possible. It is the purpose of this report to present our experience with various pathologic lesions supplied by the external carotid artery, treated by embolization using Gelfoam.

Clinical Material and Methods

This series comprises eight patients. Three had arteriovenous malformations (AVM), one had a facial hemangioma, and another had a traumatic external carotid-cavernous sinus fistula. The remaining three presented a highly vascularized tumor (Table 1). Serial angiography including both carotid and basilar systems was performed in all patients.

Technique of Embolization

The technique of embolization is essentially the same as originally described by DJINDJIAN (4, 6). Superselective catheterization of the branches of the external carotid artery was performed by the transfemoral catheter technique. All patients except two were treated under local anesthesia. Once the feeding artery had been reached by the catheter, strips of Gelfoam were injected through the catheter into the vessel. Embolization was performed stepwise under fluoroscopic monitoring. When embolization had been completed, control angiography was performed.

Table 1. Clinical material

		No. of cases
Arteriovenous angioma		3
Scalp	2	
Dural	1	
Hemangioma of the face		1
External carotid-cavernous sinus fistula		1
Tumors		3
Mengingioma	2	
Glomus tumor	1	
Total		8

Results

1. Arteriovenous Malformations of the Scalp and Dura Mater

In all three patients with AVM of the scalp or the dura, complete embolization of the feeding arteries could be achieved, making an open surgical approach superfluous. In the two patients with *arteriovenous malformations of the scalp*, the dilated occipital artery was the main feeder in one case, whereas the occipital artery as well as the superficial temporal artery fed the malformation in the other (Fig. 1). In the patient with a *dural angioma*, angiography revealed a large shunt between the occipital artery and the posterior branches of the middle meningeal artery and the homolateral transverse sigmoid sinus (Fig. 2).

2. Hemangioma of the Face (Fig. 3)

A 26-year-old femal exhibited a hemangioma involving the left facio-orbital region. She reported bruit and painful sensations. Preceding attempts to treat her with x-rays and electrocauterization remained unsuccessful. The angiographic study revealed a large hemangioma supplied by the homolateral alveolar, suborbital, and sphenopalatine branches of the internal maxillary artery, as well as by several aberrant arteries. The result of embolization was satisfactory but incomplete. Control angiography, performed 5 months later, showed a partial refilling of the malformation through the recanalized internal maxillary artery and by new collaterals from the superficial temporal artery as well as from the maxillary artery. Embolization of these feeding arteries was performed in a second session, resulting in a complete disappearance of the hemangioma on angiography.

3. Fistula Between the External Carotid Artery and the Cavernous Sinus

A carotid-cavernous fistula may be fed simultaneously by the internal carotid and by the external carotid artery (9). The most frequent feeding arteries coming from the external carotid are the meningeal and the pterygoidal branches of the internal maxillary artery as well as the ascendent pharyngeal artery (8).

Our patient, a 21-year-old student, had a traumatic internal carotid-cavernous sinus fistula. The clinical symptoms were pulsating exophtalmus, proptosis, chemosis, and amaurosis, and he reported bruit and pain in his right orbita. A trapping operation, combined with embolization of the cavernous sinus by metal spheres via the internal carotid artery, gave a good temporary result. Three months later, however, the previous symptoms were noticed to have returned. In addition, the patient complained of having recurrent epistaxis. The angiographic study revealed an external carotid-cavernous sinus fistula fed by the homolateral branches of the internal maxillary artery. Since the external carotid artery had been ligated previously in the neck, the maxillar artery filled through anastomoses from homolateral deep cervical arteries. After embolization of these, the fistula could no longer be demonstrated angiographically.

4. Hypervascular Tumors Supplied by the External Carotid Artery

Embolization of highly vascular tumors supplied by several branches of the external carotid artery was performed in one patient with a glomus tumor, in one patient with frontobasal meningioma, and in one case of frontal convexity meningioma. The *glomus tumor* was supplied by the occipital, the ascendent pharyngeal, the retroauricular, and the internal maxillary arteries. In view of this large and inoperable process localized underneath the basis of the skull, embolization was tried as a palliative measure. In contrast to this, embolization of the feeding arteries in the two *meningiomas* was performed as a first step prior to direct tumor removal. In both cases, the supplying vessels were the superficial temporal and the middle meningial arteries (Fig. 4). Selective embolization resulted in a considerable reduction of tumor vascularity and, hence, in a facilitation of the surgical procedure.

Comment

The territory of the external carotid artery represents an ideal field for therapeutic embolization of various vascular and tumoral lesions because of the possibility to obtain selective access to these vessels by newer catheterization techniques (6, 14). In agreement with other reports on larger series, our results indicate that vascular malformations and fistulas between the external carotid artery and the cavernous sinus may be suitable for artificial embolization (4). The distal occlusion of feeding arteries close to the actual hemodynamic shunt offers advantages when compared with conventional vessel ligation, because the malformation can be excluded from the circulation more effectively (10). Moreover, preservation of the proximal part of the vessel, allows repeating the procedure in incompletely treated cases, as in our patient with a hemangioma. It should be mentioned, however, that with the development of future embolization material, presently under study, this risk of recanalization of the injected vessels will be less than with our present material (13). The results in the two cases of meningioma demonstrate an additional potential application of this technique.

Recent reports indicate that superselective catheterization of cerebral vessels is possible and that there may be additional indications for therapeutic embolization of internal carotid-cavernous sinus fistulas, of arteriovenous malformations, and in selected cases of cerebral aneurysm (2, 5, 17).

Summary

Eight cases with various vascular and tumoral lesions in the distribution of the external carotid artery were satisfactory treated by embolization with Gelfoam. These cases included vascular malformations of the scalp, face, and dural sinuses, meningiomas, one glomus tumor, and one fistula between the external carotid artery and the cavernous sinus. Superselective transfemoral catheterization of branches of the external carotid artery was used for embolization. Artificial embolization seems to be an independent method of treatment in patients with angiomatous malformations and external carotid-cavernous sinus fistulas. In patients with highly vascularized tumors, embolization may be of advantage when employed prior to surgical tumor removal.

References

1. BROOKS, B.: Treatment of traumatic arterio-venous fistula. South. Med. J. 23, 100-106 (1930)
2. DEBRUN, G., LACOUR, P., CARON, J.-P., HURTH, M., COMOY, J., KERAVEL, Y.: Traitement des lésions vasculaires carotido-caverneuses par ballonnet gonflable et largable. Nouv. Presse Méd. 20, 1294-1296 (1976)

3. DILENGE, D., CLADERON, H.: Cathétérisme super-sélectif et embolization des pédicules artériels de deux méningiomes de la fosse postérieure. Neurochir. 22, 711-720 (1976)

4. DJINDJIAN, R.: III. Embolization in craniocerebral pathology. Neuroradiology 6, 143-152 (1973)

5. DJINDJIAN, R.: Superselective internal carotid arteriography and embolization. Neuroradiology 2, 145-156 (1975)

6. DJINDJIAN, R.: Super-selective arteriography of branches of the external carotid artery. Surg. Neurol. 5, 133-142 (1976)

7. DJINDJIAN, R., COPHIGNON, J., REY, J., THERON, J., MERLAND, J.J., HOUDARD, R.: Superselective arteriographic embolization by femoral route in neuroradiology. Study of 50 cases. II. Embolization in vertebromedullary pathology. Neuroradiology 6, 132-142 (1973)

8. DJINDJIAN, R., MANEFLE, C., PICARD, L.: Fistules artérioveineuses carotide externe-sinus caverneux. Neurochir. 19, 91-110 (1973)

9. FLEISCHER, A.S., BERG, D.J.: Balloon occlusion and embolization of an internal and external carotid-cavernous fistula. Surg. Neurol. 7, 145-148 (1977)

10. FRY, W.J.: Surgical consideration in congenital arteriovenous fistula. Surg. Clin. North Am. 54, 165-174 (1974)

11. HEKSTER, R.E.M., LUYENDIK, W., MATRICALI, B.: Transfemoral catheter embolization: a method of treatment of glomus jugulare tumors. Neuroradiology 5, 208-214 (1973)

12. LUESSENHOP, A.J.: Artificial embolization for cerebral arteriovenous malformations. Prog. Neurol. Surg. 3, 320-362 (1969)

13. MANAKA, S., IZAWA, M., NAWATA, H.: Dural arteriovenous malformation treated by artificial embolization with liquid silicone. Surg. Neurol. 7, 63-65 (1977)

14. MERLAND, J.J., DJINDJIAN, R.: Utilisation d'un nouveau matériel de ponction et de cethétérisme dans les explorations carotidiennes directes, globales, sélectives et supersélectives chez l'adulte. Ann. Radiol. 16, 9-10 (1973)

15. OLTEANU-NERBE, V.: Gefäßmißbildungen des Rückenmarks. Diagnostik und Therapie. Fortschr. Med. 11, 599-660 (1976)

16. REV, A., COPHIGNON, J., THUREL, C., THIEBAUT, J.B.: Treatment of traumatic cavernous fistulas. In: Advances and Technical Standards in Neurosurgery. KRAYENBÜHL, H. et al. (eds.), p. 87. Wien-New York: Springer 1975

17. SERBINENKO, F.A.: Balloon catheterization and occlusion of major cerebral vessels. J. Neurosurg. 41, 125-146 (1974)

18. STEIN, B.M., WOLPERT, S.M.: Surgical and embolic treatment of cerebral arteriovenous malformations. Surg. Neurol. 7, 359-369 (1977)

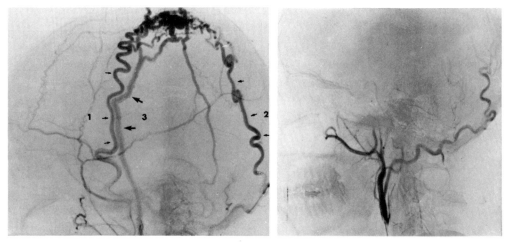

Fig. 1. Arteriovenous angioma of the scalp. Selective arteriography of the terminal branches of the external carotid artery
Left: Arterial phase with early filling veins *(3).* 1 Superficial temporal artery, 2 Occipital artery
Right: After embolization

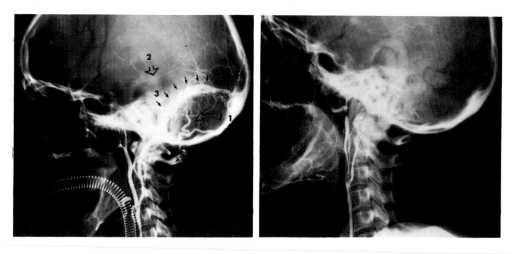

Fig. 2. Posterior fossa dural fistula. Selective arteriography of the terminal branches of the external carotid artery
Left: Before embolization
Right: After embolization. 1 Occipital artery, 2 Posterior branches of the middle meningial artery, 3 Transverse and sigmoid sinuses

Fig. 4. Frontal convexity meningioma ▷
Left: Selective arteriography of the terminal branches of the external carotid artery
Right: After embolization of the meningial arteries *(1),* of the superficial temporal artery *(2),* and of the terminal branches of the internal maxillary artery *(3)*

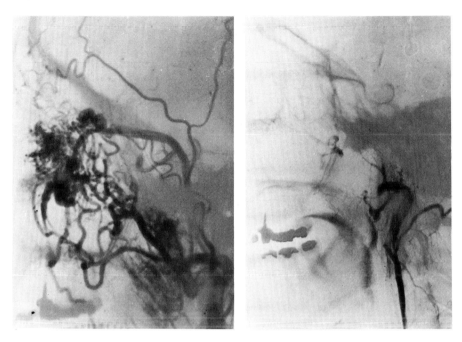

Fig. 3. Hemangioma of the face
Left: Selective arteriography of the internal maxillary artery and of the superficial temporal artery
Right: After embolization

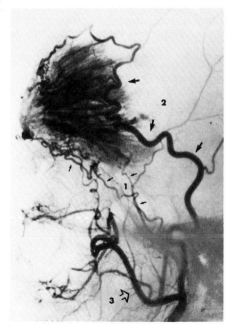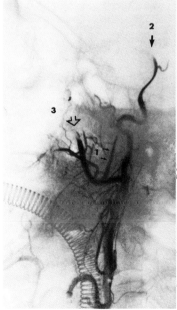

Multipurpose Bipolar Forceps[1]

J. DE PREUX

Precise hemostasis in microsurgery requires bipolar coagulation, frequent irrigation and suction of the operative field. A modified bipolar forceps which allows all these manipulations at the same time is presented.

Construction

The forceps has three elements (Figs. 1 and 2).
1. The basic element is a standard bipolar forceps.
2. On one arm of the forceps a small gauge metal tubing is fixed which is connected to an infusion bottle. This serves as an irrigator. If a high water stream is needed, a blood pressure cuff may be placed around the infusion and inflated.
3. On the other arm of the forceps, a small gauge tubing is fixed and attached to a normal suction device. This may be a rigid metal tubing or a mobile polyethylene tubing, so that the suction may be displaced more deeply or more superficially according to the type of operation.

Manipulation

When the neurosurgeon uses this forceps with the left hand he can assure a good, rapid, and precise hemostasis, so that his right hand can perform more skilled tasks (dissection, clipping, biopsy). Surgery time is markedly reduced and the surgical field clear.

---

[1] Dedicated to Professor Dr. Otto Spoerri, Director of the Neurosurgical Clinic, Göttingen.

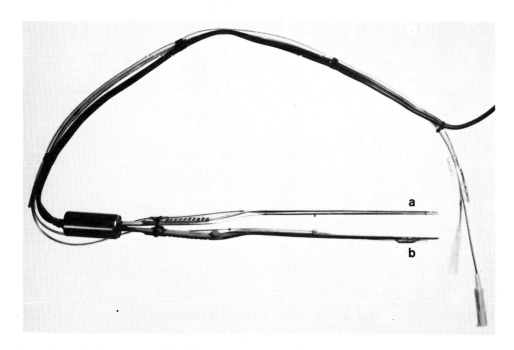

Fig. 1. Multipurpose bipolar forceps
a Irrigation, *b* suction

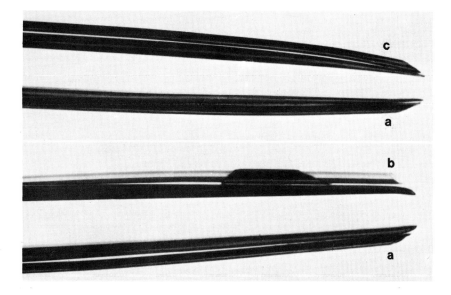

Fig. 2. Details of the forceps
a Irrigation, *b* mobile suction tip, *c* fixed suction tip

Alteration of Spinal Cord Blood Flow in the Area Surrounding an Experimental Injury

H. COLLMANN, R. WÜLLENWEBER, CH. SPRUNG, M. BOROWSKI, and R. DUISBERG

Introduction

In this morphologic and experimental work on spinal cord injury, ALLEN (1) suggested that central hemorrhagic necrosis may be the final consequence of mechanical destruction of spinal microvessels. More recent studies revealed the progressive nature of central lesions (3, 5) and favored the hypothesis of a vasogenic autodestructive process (6), which, however, has not yet been determined completely. Early changes of spinal microvasculature have been demonstrated by several methods, mainly at the point of impact (2, 3, 4, 7, 8). Our aim was to evaluate the time of onset and the reversibility of blood flow disturbances in the area surrounding an experimental traumatic lesion.

Material and Methods

Twenty adult beagle dogs were anesthetized with piritramide (Dipidolor), curarized, intubated, and artificially ventilated with a $N_2O:O_2$ mixture. Cardiovascular and respiratory functions were monitored by recording arterial and venous blood pressure, ECG, end expiratory CO_2 concentration, and by repetitive blood gas analysis. Following cervical laminectomy and incision of the dura, the spinal cord was exposed from C3 to C6. Regional spinal cord blood flow (rSCBF) was estimated using the heat clearance method: two thermoprobes were placed into the spinal cord 3-4 cm apart. Relative changes of local blood flow were continously recorded using a fluvograph. Adequate probe function was evaluated by assessing the response of blood flow to hypercapnia, induced by administration of CO_2-enriched anesthetic gas. A standardized droppe-weight trauma (450 g/cm) was then applied to the dorsal surface of the cord between the probes. Following the impact, local spinal blood flow was monitored for a period up to 5 h in the adjacent areas cranial and caudal to the lesion. The vascular reactivity to hypercapnia and to norepinephrine-induced hypertension was assessed repeatedly. In some animals, fluorescein angiography of the dorsal pial vessels was performed by injecting a bolus of 3 ml 2% sodium fluorescein into the aortic arch. At the end of each experiment, the animals were sacrificed by perfusion fixation, and the appropriate cord fragments were removed and examined microscopically in transverse or longitudinal sections.

Results

1. Following the impact, an immediate increase in systemic blood pressure was observed in virtually all cases, lasting from 2-5 min. Simultaneously, there was an immediate increase of local spinal

flow, which, however, lasted from 8-20 min, regardless of the duration of the initial increase in blood pressure.

2. Prior to the impact, artificial hypercapnia generally induced an increase of rSCBF, which returned to the control value after normalization of arterial pCO_2 (Fig. 1). Following the impact, a negative CO_2 response - a transient decrease of rSCBF during hypercapnia - was found in most cases (Fig. 1). Our interpretation of this pattern is that of a spinal steal phenomenon (9). First appearance of abnormal CO_2 response was observed as early as 4 min after the impact. Earlier CO_2 tests were not performed because the probes had not yet achieved their steady state. In all but two cases, the alteration of CO_2 response was definite and no restitution was observed.

3. Prior to the trauma there were signs of an intact autoregulation; during increase in systemic blood pressure, local spinal blood flow did not change or a slight regulatory decrease was observed (Fig. 2). We never found a breakthrough of autoregulation beyond values of 150 mm Hg MABP. Spinal cord blood flow remained constant until MABP values of 200 mm Hg. Following the impact, typical signs of loss of autoregulation appeared, usually corresponding to the negative CO_2 response; blood flow passively followed norepinephrine-induced hypertension (Fig. 2).

4. Fluorescein angiography of the dorsal superficial vessels showed the following signs of vascular alteration immediately after the trauma: a) at the point of impact and in the adjacent areas many vessels were not filled by the dye, b) circulation time was prolonged, mainly due to a prolonged passage of dye through venous vessels, c) the areas of impact was labeled by a ring of dye extravasation into the cord tissue and the subarachnoid space, indicating a circumscribed alteration of vascular permeability.

5. Central hemorrhagic necrosis at the point of impact was found in all animals. There wer multiple small hemorrhages, mainly in the posterior horns and in the gray matter adjacent to the central canal. The ventral parts of the anterior horns often remained free of hemorrhages (Fig. 3). The longitudinal extension of hemorrhagic necrosis involved one to two segments (Fig. 4).

Discussion

Signs of locally disturbed spinal cord blood flow regulation occur within a few minutes in the adjacent areas of an experimental cord lesion. The alteration of blood flow appears to be irreversible in most cases. Our observations favor the hypothesis of an early determination of the post-traumatic hemorrhagic necrosis. We can hardly support OSTERHOLM's (7) concept of a secondary vasogenic autodestructive process.

Summary

Local spinal blood flow changes in the area above and below an experimental cord lesion were monitored using the heat clearance technique. Within a few minutes after the impact, blood flow response to hypercapnia as well as autoregulation were severely affected. Fluorescein angiography of superficial spinal vessels demonstrated immediate vascular alterations at the point of impact and in adjacent areas.

References

1. ALLEN, A.R.: Remarks in histopathological changes in spinal cord due to impact: an experimental study. J. Nerv. Ment. Dis. 41, 141-147 (1914)
2. BINGHAM, W.G., GOLDMAN, H., FRIEDMAN, St.J., MURPHY, S., YASHON, D., HUNT, W.E.: Blood flow in normal and injured monkey spinal cord. J. Neurosurg. 43, 162-171 (1975)
3. DOHRMANN, G.J., WAGNER, F.C., BUCY, P.C.: The micro-vasculature in transitory traumatic paraplegia. An electron microscopic study in the monkey. J. Neurosurg. 35, 263-271 (1971)
4. KOBRINE, A.J., DOYLE, T.F., MARTINS, A.N.: Local spinal cord blood flow in experimental traumatic myelopathy. J. Neurosurg. 42, 144-149 (1975)
5. NEMECEK, St., PETR, R., SUBA, P., ROSZIVAL, V., MELKA, O.: Longitudinal spinal cord injury - evidence for two types of post-traumatic oedema. Acta Neurochir. 37, 7-16 (1977)
6. OSTERHOLM, J.L.: The pathophysilogical response to spinal cord injury. The current status of related research. J. Neurosurg. 40, 5-33 (1974)
7. OSTERHOLM, J.L., MATHEWS, G.J.: Altered norepinephrine metabolism following experimental spinal cord injury. Part I: Relationship to hemorrhagic necrosis and post-wounding neurological deficits. J. Neurosurg. 36, 386-394 (1972)
8. SANDLER, A.N., TATOR, Ch.H.: Review of the effect of spinal cord trauma on the vessels and blood flow in the spinal cord. J. Neurosurg. 45, 638-646 (1976)
9. WÜLLENWEBER, R., SCHRÖDER, F.K.: Spinal-steal in man recorded by a heat-clearance technique. In: Present Limits of Neurosurgery (Proceedings of the 4th European Congress of Neurosurgery, Prague, 1972), pp. 211-214. Amsterdam: Excerpta Medica 1972

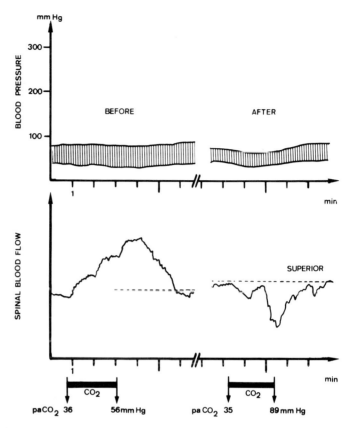

Fig. 1. Spinal cord blood flow response to hypercapnia. Positive CO_2 response before, negative CO_2 response (spinal steal) after trauma

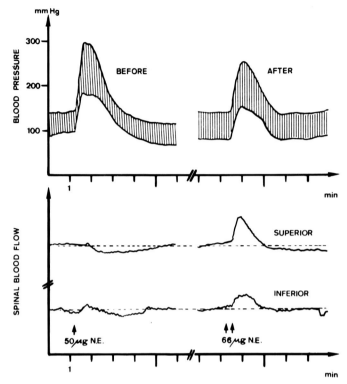

Fig. 2. Autoregulation of spinal cord blood flow. Intact autoregulation before, loss of autoregulation following trauma

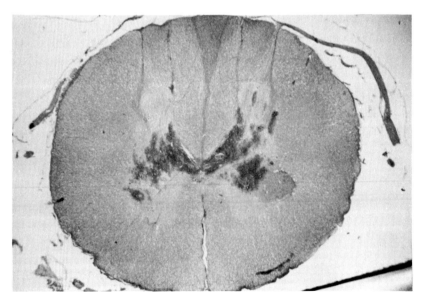

Fig. 3. Central hemorrhagic necrosis following experimental spinal cord trauma

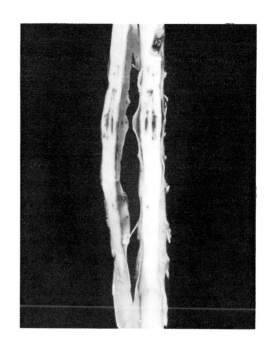

Fig. 4. Central hemorrhagic necrosis following experimental spinal cord trauma. Longitudinal section

Histologic Findings in Graded Experimental Spinal Cord Compression in the Cat

J. Schramm, K. Hashizume, H. Takahshi, and T. Fukushima

The acute concussive spinal cord injury model has been used extensively for the histologic and neurophysiologic evaluation of spinal cord injury (2, 3, 5, 9, 11, 12). The sequential morphologic alterations following acute concussive injuries are well-known (2, 3, 4, 5, 10, 11, 12). Only little has been said about histologic changes following graded cord compression (6, 7). In this investigation, the histologic alterations following graded subacute compression are compared with those following acute injury. Differences between dorsal and ventral and fast and slow compression are discussed.

Material and Methods

Twenty-eight cats (mean weight 2.4 kg) were anesthetized and artificially ventilated. Laminectomies were performed at T6 and T13. Cortical (CoSEP) and spinal (SpSEP) somatosensory evoked potentials were recorded epidurally. A fast and a slow compression group were studied with 10- and 30-min intervals between compression steps. The spinal cord was gradually compressed by means of a compression screw at T13 in 250 µm steps. Two groups of animals were studied, one with dorsal and one with ventral compression. Compression was carried on until CoSEP showed blocked conduction. Then, decompression took place and, following reappearance of CoSEP, the animal was sacrificed by means of intracardiac perfusion with 10% formalin. In 23 cases, the specimens were removed with surrounding normal tissue, serially but at 2-mm intervals and stained with hematoxylin and eosin, Nissl, and sudan black.

Results

Tissue damage was microscopically graded as follows if one or more criteria was fulfilled: *grade 0*: no change; *grade 1*: mild or moderate edema, little diapedetic bleeding; *grade 2*: extensive edema, numerous diapedetic hemorrhages, some petechiae; *grade 3*: numerous petechiae, some coalescing petechiae, small or moderate hemorrhage; *grade 4*: extensive hemorrhage, moderate or large hemorrhagic necrosis.

Starting in the dorsal central *grey matter* edema rich in protein, diapedetic hemorrhages and small petechiae were found in less severely damaged cords. In more severe cases, hemorrhages and hemorrhagic necroses were found, involving the dorsal and ventral horns or the entire grey matter. The cell bodies showed chromatolysis, vacuolization, and shrinking, with distension or pericellular spaces. Small vessel distension and stasis and, in later stages, polymorphonuclear infiltration of vessel walls was seen (Fig. 1).

The *white matter* was edematous to a varying degree in all cases. In nine cases, edema and/or axonal swelling was the only finding. Petechiae and large hemorrhages occurred less frequently than in grey matter (Table 1). From what was seen in less extensively damaged cases, grey matter alterations preceded those in white matter. In all cases except one, grey matter was more severely affected than white matter (Fig. 2).

Table 1

	Grade 0	Grade 1	Grade 2	Grade 3	Grade 4
Grey matter	0	1	6	7	9
White matter	0	10	6	5	2

There was no definite difference between findings following dorsal and ventral compression. There was, however, a tendency toward more severe ventral white matter damage following ventral compression (Fig. 2A). Thus, in ventral compression, the same type and sequence of histologic alteration was seen, although with a different distribution. No significant difference was found between fast and slow compression groups (Fig. 2B), despite a tendency toward greater white matter damage in the fast compression group. Although the compression was performed until conduction block for CoSEP occurred, histologic findings in dorsal columns did not correlate well with SEP findings. In most cases, only moderate to severe edema developed. Less frequently, diapedesis (three cases), small hemorrhages (two cases), and petechiae (one case) were also seen. In all but one case, CoSEP returned within 5-25 min after compression, despite the above-mentioned white matter changes and severe hemorrhage or even total hemorrhagic necrosis of grey matter (Fig. 3). No correlation between grey matter damage and SEP could be demonstrated.

In summary, the following conclusions may be drawn:
1. The sequence and type of histologic change in *graded* spinal cord compression does not differ from that already described in *acute* concussive injury.
2. Comparison between dorsal and ventral compression shows a tendency toward more pronounced ventral white matter damage in the presence of ventral compression.
3. Comparison between the slow and fast graded compression inconstantly reveals more severe white matter damage in the fast compression group.
4. Conduction failure in CoSEP occurred even without gross histologic changes in dorsal columns.

Comment

Our findings confirm those of other authors (3, 5, 6, 10) that grey matter damage nearly always precedes and is more severe than white matter damage. Regarding white matter damage, HUJUDA (7) described a preferential involvement of ventral white matter, although much less pronounced, in subacute ventral compression studies. D'ANGELO (1) has proposed that evoked potential changes correlate with the severity of spinal cord damage, since blocked conduction was seen if white matter hemorrhage or destruction had occurred. MARTIN (8) drew similar conclusions in chronic preparations. Our data and those of GRIFFITHS (6), however, showed that conduction failure occurs even without gross histologic change in dorsal columns. We conclude that direct pressure to neuronal structure also plays a role in the abolition of the evoked cortical potential.

Summary

The histologic changes that follow subacute graded dorsal and ventral spinal cord compression in 23 cats are described. These changes are compared between four groups: dorsal, ventral, fast, and slow compression. Histologic data are correlated with the cortical somatosensory-evoked response.

References

1. D'ANGELO, C.M., VANGILDER, J.C., TAUB, A.: Evoked cortical potentials in experimental spinal cord trauma. J. Neurosurg. 38, 332-336 (1973)
2. DUCKER, T.B., ASSENMACHER, D.: The pathological circulation in experimental spinal cord injury. Proc. 17th Spinal Cord Injury Conference, pp. 10-11 (1969)
3. DUCKER, T.B., KINDT, G.W., KEMPE, L.G.: Pathological findings in acute experimental spinal cord trauma. J. Neurosurg. 35, 700-708 (1971)
4. FAIRHOLM, D.J., TURNBULL, I.M.: Microangiographic studies of experimental spinal cord injuries. J. Neurosurg. 35, 277-286 (1971)
5. GOODKIN, R., CAMPBELL, J.B.: Sequential pathologic changes in spinal cord injury, a preliminary report. Surg. Forum 20, 430-432 (1969)
6. GRIFFITHS, I.R.: Vasogenic edema following acute and chronic spinal cord compression in the dog. J. Neurosurg. 42, 155-165 (1975)
7. HUKUDA, S., WILSON, C.B.: Experimental cervical myelopathy: Effects of compression and ischemia on the canine cervical cord. J. Neurosurg. 37, 631-652 (1972)
8. MARTIN, S.H., BLOEDEL, J.R.: Evaluation of spinal cord injury using cortical evoked potentials. J. Neurosurg. 39, 75-81 (1973)
9. NEMECEK, S., PETR, R., SUBA, P., ROZSIVAL, V., MELKA, O.: Longitudinal extension of oedema in experimental spinal cord injury. - Evidence for two types of post-traumatic oedema. Acta Neurochir. 37, 7-16 (1977)
10. WAGNER, F.C., Jr., DOHRMANN, G.J., BUCY, P.C.: Histopathology of transitory traumatic paraplegia in the monkey. J. Neurosurg. 35, 272-276 (1971)
11. WAGNER, F.C., DORHMANN, G.J., TASLITZ, N., ALBIN, M.S., WHITE, R.J.: Histopathology of experimental spinal cord trauma. Proc. 17th Spinal Cord Injury Conference, pp. 8-9 (1969)
12. WHITE, R.J., ALBIN, M.S., HARRIS, L.S., YASHON, D.: Spinal cord injury sequential morphology and hypothermia stabilazation. Surg. Forum 20, 432-434 (1969)

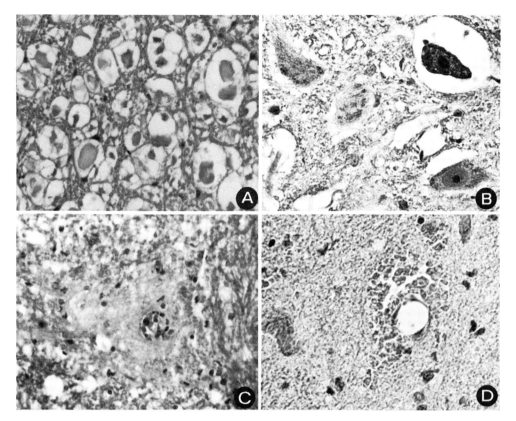

Fig. 1
A Photomicrographs showing axonal swelling in ventral white matter (x 250)
B Neuronal change in pericentral grey matter (x 250)
C Perivascular fibrinoid exudate and polymorphonuclear infiltration of vessel wall (x 250)
D Petechial hemorrhage in dorsal central grey matter with ruptured thin-walled vessel in center (x 40) (hematoxylin and eosin stain)

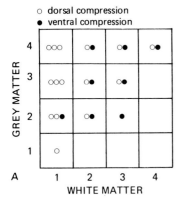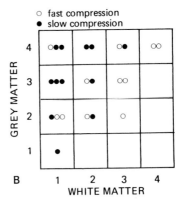

Fig. 2. Relationship between histologic alterations in grey and white matter following
A Dorsal and ventral
B Fast and slow compression
The grade of severity is indicated by numerals

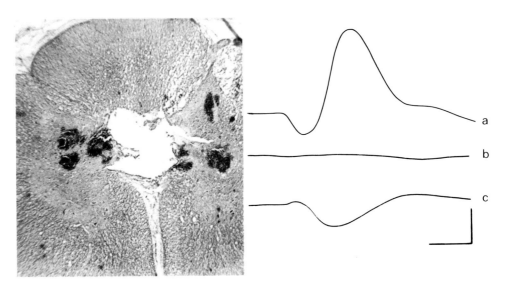

Fig. 3. Cat No. 18. On the left, microscopic view of maximum damage to spinal cord at injury site (x 25). On the right, CoSEP before compression (*a*), at conduction block (*b*), and 6 min after decompression (*c*). Note change in amplitude and peak latencies which were observed in all animals in which CoSEP recovered. Horizontal bar indicates 20 ms, vertical bar 25 µV. Positivity is upward

Epidural Temperature Changes During Anterior Cervical Interbody Fusion With Polymethylmethacrylate

K. ROOSEN, W. GROTE, J. LIESEGANG, and U. LINKE

For anterior cervical interbody fusion, we use a plastic dowel of a polymeric material based on polymethylmethacrylate, a rapidly hardening plastic cement (Palacos R°).

A series of experimental and intraoperative temperature measurements was performed in order to study the occurrence of thermic necrosis caused by polymerization heat in the adjacent neuronal tissue. Initially, 2 cm^3 of the polymer-monomer mixture (constant ratio) were poured into a cylindric aluminium case, 16 mm high, 18 mm in diameter, and with a wall thickness of 0.5 mm.

The temperatures were measured by flexible thermoelements made of iron conctantan with a diameter of only 2 mm. The following parameters were measured at constant room temperature:

1. Surface temperature of the dowel in air.
2. Temperatures at the surface at 1 mm depth and in the center of the plastic cylinder (Fig 1).
3. So as to reproduce operative conditions, temperature changes were measured at the backside of 4-5 mm and 8-10 mm layers of Gelfoam applied to the surface (Fig. 1) of the polymer, also in aqueous medium.

The highest average temperature (84.5°C) was found in the center of the plastic dowel; 95.3°C was measured only once. The lowest temperatures were recorded at the backside of Gelfoam.

The mean maximal surface temperature of the dowel in air was 76.7°C (absolute maximum was 83.7°C). In circulating water (37°C), we did not measure more than 41.6°C, respectively 43.2°C. The temperatures return to normal faster within the water bath than in air (Fig. 1). As described by others (1, 2, 3, 5, 7, 8, 9), our results indicate that the changes of surface temperature depend essentially on the thermal conductivity of the surrounding medium.

In the course of 16 cerival anterior intervertebral body fusions, the thermometer tip was placed on the spinal dura mater following total removal of the intervertebral disc. The probe was fixed to the lateral bony structures. Room and body temperature were continuously measured. As to the operative technique (4), the intervertebral space is covered dorsally and on both sides with 2 mm layers of Gelfoam just prior to application of the viscous cement. The average amount of methylmethacrylate used was 1 cm^3 (1.6 cm^3 at the most). Correct positioning of the probe was controlled by fluoroscopy.

Figure 2 shows the changes in epidural temperatures during the hardening process, as well as the recorded peak values. Maximum temperatures averaged 40.6°C. The level of polymerization heat definitely depends on the amount of monomer fluid used, being about 13-30 kcal/mol (1.6).

Our results allow the following conclusions. In analogy to the aqueous medium, thermal conductivity of the circulating blood and of the adjacent body tissue prevents a temperature increase beyond 40.6°C. The temperature of 56°C, usually regarded as necessary for protein coagulation, is by far not reached. On the other hand, the operative precautions, small amount of monomer fluid and the Gelfoam protection, are a safe prevention from thermonecrosis of the spinal cord and the meninges.

Summary

An experimental and clinical study which demonstrates the temperature changes measured in the epidural space of the cervical spine during anterior interbody fusion is reported. A rapidly hardening plastic cement, polymethylmethacrylate is used. The results indicate that there is no risk of thermonecrosis by polymerization heat in the adjacent neuronal tissue.

References

1. BIEHL, G., HARMS, J., HANSER, U.: Experimentelle Untersuchungen über die Wärmeentwicklung im Knochen bei der Polymerisation von Knochenzement. Arch. Orthop. Unfallchir. 78, 62-69 (1974)
2. DEBRUNNER, H.U.: Die Erwärmung von Knochenzement bei der Polymerisation. Arch. Orthop. Unfallchir. 78, 309-318 (1974)
3. DEBRUNNER, H.U., WETTSTEIN, A.: Die Verarbeitungszeit von Knochenzementen. Arch. Orthop. Unfallchir. 81, 291-299 (1975)
4. GROTE, W., BETTAG, W., WÜLLENWEBER, R.: Indikation, Technik und Ergebnisse zervikaler Fusionen. Acta Neurochir. 22, 1-27 (1970)
5. HUPFAUER, W.: Möglichkeiten und Problematik der Anwendung von Polymethylmethacrylaten ("Knochenzement") in der Orthopädie. Habilschr. Essen (1973)
6. KROESEN, A.: Experimentelle Untersuchungen zur Bestimmung der Oberflächentemperaturen des auspolymerisierenden Knochenzementes Palacos. Inaug.-Dissertation, Köln (1970)
7. PETERS, G., BIEHL, G., HANSER, U.: Experimentelle Untersuchungen über die Wärmeentwicklung im Knochen bei der Polymerisation von Polymethyl-Methacrylat. Saarländ. Ärztebl. 11, 637-639 (1970)
8. WILLERT, H.-G., PULS, P.: Die Reaktion auf Knochenzement bei der Allo-Arthroplastik der Hüfte. Arch. Orthop. Unfallchir. 72, 33-71 (1972)
9. WILLERT, H.-G., SCHREIBER, A.: Unterschiedliche Reaktionen von Knochen und Weichteillager auf auspolymerisierende Kunststoffimplantate. Z. Orthop. 106, 231-252 (1969)

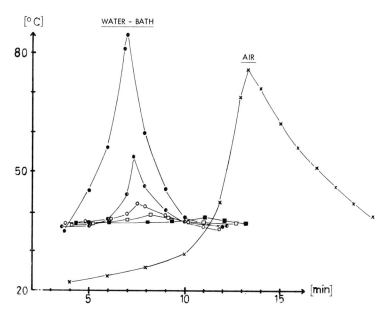

Fig. 1. Experimental temperature measurements
Air: x————x on the surface of the plastic dowel
Water bath: At the graft O————O surface, ◐————◐ 1 mm below surface, ●————● center; Gelfoam in between the dowel and the thermoelement
□————□ 4-5 mm layer, ■————■ 8-10 mm layer

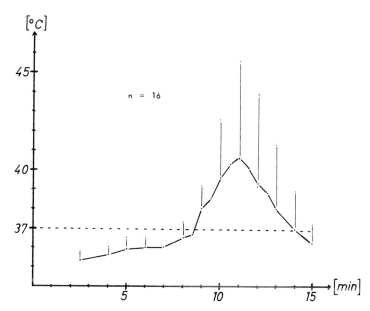

Fig. 2. Clinical temperature measurements in the epidural space

Value of EMG Monitoring in Percutaneous Cordotomy
J. WICKBOLDT and F. MILTNER

The site of coagulation in high cervical lateral cordotomy is generally determined according to the criteria of MULLAN et al. (8), ROSOMOFF et at. (9), HEKMATPANAH (4), and TAREN et al. (11). Additional control of the target point seems desirable, especially in the uncooperative patient. MULLAN et al. (8) and TAREN et al. (11) considered the examination of the afferences by somatosensory cervical and cortical evoked potentials to be useful. First results were reported by LIBERSON et al. (6). ENTZIAN et al. (3), TASKER et al. (12), and AMANO et al. (1).

We studied the motor efference by electromyographic methods during this procedure. The results obtained up to now revealed considerable safety in avoiding pareses. In case of incorrect positioning of the electrode, usual stimulation with right-angle impulses (100 Hz, increasing amplitude) shows an increasing activation in the leg muscles ipsilateral to the side of the operation, while the contralateral muscles are not influenced (Figs 1B and 4A). In cases of correct positioning of the electrodes, the ipsilateral and contralateral leg muscles are not activated, there being a usually bilateral inhibition of possibly existing spontaneous activity. Inhibition can last longer than stimulation (Figs. 1A, 2, and 4C).

The following findings demonstrate the special value of this additional control. Although the patient only indicates subjective sensation of spinothalamic tract stimulation, an activation of the ipsilateral leg muscles can be noticed electromyographically. Objectively noticeable, but not recognized by the patient, contraction of the leg muscles results only when the spinothalamic tract sensations have become nearly insupportable (Figs. 3 and 4B). In such cases, coagulation may lead to an ipsilateral paresis, although the information given by the patient may lead one to think of a correct position of the electrode.

With increasing nearness to the ideal coagulation point, the averaged EMG potentials induced by single shocks, also investigated by continuous EMG recording, show a decrease with a constant latency of the initial baseline deflection generally between 14-18 ms (stimulation point C1/C2 in the middle of the quadriceps femoris muscle (Fig. 4a, b, b'). When the ideal target point is attained, there are stimulation-dependent answers and symmetric potentials with an initial baseline deflection latency over 10-25 ms and of very low amplitude (Fig. 4C).

The disturbance of motricity, especially the appearance of ipsilateral paresis, even if transient, is the most frequent (4%-17% (7)) and, at the same time, the most important complication of unilateral percutaneous cordotomy. The reason for this is the extension of the lesion and, possibly, an edema caused by coagulation as well as the individual variations of the spinal pathways (11). Possibly due to this variation and also to the neighborhood of the pyramidal tract, there is a partial lesion of the efferent motor pathways. We are convinced that lesions of the motor pathways can be avoided by EMG control, since we have observed no more postoperative pareses. However, we often see shortlasting and fully reversible ataxic disturbances due to the inavoidable concomitant lesion of the spinocerebellar tract, which partly covers the spinothalamic tract. Probably this is also the cause of the inhibitory effect on the cortex, the mesencephalic, and the cerebellar structures (2, 10, 14). Possibly this interpretation of the long-loop inhibition explains the long latency of the low-aplitude potentials of the averaged potentials, pushing the J-motoric. The inhibition, however, can also be interpreted as direct stimulation of the reticulospinal tract and its shortway polysynaptic connections (5).

As to our findings and clinical results, we consider simultaneous EMG control indispensable. It provides further objective data and increased safety. The lesion is performed only when no activation results and can be performed without serious motor consequences if an inhibition of the spontaneous discharge upon stimulation takes place.

References

1. AMANO, K., KITAMURA, K., KAWAMURA, H. TANIKAWA, T., KAWABATAKE, H., NOTANI, M., IZEKI, H.: A study on the lateral spinothalamic tract in man. Cerebral evoked response by stimulation of the lateral spinothalamic tract in 50 cases of percutaneous cervical cordotomy. In: Six International Congress of Neurological Surgery, p. 26. Amsterdam-Oxford: Excerpta Medica 1977

2. ECCLES, J.C., ITO, M., SZENTAGOTHAI, J.: Inhibitory action of the Purkinje cell axons. In: The Cerebellum as a Neuronal Machine. p. 124. Berlin-Heidelberg-New York: Springer 1967

3. ENTZIAN, W., LINKE, D., GEHLEN, W.: Experiences with percutaneous cordotomy. The problem of localisation of the spinothalamic tract by recording evoked potentials in the EEF after intramedullar stimulation. In: Six International Congress of Neurological Surgery, p. 26. Amsterdam-Oxford: Excerpta Medica 1977

4. HEKMATPANAH, J.: Techniques and results of percutaneous cordotomy. Med. Clin. 52, 189-201 (1968)

5. HENATSCH, H.D.: Bauplan der peripheren und zentralen sensomotorischen Kontrollen. In: Sensomotorik, Physiologie des Menschen, Vol. 14. GAUER, O.H., KRAMER, K., JUNG, R. (eds.), p. 193. München-Berlin-Wien: Urban & Schwarzenberg 1976

6. LIBERSON, W.T., VORTIS, H.C., UEMATSU, S.: Recording of evoked potentials in the spinal cord during 'closed' cervical cordotomy. In: Fourth International Congress of Neurology, p. 141. Amsterdam-Oxford: Excerpta Medica 1969

7. LORENZ, R., GRUMME, Th., HERRMANN, H.-D., PALLESKE, H., KÜHNER, A., STEUDE, U., ZIERSKI, J.: Percutaneous cordotomy. In: Advances in Neurosurgery, Vol.3. PENZHOLZ,H., BROCK,M., HAMER,J., KLINGER,M., SPOERRI,O. (eds.), p.178. Berlin-Heidelberg-New York: Springer 1975

8. MULLAN, S., HEKMATPANAH, J., DOBBEN, G., BECKMAN, F.: Percutaneous, intramedullary cordotomy utilising the unipolar anodal electrolytic lesion. J. Neurosurg. 22, 548-553 (1965)

9. ROSOMOFF, H.L., CARROL, F., BROWN, J., SHEPTAK, P.: Percutaneous radiofrequency cervical cordotomy: technique. J. Neurosurg. 23, 639-644 (1965)

10. STRATA, P.: Das Kleinhirn. In: Sensomotorik, Physiologie des Menschen, Vol. 14. GAUER, O.H., KRAMER, K., JUNG, R. (eds.), p. 421. München-Berlin-Wien: Urban & Schwarzenberg 1976

11. SWEET, W.H.: Recent observations pertinent to improving anterolateral cordotomy. Clin. Neurol. 23, 80-95 (1976)

12. TAREN, J.A., ROSS, D., CROSBY, E.C.: Target physiologic corroboration in stereotaxic cervical cordotomy. J. Neurosurg. 30, 569-584 (1969)
13. TASKER, R.R., ORGAN, L.W., HAWRYLYSHYN, P., SMITH, K.C.: Results in 350 consecutive percutaneous cordotomies for the relief of pain using physiological control of lesion site. In: Six International Congress of Neurological Surgery, p. 26. Amsterdam-Oxford: Excerpta Medica 1977
14. WIESENDANGER, M.: Pathophysiology of muscle tone. Berlin-Heidelberg-New York: Springer 1972

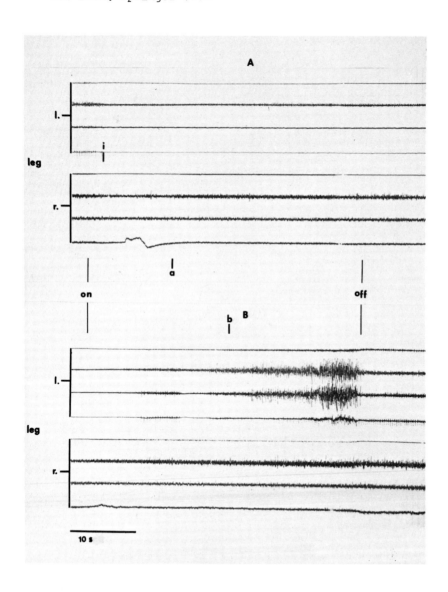

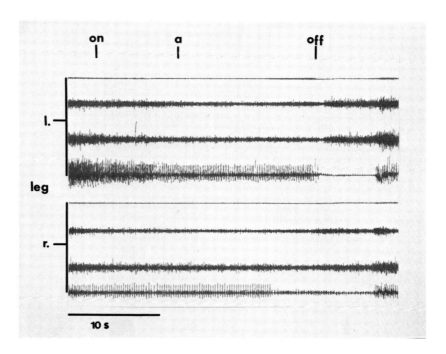

Fig. 2. Left-sided percutaneous cordotomy. Correct position of electrode. Inhibition of spontaneous EMG rate in both legs. Cold feeling in the right leg at 0.2 V (a)

◁

Fig. 1. High left-sided percutaneous cordotomy. Continous recording of EMG in different muscles of the left and right leg during intramedullary stimulation. Amplitude of stimulation (100 Hz, 1 ms, right angle pulses) increasing from 0-0.5 V (on-off)
A Correct position of electrode. Ipsilateral inhibition of spontaneous activity at 0.15 V (i). Warm feeling in the right hand at 0.25 V (a)
B Incorrect position of electrode. Activation of EMG only on the left side. Contraction of leg muscles visible at 0.35 V (b)

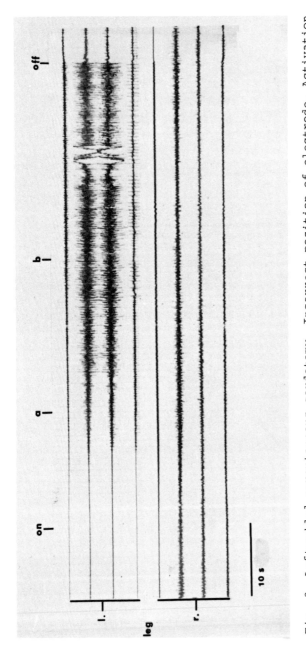

Fig. 3. Left-sided percutaneous cordotomy. Incorrect position of electrode. Activation of EMG activity in the left leg by increasing stimulus amplitude. Burning feeling in right forearm at 0.25V (a); EMG activation still visible. Muscle contraction at 0.4 V, but the patient does not notice it

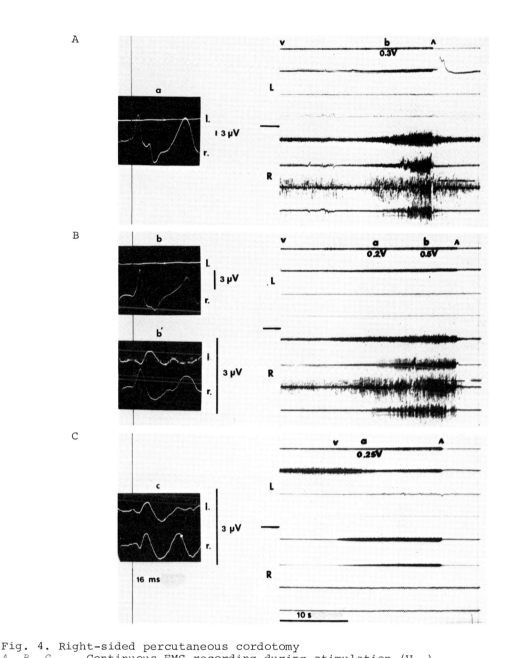

Fig. 4. Right-sided percutaneous cordotomy
A, *B*, *C*   Continuous EMG recording during stimulation (V-)
a, *b*, *b'*, *c* Averaged EMG potentials evoked by single shocks
               (1 mV right-angle pulse)
A, *a*   Incorrect position
B, *b*, *b'*   Incorrect position
C, *c*   Correct position
Ab, *Bb*   Muscle contraction visible in right leg
Ba, *Ca*   Patient indicated sensations from stimulating the spino-
               thalamic tract, at the averaged potentials belonging to B.
               In b cold feeling in the left leg and in b' warm feeling
               in the left forearm

Value of the F Wave in the Diagnosis of Cervical and Lumbosacral Root Compression Syndromes[1]

H. TAKAHASHI, M. STRASHILL, and L. KÜTER

Introduction

The F wave is a small muscle potential which follows the direct M response on supramaximal stimulation of a nerve (10) (Fig. 1). Originally, the F wave was regarded as a reflex response (10). DAWSON, MERTON, and other investigators convincingly demonstrated that the F wave resulted from antidromic activation of the spinal motor neurons (3, 5, 6, 7, 8, 9, 10, 12, 14). Thus, the F wave travels at first from the stimulating point to the spinal cord via motor fibers and activates anterior horn cells antidromically, which results in the delayed muscle potential. The F wave changes may thus reveal lesions of proximal nerve segments (anterior root, plexus, etc.), which are not accessible to conventional nerve conduction studies (4).

The H reflex can also bee used in order to diagnose lesions of the proximal nerve segments (2, 1), but in normal cases the H reflex can be elicited only from S1 myotomes. The present investigation was undertaken in search of possible changes of the F wave parameters in spinal root compression syndromes.

Material and Method

Fifty-nine patients with lumbosacral root compression syndromes and 20 patients with cervical root compression syndromes were examined. Additionally, 28 control subjects without neurologic signs were examined. The F waves were recorded from M. flexor hallucis brevis (S1), M. extensor hallucis longus (L5), thenar (C7, 8), and hypothenar muscles (C8, Th1) after electric stimulation of the corresponding nerves, at the ankle (N. tibialis), the knee (N. peroneus), and the wrist (N. medianus, N. ulnaris).

Supramaximal electric stimuli were delivered percutaneously, and using the surface electrodes, the action potentials were recorded by storage oscilloscope. Data were photographed instantly and subsequently analyzed. At least eight F waves were recorded in each myotome to determine their minimum latency, maximum latency, mean latency and mean potential amplitude. The following parameters were analyzed:

1. Delta L: latency difference between the right and left side of the same nerve in each control subject and latency difference between the pathologic and intact side in patients with spinal root compression syndromes.
2. Delta A: amplitude difference defined analogously as delta L. The rejection limit (5% level) of the control delta L was calculated in order to know the normal range of the delta L. The Wilcoxon test (5% level) was applied for verification of paired differences in the patient group.

---

[1] Supported by a grant of the Deutsche Forschungsgemeinschaft.

Results

1. Amplitude Differences (Delta A)

Despite a certain tendency to decrease on the pathologic side, amplitude differences were not significant at the 5% level.

2. Latency Differences (Delta L)

In order to determine the most reliable and sensitive parameter, three kinds of latency differences were compared: delta L of the mean latency, delta L of the maximum latency, and delta L of the minimum latency. Of these, delta L of the minimum latency has the smallest mean value and smallest standard deviation in the control subject, which means the smallest latency differences between the right and left side. Thus, we concluded that the latency difference of the minimum latency is the best parameter for clinical application and we use only this delta L for the following analysis. By a screening statistical test at the 5% level, we found that the cases with only subjective complaints and with bilateral spinal root compression syndromes showed no significant delta L. We then analyzed the cases with unilateral neurologic, myelographic, and operative findings of spinal root compression in detail.

a) Tibial Nerve F Wave (21 Cases, Fig. 2)

The cases with neurologic signs of S1 root compression showed significant latency differences between the pathologic and intact side, i.e., the F wave of the pathologic side was significantly delayed. The myelographic and/or operative findings also correlate with the significant F wave delay, but two cases who had myelographic findings without neurologic signs showed no significant delay in pathologic sides. The delay (delta L) was greater in cases with motor deficits than in those with only sensory signs.

b) Peroneal Nerve F Wave (Ten Cases, Fig. 2)

The result is the same as that of the tibial nerve. Neurologic, myelographic, and operative findings of L5 lesions correlate well with the significant delay of the F wave in the pathologic side. There is also good correlation between the delay (delta L) and neurologic severity of L5 symptoms.

c) Median Nerve F Wave (Ten Cases, Fig. 3)

The correlation between findings of C7 and/or C8 root compression and the F wave delay was not statistically verified. Only three out of ten cases showed the F wave delay (delta L) greater than 2 ms.

d) Ulnar Nerve F Wave (Six Cases, Fig. 3)

The cases with unilateral root compression syndromes of C8 and/or Th1, diagnosed by neurologic, myelographic, and operative findings, were only six. Five cases showed F wave delays on the diseased side, ranging from 2.1-4.3 ms. One case had no latency difference (delta L = 0). The total number of cases is too small for statistical analysis, but the F wave of the diseased side showed a great tendency to delays longer than 2 ms.

3. Normal Limit of Delta L (Figs. 2 and 3)

The statistical rejection limit of the normal control delta L at the 5% level was calculated in order to determine the demarcation between normal and pathologic findings (Figs. 2 and 3). Tibial peroneal, and ulnar nerve F waves had an increased delta L in cases with unilateral S1 (67%), L5 (70%), and C8 and/or Th1 (83%) syndromes. In cases with C7 and/or C8 syndromes, only 30% of the median nerve F wave showed a delay greater than this limit.

Discussion

We tested various parameters of the F wave statistically and concluded that delta L of the minimum latency is the most reliable and sensitive parameter for detection of a pathologic state. Delta L can be obtained easily, as compared to the F wave conduction velocity, which some authors determined in various neuropathies or in children and infants (6, 7, 8, 9). Furthermore, delta L allows the elimination of differences in recording conditions, failures of approximating nerve length, age differences, etc., which influence nerve conduction velocity (4). The value of the rejection limit (Figs. 2 and 3) suggested that a difference of approximately 2 ms or such a delay on one side may be the limit between the normal variation and pathologic delta L. Using these limits, false-positive may be about 5% and false-negative may be approximately 30% in the presence of unilateral S1, L5, or C8 and/or Th1 syndromes.

GÖRKE (6) measured the latency differences of the tibial and ulnar nerve F waves in children and infants without neurologic signs. Maximum latency differences were 2 ms for the ulnar and 4 ms for the tibial nerve F wave. The range of differences is larger than ours, probably because he described the range of the maximum values of differences, because the F wave was not elicited by supramaximal stimuli, and because the subjects were all children and infants.

The delay of tibial and peroneal nerve F waves correlated well with neurologic (especially motor) signs, as well as with myelographic and operative findings. The study of the F wave can thus be of diagnostic help in cases of unilateral lumbosacral root compression syndromes. The median nerve F wave showed no significant delay in cases of unilateral C7 and/or C8 syndrome, probably because multisegmental innervation to thenar muscles is more distinct than to the other muscles (13) or because of the small number of cases with definite motor deficits.

As to the ulnar nerve F wave, the delay (delta L) on the diseased side correlated well with the findings of C8 and/or Th1 root compression, despite the small number of patients. The precise causes for the differences in results between the median and the other nerves must be clarified by further studies.

Summary

1. In patients with unilateral cervical or lumbosacral root compression syndromes, the F waves were elicited in the corresponding myotomes.
2. As compared to the intact sides, the F waves were significantly delayed in the corresponding myotomes in the presence of S1, L5, and C8 and/or Th1 root compression syndromes.
3. The F wave latency delay recorded from thenar muscles did not statistically correlate with C7 and/or C8 syndromes.
4. The rejection limit of the control delta L was considered to be the 5% level and represents the approximate limit of normality.

References

1. BRADDOM, R.I., JOHNSON, E.W.: Standarization of H reflex and diagnostic use in S1 radiculopathy. Arch. Phys. Med. Rehabil. 55, 161-166 (1974)

2. DESCUS, P., COLLET, M., RESHE, F., LAJAT, Y., GUIHENEUC, P., GINET, J.: Intérêt du réflexe de Hoffmann dans l'exploration des lésions radiculaires lumbo-sacrées d'origine discrale. Neurochirurgie 19, 627-640 (1973)

3. DAWSON, G.D., MERTON, P.A.: "Recurrent" discharges from motor neurons. Twentieth International Congress of Physiology. Brussels: Abstract of Communications, 221-222 (1956)

4. DOBBELSTEIN, H., STRUPPLER, A.: Die Nervenleitgeschwindigkeit als diagnostisches Kriterium bei peripheren neurologischen Störungen. Fortschr. Neurol. Psychiatr. 31, 616-636 (1963)

5. GASSEL, M.M., WIESENDANGER, M: Recurrent and reflex discharges in plantar muscles of the cat. Acta Physiol. Scand. 65, 138-142 (1965)

6. GÖRKE, W.: Die F-Welle im Kindesalter. Z. E.E.G.-E.M.G. 5, 159-164 (1974)

7. KIMURA, J.: F-wave velocity in the central segment of the median and ulnar nerves. Neurology 24, 539-546 (1974)

8. KIMURA, J., BOSCH, P., LINDSAY, G.M.: F-wave conduction velocity in the central segment of the peroneal and tibial nerves. Arch. Phys. Med. Rehabil. 56, 492-497 (1976)

9. KING, D.: Conduction velocity in the proximal segments of a motor nerve in the Guillain-Barré syndrome. J. Neurol. Neurosurg. Psychiatry 39, 538-544 (1976)

10. MAGLADERY, J.W., McDOUGAL, D.B. Jr.: Electrophysiological studies of nerve and reflex activity in normal man. 1. Identification of certain reflexes in the electromyogram and the conduction velocity of peripheral nerve fibres. Johns Hop. Hosp. Bull. 86, 265-290 (1950)

11. MAYER, R.F., FELDMANN, R.G.: Observation on the nature of the F-wave in man. Neurology 17, 147-156 (1967)

12. McLEAD, J.G., WARANG, H.S.: An experimental study of the F-wave in the baboon. J. Neurol. Neurosurg. Psychiatry 29, 196-200 (1966)

13. SCHLIAC, H.: Wurzelläsionen. In: Läsionen peripherer Nerven. 2. Aufl. MUMENTHALER, M., SCHLIAC, H. (Hrsg.), S. 126-170. Stuttgart: Georg Thieme 1973

14. TRONTELJI, J.V., TRONTELJI, M.: F-response of human facial muscles - a single motoneurone study. J. Neurol. Sci. 20, 211-222 (1973)

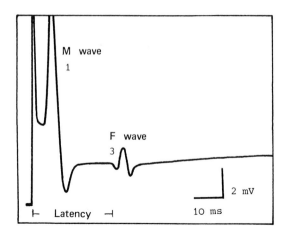
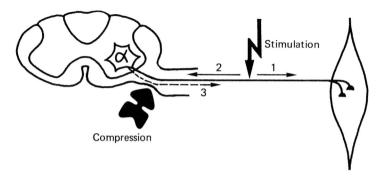

Fig. 1. *Upper panel*: Photograph of the M and F waves recorded from thenar muscles. The initial deflection followed by the M wave is the artifact due to stimulation
Lower panel: Scheme of the passage of the M and F waves. Following supramaximal stimulation of the motor nerve, the orthodromic impuse (*1*) causes the M wave (*1* in the upper panel). On the other hand, the antidromic impulse (*2*) activates the anterior horn cell, which again causes the orthodromic impulse (*3*) and the F wave (*3* in the upper panel)

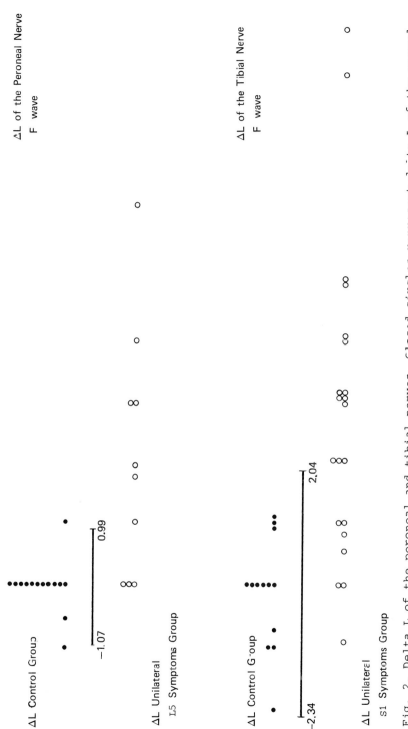

Fig. 2. Delta L of the peroneal and tibial nerves. Closed circles represent delta L of the normal control subjects and open circles are the delta L of the patients. The figures and the horizontal lines show the calculated normal range at the 5% level

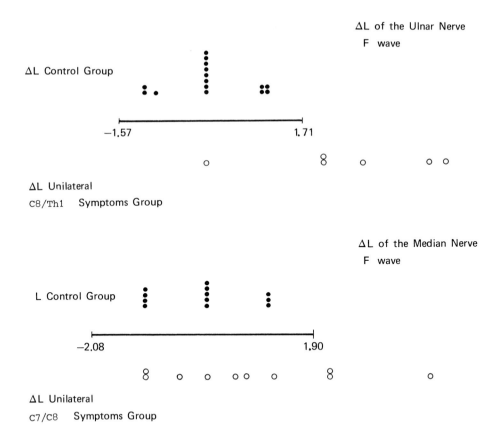

Fig. 3. Delta L of the median and ulnar nerve (symbols as in Fig. 2)

Diagnostic Value of the Somatosensory Evoked Response (SER) in Peripheral Nerve Lesions

H. ASSMUS

Common sensory function tests such as the two-point discrimination, sweating pattern, and picking-up tests, depend on many subjective factors and on the readiness of the patient to collaborate and are, therefore, often unreliable. Assessment of the sensory nerve action potential (NAP) provides an objective tool in measuring the sensory function. This method, however, fails in severe sensory disturbances, e.g., in early stages of sensory reinnervation and in proximal nerve lesions. Even weak afferent volleys, however, usually evoke cortical potentials, which can be detected by averaging techniques. Several studies on the SER in a few cases of peripheral nerve lesions have been reported in the literature (1-6). Our intention was to test the clinical value of this method (with a somewhat modified technique) in a larger number of patients.

Methods and Results

Median and ulnar nerves were stimulated with short electric square impulses (0.2-0.6 ms) delivered to finger nerves and nerve trunks at different levels. In contrast to other investigators, we used relatively frequent stimuli at a rate of 4-5/s. Thus, the recording time could be significantly reduced. The SER was recorded by subcutaneous needle electrodes placed over the hand field of the contralateral primary cortex (different electrode) and the midline of the forehead (indifferent e.); 512 responses were averaged using an EMG amplifier (MEDELEC or TÖNNIES with a band width of 2 or 15-1000 Hz) and a NICOLET 527 averager. Since the analysis time was 100 ms, only the first components of the SER were evaluated. Normally, the first components consists of negative (N1)-positive (P1)-negative (N2) deflections, i. e., the initial complex, followed by a larger positive wave (P2). (Fig. 1). There are, however, individual variations in wave form, especially doubled peaks.

The evaluated material consists of 72 patients, most of whom have been followed up for 1 year or more. They suffered from median nerve lesions treated by suture or nerve transplantation (25 cases), carpal tunnel syndrome (CTS) (28 cases), sulcus ulnaris syndrome (SUS) (ten cases), and radicular or brachial plexus lesions (nine cases).

The results are summarized as follows. Patients with mild and moderate sensory disturbances, e.g., in cases of CTS, showed increased N1 latencies up to 28-30 ms and a reduction in amplitude of the initial N1/P1 complex. Similar findings were recorded in cases of nerve suture, especially in children with good clinical results. In patients with severe sensory loss, usually no initial complex could be detected. In such cases, the first component seen was a large P2 wave with a peak latency of 50-60 ms. This was also true for early stages of reinnervation, when pinprick was felt but no further differentiation was possible and no motor response could be obtained (Fig. 2a). Follow-up studies of regenerating nerves, e.g., postoperatively, revealed an improvement of the N1 latency and in amplitude of the initial complex, while the wave form of the SER was rather constant in an individual patient. These changes in latency and amplitude were parallel to the clinical improvement as tested by two-point discrimination (Fig. 2a, b). In patients with mild sensory disturbances, especially of radicular origin, changes could be detected only by comparing with the contralateral SER. Gradual decline of sensibility reaching as far as analgesia, could be observed in a case of C8 syndrome and verified by the SER. In accordance with the clinical sensory test, the SER revealed increasing abnormalities from the second to the fifth finger (Fig. 2c). In compression syndromes, the SER recorded upon stimulation proximal to the lesion was always normal (Fig. 2d).

Conclusions

The magnitude of the initial components of the SER correspond well to the the magnitude of synchrony of the afferent input. Desynchronization of the afferent volleys due to decreasing conduction velocity and loss of fibers affects latency and form of the SER. On the other hand, a linear correlation between the initial complex of the SER and the intensity of sensation cannot be assumed in pathologic cases. A possible correlation of this kind cannot be excluded, on the basis of this study, for the later components. Therefore, further studies using psychophysical methods are planned.

SER is of high diagnostic value for routine clinical assessment of sensory nerve function, especially for evaluating early and late stages of reinnervation following nerve repair, in forensic medicine, and in the presence of radicular lesions, where the sensory nerve action potential is always normal. The test, which completes nerve conduction studies, is easily performed in about 10-15 min and can be repeated as often as necessary.

References

1. BERGAMINI, L., BERGAMASCO, B., GANDIGLIO, G., MOMBELLI, A.M., MUTANI, R.: Somato-sensory evoked cortical potentials in subjects with peripheral nervous lesions. Electromyography 5, 121-130 (1965)
2. DEBECKER, J., NOEL, P., DESMEDT, J.E.: The use of average cerebral evoked potentials in the evaluation of sensory loss in forensic medicine. Electromyography 11, 131-135
3. DESMEDT, J.E., FRANKEN, L., BORENSTEIN, S., DEBECKER, J., LAMBERT, C., MANIL, J.: Le diagnostic des ralentissements de la conduction afférente dans les affections des nerfs périphériques: intérêt de l'extraction du potentiel evoqué cérébral. Rev. Neurol. 115, 255-262 (1966)
4. GIBLIN, D.R.: Somatosensory evoked potentials in healthy subjects and in patients with lesions of the nervous system. Ann. N.Y. Acad. Sci. 112, 93-141 (1964)
5. JÖRG, J.: Die elektrosensible Diagnostik in der Neurologie. Schriftenreihe Neurologie, Bd. 19. Berlin-Heidelberg-New York: Springer 1977
6. SCHRAMM, J., HASHIZUME, K.: Somatosensory evoked potentials (SEP) in patients with peripheral, spinal and supraspinal lesions of the sensory system. In: Advances in Neurosurgery, Vol. 4. WÜLLENWEBER, R., BROCK, M., HAMER, J., KLINGER, M., SPOERRI, O. (eds.), pp. 250-255. Berlin-Heidelberg-New York: Springer 1977

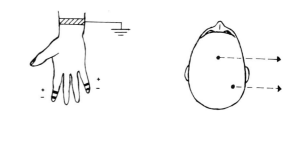
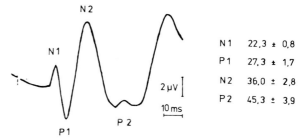

Fig. 1. Equipment used for averaging and recording (*left*). Sites of stimulation and recording (*upper right*) and wave form and normal values of the first components of the SER elicited by stimulating median nerve fibers at the second finger (*lower right*)

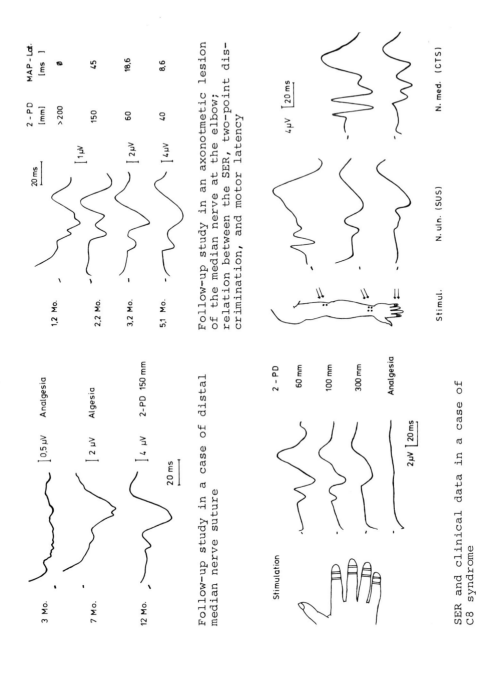

Fig. 2. SERs in cases of peripheral nerve lesion

Subject Index

Agenesis of temporal lobe 297
Aneurysm 351
-, false 123
-, iatrogenic intracerebral 124, 127
-, traumatic 118, 125, 130
Angioblastoma 160, 161
Angiography, cerebral 1, 119, 128, 260
Angiotomography 229
-, posterior fossa 229
Anti-parkinsonian drugs 83
--, EEG activity 84
--, Glasgow coma scale 87
Apallic syndrome 44, 92
Aqueduct, catheterization 216
Arnold Chiari see malformation
Arteriovenous fistulas 118
- malformations 354

Biology of medulloblastoma 232
Blood vessel injuries 113
Brain contusion 117
- death 1, 52, 84, 346
- edema 336
- nerves 221
- stem see tumor
- tumors 279, 285, 289
--, chemotherapy 289, 292
--, classification 279
--, malignancy 285
--, proliferation 285

Carotid artery, traumatic occlusion 118
Carotid-cavernous sinus fistula 122, 354
Catecholamines 83, 85
Catheterization of superior vena cava 349
Cavernous sinus 122, 264, 354
Cerebellar hematomas 168
- infarctions 168
- tumor 159, 266
--, astocytomas 267
--, catamneses 266
--, ICP 179
Cerebellopontine angle, endoscopy 269
--, tumor 271
Cerebral angiography 1
- concussion, standardized 138
- contusion 27, 56
- death 1, 52, 84, 346
- trauma see head injury
Cerebrospinal fluid see CSF and ICP
Cervical fusion 373
Chemotherapy of brain tumors 289, 292
Child abuse 91
-, head injury 91, 98, 102
Chronomorphology of brain death 346
Circulation, intracranial 1
Classification of brain tumors 279
- of severe head injury 16, 140
Coma 12, 16, 54
-, classification 12, 16, 54
-, length 12, 16, 98, 101, 105
-, levels 16, 83
-, scale 13, 16, 87, 133
-, -, Glasgow 87
Computerized tomography (CT) 27, 31, 52, 62, 116, 159, 166, 171, 176
--, artifacts 166
--, basilar artery 176
--, brain death 52
--, brain stem 167
--, cervical spine 171
--, differential diagnosis 167
--, head injury 27, 31
--, intracerebral hematomas 62
--, limitation 166
--, posterior fossa 171
Consciousness, disturbance 16, 102
-, loss of 92
Contrast medium see ventriculography
Contusion, cerebral 27, 56, 138
Cordotomy 376
Cranial circumference 320
Craniocerebral injury see head injury
CSF, electrophoresis 136
CSF-lactate 181
-, disorders of circulation 199
-, drainage see ICP
CSF lipids 139

CSF, pressure see ICP
CSF proteins 133

Death, brain 1, 52, 84, 346
Densitogram, lipid 142
DNA in brain tumors 285

Ear, middle 259
EEG 36, 44, 313, 336
-, comatose patients 83
-, computer evaluation 336
-, frequency analysis 36
-, head injury 36, 44
-, secondary mesencephalic lesions 313
Embolization 354
EMG 221, 376, 382, 389
-, posterior fossa processes 221
Empyema-interhemispheric subdural 302
Endoscopy of the cerebellopontine angle 269
Ependymoma 160, 161, 217, 266
Epidermoid 160, 162
Epidural hematoma 117
Epilepsy, posttraumatic 92
Extremity fractures 112

F-wave 382
Fall-asleep-syndrome 102
-, EEG 103
Fibrinogen 133
Forceps, bipolar 360
Fractures, extremity 112
Frontobasal head injury 78, 79, 80
---, brain edema 78
---, catamnestic results 79, 82
---, consciousness, state 81
---, CSF fistula 78
---, early surgical treatment 78
---, meningitis 78
---, time of operation 80

Globulins, α-2 132, 136
Glomus jugulare tumors 259

Haptoglobulin 133
Head injury 1, 5, 12, 16, 27, 31, 36, 44, 71
--, aphysia 88
--, biochemical data 132
--, children 44, 91, 98, 102
--, classification 16, 31, 140
--, computer tomography 27, 31
--, EEG 36, 44
--, electroencephalogram 88, 89
--, employment 89
--, epidemiology 31
--, experimental 132, 138, 141
--, hemiparalyse 89
--, infancy 91, 98, 102
--, -, EEG results 92
--, -, follow-up studies 98
--, -, intelligence quotient 92
--, -, neurologic symptom 98
--, -, permanent damage 94
---, -, prognosis for survival 99
--, -, psychopathologic deficit 92
--, -, sequelae, late 91
--, long-term observation 88
-- in North America 108
--, mortality rate 108
--, prognosis 1, 12, 16, 31, 36, 52
--, safety helmets 72, 75
--, severe 16, 91, 102, 107
--, social consequences 89
--, symptoms 27
--, unconsciousness 88
--, young motorcyclists 71
Hemangioblastoma 266, 268
Hemangioma 354
Hematoma 56, 62, 68
-, autopsies 68
-, cerebellar 168
-, clinically nonmanifest 68
-, computerized tomography 62
-, epidural 68, 117
-, intracerebral 56, 62, 68
-, subdural 68, 117
Hydated cyst 306
Hydrocephalus 259, 331
Hyperventilation 336

ICP 179-208
-, B-waves 189
-, cerebellar tumors 179
-, circadian waves 188
-, plateau waves 189
-, ramp waves 189
Immunoelectrophoresis 236
Infarction, cerebellar 168
Injury, head see head injury
-, spinal cord 362, 368
Intensive therapy 349
Intracranial circulation 1
- hematomas 56, 62, 68
- pressure 1, 5, 179, 194, 199, 331, 336
--, circadian waves 188
--, continuous measurements 179, 188, 194, 211
--, decompensation 203
--, hydrocephalus 178
--, -, occlusus 179, 194
--, long-term measuring 179
--, ventriculoauricular shunt 194

Jugular vein   260

Laceration   18
Lindau's disease   266
Lipid metabolism   138
Long-term measuring of ventricular CSF   179

Malformation, Arnold Chiari   150, 217
-, basilar artery   176
Measurement of cranial circumference   320
Measuring, long-term of ventricular CSF   179
Medulloblastoma   159, 160, 239, 245, 257, 266
- of childhood   257
-, clinic   239
-, prognosis   245, 257
-, treatment   245, 253, 257
Memory, disturbances   105
Meningeoma   162
Meningitis   78
Metastases   159, 217
Metrizamide   150, 174
Mnestic disturbance   105
Mortality of multiple injuries   114
Motorcyclist, accident   71
Multiple injuries   112

Nerve lesions   389
Neuroblastoma   217
Neuroma   159, 160, 161

Oligodendroglioma   217
Open head injuries   117
Orbital phlebography   260
Osmotherapy   336
Osteoblastoma   311
Osteogenic sarcoma   311

Parapontine tumors   224
Peripheral nerves   389
Phlebography, orbital   260
Platelets   133
Posterior fossa   211 ff.
--, catheterization of aqueduct   216
--, CSF measuring   179
--, CT see Computer tomography
--, decompression   217
-- tumors   159, 194, 203, 211, 216, 221, 224, 229, 232, 239, 253, 257; see also medulloblastomas
---, angiography   229
---, EMG of brain nerve reflexes   221
---, immunoelectrophoretic evaluations   236

---, medulloblastomas   232, 239, 245, 253, 257
---, parapontine   224
---, prepontine   224
Prepontine tumors   224
Pressure, intracranial   1, 5
Prevention of head injury   71, 75
Prognosis of head injury   1, 12, 16, 31, 36, 52, 132

Radiation   155
Resorbable contrast media see ventriculography
Reticular activating system   83

Safety helmets see head injury
Sarcoma   159, 160, 161, 217
Schedule of treatment   112
Selective angiography   262
Serum lipids   140
- urea   133
Shunt see ventricular shunt
-, ventriculoauricular   194, 199, 209
Sinugraphy   260
Sodium retention   133
Spinal cord   362, 368, 373, 382
--, blood flow   362
--, cervical fusion   373
--, compression   368
--, histologic findings   368
--, injury   362
--, root compression   382
Spongioblastoma   159, 217
Stupor, posttraumatic in children   102
Subdural hematoma   117
Survival rate, head injury   17

Temporal lobe, agenesis   297
Trauma, cerebral see head injury
Traumatic aneurysm   124
Treatment, aneurysm   351
-, arteriovenous malformation 354
-, brain edema   336
-, brain tumors   289, 292, 324
-, carotid-cavernous sinus fistula   354
-, hemangioma   354
-, lesions of the base of the skull   324
-, multiple injuries   113
-, schedule of   112
Tumor, brain stem   155, 217
-, cerebellar   155, 159, 166, 179, 216
-, classification   279
-, midline   155
-, radiation   157
- surgery   324

Unconsciousness, duration 16, 98, 101, 105
Urea 134

Vascular injury 116, 119
- surgery 351
Ventricular shunt 199, 209
--, drainage 203, 209, 211
Ventriculography 147, 150, 155
-, amipaque 150
-, dimer-X 155
-, positive 174-178
Vermian pseudotumor 167

Advances in Neurosurgery

Volume 1

Brain Edema

Pathophysiology and Therapy
Cerebello Pontine Angle Tumors
Diagnosis and Surgery

Editors: K. Schürmann, M. Brock, H.-J. Reulen, D. Voth

1973. 187 figures. XVII, 385 pages
ISBN 3-540-06486-9
Distribution rights for Japan: Nankodo Co. Ltd., Tokyo

Contents: Pathophysiology of Brain Edema. – Clinical Therapy of Brain Edema. – Intracranial Pressure, Cerebral Blood Flow and Metabolism. – Diagnosis of Cerebello-Pontine Angle Tumors. – Surgery of cerebello-Pontine Angle Tumors. – Miscellaneous.

Volume 2

Meningiomas

Diagnostic and Therapeutic Problems
Multiple Sclerosis
Misdiagnosis
Forensic Problems in Neurosurgery

Proceedings of the 25th Annual Meeting of the "Deutsche Gesellschaft für Neurochirurgie" Bochum, September 22 - 25, 1974

Editors: W. Klug, M. Brock, M. Klinger, O. Spoerri

1975. 200 figures, 86 tables. XXI, 444 pages
ISBN 3-540-07237-3
Distribution rights for Japan:
Nankodo Co. Ltd., Tokyo

Contents: Meningiomas. – Multiple Sclerosis. – Forensic Problems in Neurosurgery. – Free Communications.

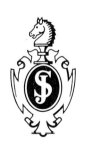

Springer-Verlag
Berlin
Heidelberg
New York

Volume 3

Brain Hypoxia
Pain

Proceedings of the 26th Annual Meeting of the "Deutsche Gesellschaft für Neurochirurgie" Heidelberg, May 1 – 3, 1975

Editors: H. Penzholz, M. Brock, J. Hamer, M. Klinger, O. Spoerri

1975. 160 figures, 110 tables.
XIX, 460 pages
ISBN 3-540-07466-X
Distribution rights for Japan:
Nankodo Co. Ltd., Tokyo

The mechanisms involved in physiological and pathological oxygen supply to the central nervous system are of fundamental theoretical and clinical importance. In the first section of this volume, the basic aspects of this problem are extensively discussed by scientists of international fame.

Pain is older than mankind. Its neuroanatomical and neurophysiological substrates have always attracted the attention of neuroscientists. The treatment of pain has gained new impulses from recent stimulation techniques. In the second section the classical methods of pain treatment are reviewed and the latest procedures are presented and discussed.

The last section of this book contains contributions on various aspects of current neurosurgical diagnosis, therapy and research.

Volume 4

Lumbar Disc
Adult Hydrocephalus

Editors: R. Wüllenweber, M. Brock, J. Hamer, M. Klinger, O. Spoerri

1977. 154 figures, 67 tables.
XXIII, 338 pages (8 pages in German)
ISBN 3-540-08100-3
Distribution rights for Japan:
Nankodo Co. Ltd., Tokyo

Volume 4 of *Advances in Neurosurgery* is dedicated to two subjects which constitute a daily challenge to the neurosurgeon.

The first part of this volume deals with the *Lumbar Disc*. Special consideration was given to the problems of recurrences and of disc heriation in youngsters and elderly patients. Prognostic and catamnestic aspects have been evaluated through an extensive joint statistic inquiry.

In the second part, attention is focused on *Adult Hydrocephalus*. The various diagnostic procedures presently employed – including those of nuclear medicine – are analyzed as concerns their significance for therapy and prognosis. The clinical applications of continuous intracranial pressure monitoring, and the pathophysiologic importance of the obtained data are discussed.

The third part of this volume contains a series of contributions on neurotraumatology (head injuries, brain edema, intensive care and on neurophysiological topics.

Springer-Verlag Berlin Heidelberg New York